TABLE OF CONTENTS

Volume I

THE AIDS READER

Edited by
Loren K. Clarke
and
Malcolm Potts

Branden Publishing Company

Library of Congress Cataloging in Publication Data
The AIDS reader.

Bibliography: p.
Includes index.
1. AIDS (Disease) I. Clarke, Loren K., 1936-
II. Potts, Malcolm, 1935-.
RC607.A26A3489 1988   614.5'993   87-31990
ISBN 0-8283-1918-9 (pbk. : v. 1)

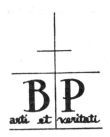

Branden Publishing Company
17 Station Street
Box 843 Brookline Village
Boston, MA 02147

".... during the Plague people were more addicted to prophecies and astrological conjurations, dreams and old wives' tales than ever before or since."

Daniel DeFoe, 1722

".... Woe to those who invest illness with moral judgement."

Graffiti on a Church wall

Through The AIDS Reader, *many voices speak with one purpose: information and understanding. The selections are all well chosen, readable and will be of interest to a wide audience. Gathering so many relevant articles into a single publication provides a fresh and stimulating perspective. This perspective is often lacking in other AIDS books which rely upon a single author's interpretation rather than primary sources.*

Dr. Robert C. Gallo
Chief, Laboratory of Tumor
and Cell Biology,
National Cancer Institute,
NIH, Bethesda, Maryland

Dr. Howard Z. Streicher
Senior Staff Fellow
Laboratory of Tumor and
Cell Biology,
National Cancer Institute,
NIH, Bethesda, Maryland

Within the seven years since its recognition, AIDS has become a global pandemic with cases present in over 130 countries. Without the availability of an effective treatment or vaccine, our best efforts to contain this disease are based solely on the principles of education. In The AIDS Reader, *Clarke and Potts have compiled significant articles covering the basic science of the virus, its epidemiology, transmission characteristics, future projections, epidemiologic trends, therapy and preventive strategies, as well as the societal impact of this disease and its implications in our culture. These articles provide significant insight into the development and rapid spread of the disease and provide the necessary information required for effective prevention and control strategies.*

Dr. Thomas C. Quinn
Senior Investigator,
Laboratory of Immunoregulation
National Institute of Allergy
and Infectious Diseases,
NIH, Bethesda, Maryland

FOREWORD

The mystery and fear which have accompanied the disease known as AIDS, have spawned an avalanche of printed material on the subject. As many of the efforts to understand the disease and its profound implications have been advanced, and our understanding and acceptance improved, so too has the quality of the material.

This book is one of the first to take a comprehensive view of the new virus and will substantially contribute to public understanding of the virus, the disease and the epidemic. It provides, for the first time, a collection of material which both traces the evolution of the disease, and places it in the present perspective of what we know and what we do not. The authors have done a superlative job of culling the mountains of literature to select a group which provides perspective, compassion, and insight.

My organization answers more than 75,000 telephone calls each month to our National AIDS Hotline from people concerned about AIDS. If each of them had this book on their shelf, few of those calls would be needed.

Dr. Michael Rosenberg
Executive Director
American Social Health Association

PREFACE

We hope this is a balanced book — since balance is what seems to be lacking in the mystery, confusion and panic surrounding the attack which is being mounted against humanity by the virus which causes the disease called AIDS.

The book begins with a detailed and technical journey into the laboratories where the keys to the understanding of the virus were forged in the early years of the search for the infectious agent of AIDS. The discovery of the virus, which was originally called HTLV-III/LAV and which became known as HIV (Human Immunodeficiency Virus), is only a small part of the saga.

The main story — and the story which occupies the major portion of this book — is the tracing of the path of the virus from whence (wherever) it came through the biological alleys and dark pathways of human understanding into the future to which (wherever) it is going. It is a document which captures a photograph of the epidemic through the window of the first seven years since its discovery in 1981. It ends, as all books on AIDS must, poised on the edge of the next frightening revelation — where is it going to appear next and how will the scientists, the politicians, the policymakers and the public react to it? Will it disrupt the public health mechanisms of the developed and the developing nations? Will it plunder the public resources of the technological system which has been built around the idea of cure, or will we all become more acutely aware of perhaps the most necessary part of public and personal health — prevention!

Epidemiologists are the Monsieur Poirots of science. However, not every epidemiologist acts in such a strict framework as an Agatha Christie mystery novel. The real-life virus detective must work in the muddled, unforgiving and relentless jungles, savannahs and file storage rooms of the world in order to get back to the origin of this disease. We have at least learned one important thing from the AIDS virus already, and that is, that it is a *new* disease. Medical people, politicians, journalists and the public in general are putting enormous pressures on scientists to "find out where it began." Knowing where it began is not the real issue when society is mobilizing against a giant as menacing as the AIDS epidemic. However, the most pressure is being placed by the politicians who want to know where it started so that they can point at "them" and reassure "us" that we are victims rather than executioners.

Meanwhile, as the epidemic wreaks its havoc across the borders of practically every sovereign nation in the world, there are those who "know" that it is obviously sent by an angry and heterosexual middle-class God to punish the wicked and sinful children who strayed from the "straight" and narrow pathway outlined by Moses. These people are the hand-wringers who populate candle-light vigils and who pray for divine intervention to end the suffering. Since so very few miraculous cures via divine intervention have been reported in the scientific literature, this book contains no article on the topic. We do, however, offer some of the rationalizations for the recognized impotence of both human and divine treatments in the face of the inexorable march of a biological phenomenon through the living body of a humanity which — in some ways — is obviously not prepared to cope at this point.

We also afford a rare opportunity to the general reader to listen in on the conversations of scientists — via the hallowed tradition of "Letters to the Editor". In the early days of any new phenomenon, the scientific establishment struggles against the exigencies of a sometimes fickle and always enigmatic Nature in the attempt to "get a handle" on the problem. It has always been, of course, the opinion of scientists that absolutely anything can be solved with the correct application of the tools of the trade and chemicals in the pharmacopia. One can see in the letters which are the record of the early conversations among various disciplines that this historical confidence has been shaken by the ambiguity and maliciousness of the HIV virus.

There are still a few "flat-earthers" in the profession who want to tear down all the theories and rebuild the structure around a new and novel idea. This may be an indication that at least nothing is being done in vain: but of course, maybe everything is being done in vain.

And then there is Africa. We call it the Agony of Africa in a section which is intended to show a broad spectrum of the dilemma over the continent. We show the fingers pointing both ways — Africans blaming the North saying that AIDS is an airborne plague — brought to Africa by thousands of Western businessmen via PanAm, Lufthansa and British Air. We also show the view out the laboratory window of a virus which has very close links with viruses found in the higher primates which live mostly in the central African AIDS belt. Who is right and who is wrong may mean something someday in the History of Medicine Textbooks which will be read by fledgling epidemiologists and virologists. But the discussion has no place on the mean back streets and dusty rural roads where young, productive men and women are being struck down in increasingly alarming numbers by a plague which came from "somewhere".

When all the histories of infectious diseases are written and collected together into one massive medical research library, we may begin to see how much more death and devastation can be spread by the typhus louse, the plague flea, the yellow-fever mosquito and the tiny AIDS virus, than has ever been dealt by the sword, lance, machine gun, and even atomic bomb. Civilizations have retreated before the onslaught of malaria, and armies have crumbled into rabble in the pathway of cholera, or of dysentery and typhoid bacilli. Huge areas of the world have been devastated by a trypanosome that travels on the wings of the tsetse fly and generations have been harassed by the syphilis of the itinerant lover. Maybe the conclusion that a standing cock has no conscience is a fitting metaphor for this modern disease which, while travelling by sperm and blood, can — in the act of love between two human beings — kill them both!

I. What Is Aids?

Introduction
The Most Presumptuous Pox

Malcolm Potts
December 1, 1987

The last case of smallpox occurred in October 1977 in the seaport of Merca, Somalia. Ten years earlier, smallpox was causing two million deaths a year.

Syphilis was the Great Pox of the 16th Century, called by one contemporary "the most presumptuous pox." In the 1930's, the U.S. Surgeon General claimed it infected one in every ten adult Americans. Probably that was an exaggeration, but between the two World Wars up to 60,000 babies a year were born suffering from congenital syphilis. Advertisements were used to warn the public of the dangers of venereal diseases. After the introduction of penicillin in 1943, the disease virtually disappeared in the US.

Is the Acquired Immunity Deficiency Syndrome (AIDS) a new pox to be ranked beside prior human plagues? Will it be brought under control by some vaccine like smallpox, or some therapy like syphilis? Will it lead to massive changes in sexual and social behavior, as some earlier epidemics appear to have done?

In the six years since Dr. Michael Gottlieb treated five cases of *Pneumocystis carinii* in previously fit, young gay men, and Dr. Bruce Voeller first coined the acronym AIDS, more than 20,000 Americans have died of the disease and between 0.5 to 1.7 million have caught the virus.

Research has traced what appeared to be antibodies to AIDS virus in blood stored since 1959 in Zaire. It is interesting, although of no public health importance, to know where AIDS has come from; what is important is to understand where it is going.

A reasonable explanation of the origin of the virus is that it evolved in a primate and was somehow transferred to people. Which primate — why not the most promiscuous, the chimpanzee? It is possible to infect chimpanzees with HIV, but they do not appear to manifest the disease. Could the virus have escaped from a laboratory and in a way are other primates reaping a terrible revenge on us for the experiments we have, without sufficient thought performed on them?

Over the next five years, 235,000 new cases of AIDS are expected, or one in 1000 of the U.S. population. The care and treatment of this number of victims will cost $8 — 16 billion a year. By 1991, more Americans will have died of AIDS than were killed in ten years of the war in Vietnam. AIDS itself has not yet really escaped beyond the well-known high risk groups. But the virus has already infected one in 300 army recruits in Wisconsin, one in 200 couples marrying in California, one in 40 pregnant women from the urban ghettos of New York, and one in 20 of the total population of San Francisco. And all those who are seropositive remain under sentence of death, even though we do not know fully the rate at which the symptoms are going to appear. In 1981, there were 90 cases of AIDS in homosexual Americans; today the gay community is reeling under the attack by the virus and at the same time must suffer increasing assaults by purveyors of prejudice and fear.

The situation in developing countries is even more grim. Today, in high prevalence areas of Central Africa, between one in 1000 and one in 2000 is developing AIDS each year. The annual incidence of AIDS virus infection approaches one percent in a few areas and in Zaire, up to 12% of pregnant women coming to urban hospitals carry the virus. Up to 18% of blood donors in Rwanda and Zambia have the HIV, and the rates in some other countries are even higher. A quarter to 88% of prostitutes in some large cities now have antibodies to the disease. Perhaps five to ten million people have the disease. Cases have occurred in Bombay and Bangkok; it is as if in a street of flimsy wooden houses each one already has one corner alight. The worldwide death toll in the 1990's could be 10 million or more, with higher numbers if the epidemic is not contained.

Eight out of 10 cases of AIDS in the US are the result of sexual contact. Sexual activity has been demonstrated to transmit infection between homosexual men, from man to woman, and woman to man. Transmission through oral-genital contact, while possible, is rare. Among gay men, the recipient of anal sex is more likely to get the disease. For the developing world, where breastfeeding itself is often a matter of life and death, data are urgently needed on the risk of transmitting the virus through breastmilk.

Is it the pattern of concomitant diseases, genital lesions, the use of contaminated needles for injections, malnutrition, or some other factor, that makes the male:female ratio of victims one to one in Africa? As many men have intercourse with other women, but a few women have intercourse with an exceedingly large number of men, one would not expect the ratio of male:female cases to be one to one, even if the disease was spread exclusively by heterosexual intercourse. And why are Oriental American populations under-represented among U.S. victims? Why are most US hemophiliacs seropositive, but manifest AIDS at a lower than expected rate? Questions are many, including questions about possible interactions between AIDS and various methods of family planning.

The bad news about the human immunodeficiency virus (HIV) is that, like the influenza virus, it can change its protein coat rapidly; unlike smallpox or influenza, but like polio, the victim can appear perfectly healthy and still spread the disease; and, like rabies, once symptomatic, it is invariably fatal.

The good news about HIV is that it is fragile and can only be transmitted by direct contact between bodily fluids. Heating to 66 degrees C is sufficient to kill it, although it can survive air drying for many days. The virus can probably be transmitted inside white cells — to use a metaphor — we not only need to find and kill the terrorists who carry a bomb onto an airplane, but we must detect the bomb even when he has swallowed it. We are lucky it is a disease transmitted by sexual intercourse: imagine what the world would be like if the same virus was transmitted by airborne droplets like the common cold or pneumonic plague — we would all be wearing masks and spacesuits.

In projecting how many people AIDS may kill eventually, we need to guess how long the average person will live with HIV infection before manifesting the syndrome — what is the half life of a victim? When we do this a macabre paradox arises — the longer an individual lives, the more people he or she can infect, the more rapidly the disease spreads and the more people die in the end. From an epidemiologists's point of view, AIDS does not kill rapidly enough.

AIDS testing is now compulsory in the U.S. military but strongly resisted elsewhere. Paradoxically, most U.S. states require premarital screening for syphilis — in California, for example, the program costs $240,000 per case found. All other considerations apart, either premarital testing for STD's should be abandoned or AIDS testing mandated. Sadly, medical confidences are all too frequently broken and knowledge of a person who is seropositive gets into computers, and some individual men have lost their jobs, or their medical insurance, or both, after a positive ELISA test. An American soldier has been arrested in West Germany for knowingly spreading AIDS under a law that prohibits causing "bodily harm" with a weapon. As with family planning, so with AIDS, ethics are going to be almost as important as the technology.

The cost of health care for AIDS victims is horrific and is splitting the world of health into the privileged and the underprivileged, even more cruelly than other measures of development. Jonathan Mann and his colleagues have written, "the cost of caring for ten AIDS patients in the United States (approximately $450,000) is greater than the entire budget of a large hospital in Zaire, where up to 25% of the pediatric and adult hospital admissions have HIV infection." Even detection is impossibly expensive in Third World countries. One ELISA test for AIDS costs more than some African governments spend on health per capita per year. One confirmatory Western Blot test is equivalent to six months total income of someone from Guinea-Bissau. Cheaper tests are needed but may be difficult to perfect. The individual identification of cases will remain impossible in many countries. Where screening is possible, it should be focused on the blood transfusion services.

The risk of getting gonorrhea during a single act of intercourse is approximately 25% for female to male transmission and 50% for male to female infection. No one knows what the absolute risk of infection with AIDS is for a single act of sex. So far, about one in 10 wives of seropositive hemophiliacs have become infected. One study followed 47 seronegative spouses of infected partners for 18 months and found 17 developed HIV antibodies. So the risk of transmission at one intercourse may well be lower than that of bacterial STD's.

The threat of AIDS has already changed the sexual behavior of many in the homosexual community, gonorrhea rates have fallen, and the seroconversion rate for AIDS has fallen fourfold in San Francisco. AIDS is equally certain to change the life styles of heterosexuals. The trade of bar girls in Tokyo fell dramatically after one Japanese prostitute died of the disease. But we can also be sure no country will ever become totally chaste and fully and mutually monogamous. The immediate need is to slow the rate of spread of the disease.

If we do not know who has the disease all we can do is to promote general educational and "safer sex" measures. As with family planning, education is going to be a battle between commonsense and innate, sexual conservatism. Everybody knows prisoners engage in homosexuality, but as it is against the rules in English prisons, the idea of distributing condoms to inmates has been rejected.

But if people are prepared to take precautions, what should they use? An intact condom is an effective barrier against the passage of the virus. Experiments with dildos, condoms, Herpes 2 and HIV, confirm latex condoms are an effective physical barrier. Condoms made from animal intestine, however, have not been proven a safe barrier. Fischl found that 14 out of 17 partners of seropositive men who did not use condoms caught the virus, while only 3 out of 18 who used condoms seroconverted. Condoms are more likely to tear during anal intercourse and a tougher brand for sale to gay men is about to be marketed in the US. Plastic condoms, which were developed experimentally in the 1960's, urgently need to be explored as perhaps an even better prophylactic against AIDS than latex. The use of condoms in most developing countries is pathetically low.

In the laboratory, nonoxynol-9 kills herpes, chlamydia, gonorrhea, syphilis and the AIDS virus. Clinical observation confirms nonoxynol-9 reduces the transmission of gonorrhea and chlamydial infection, including a study by Family Health International among massage parlor girls in Bangkok who used the *Today Sponge* loaded with 1 gram of nonoxynol-9. However, to date, there is no large-scale clinical confirmation that the use of spermicides or condoms slows the spread of AIDS in a real life situation.

I would like to claim to have shown a great perspicacity and clairvoyance when I conducted the world's first clinical trials of the acceptability of spermicidally lubricated condoms in the early 1970's, but I can't. I merely saw making an incremental improvement in a common sense and useful method which had been neglected by many who work in family planning clinics. But today, in view of the unique killing ability of the disease, the pattern of spread, and what we know from laboratory observations, it seems to me that the single best advice to give someone who believes they may be exposed to AIDS, and who still knowingly engages in intercourse, is to use a spermicidally lubricated condom. Like lifeboats on an ocean liner, a spermicide cannot guarantee survival but it is reassuring to have it available.

In an *in vitro* experiment in which spermicidally lubricated condoms were deliberately ruptured, HIV could not be detected in the test fluid. Problems of disposing of condoms infected with HIV have been raised, and if a spermicide did nothing else it would make a used condom non-infective.

AIDS is a rapidly changing field, but sadly we can be sure neither a vaccine nor an effective cure is going to be developed in the short term. It is even biologically plausible that a vaccine may never be developed due to the peculiar nature of the virus — then we would have the potential of a plague to rival the Black Death.

The only "vaccine" we have against AIDS is the condom, and every case of AIDS we can prevent today will prevent 2, 4, 8, 16, 32, 64, 128 and so forth tomorrow. I feel confident and emphatic that condoms, spermicides, and perhaps especially spermicidally lubricated condoms, can and must be aggressively promoted.

Abstinence, cuddling, what the Americans call necking and petting, and mutual masturbation do not transmit AIDS and must be encouraged. Perhaps AIDS will turn back the cruelly early age at which many youngsters in the West begin their sexual careers. The trouble with AIDS is that it is spread not by who you are, but by what you do. An individual who has unprotected intercourse is not having intercourse with one person but with all the partners of that person over the last several years.

For education to work, it must convince people of three things: 1) they are at risk; 2) that a lethal disease can be asymptomatic; and 3) that "safer sex" practices offer worthwhile protection. If any link in this chain is broken, then educators will be unable to haul a reluctant public out of the path of the disease.

Many people will be wise and cautious. Thirty out of 50 London prostitutes interviewed at the Praed Street clinic said they had changed their sexual habits as a result of fear of AIDS, now insisted on condom use, and had stopped offering oral intercourse. But some people will always take appalling risks out of ignorance or malice. Some seropositive women knowingly conceive a child, even though warned the baby will have a better than 50:50 chance of having the disease. A few seropositive gay men indulge in a fatalistic orgy of unprotected intercourse. Ten percent of the prostitutes interviewed at the Praed Street clinic said they would continue to work even if they caught the virus.

Prostitutes are a high risk group for AIDS infection, and some are also IV drug users. Some always use condoms with clients but never with their husbands and boyfriends, but HIV does not distinguish between an act of love and a business transaction. In most of the developing world, prostitution is simply a reflection of poverty and gross inequality in income, and prostitutes deserve more humane care and realistic advice than they often receive. We need to know whether Third World prostitutes can persuade their customers to use condoms, or they themselves will use nonoxynol-9, and if so, which of the several formulations available is most appropriate? Better still, most Third World prostitutes do their jobs for reasons of poverty and governments and the international community need to ask if they cannot pay them a wage to quit working.

Risk-taking is encouraged by ignorance, stupidity and, saddest of all, by the type of scientific illiteracy so common in America, and not altogether unknown in Europe. Some already see AIDS as a punishment sent by God for homosexuals. "They have declared war on nature, and now nature is exacting an awful retribution," said one American commentator. And the American extremist politician Lyndon la Rouche calls AIDS a plot by the "Soviet War Machine," while some Third World countries blame AIDS on American accidents in germ warfare factories. Such nonsense erodes social policy and encourages individual risk taking.

When Daniel DeFoe wrote *A Journal of the Plague Year* about the events of 1665 in London, he described how the people "were more addicted to prophecies and astrological conjurations, dreams and old wives' tales than ever they were before or since." Let us hope this will not prove true of the AIDS plague.

The experience of family planning workers attempting to interpret the risks of oral contraceptives or public health workers warning individuals about cigarettes suggests that many people are ill-prepared to make sensible decisions about anything other than certain death. Risk-taking and AIDS are not unlike risk-taking and pregnancy — neither infection nor fertilization are certain, the gambler often survives, and the penalty is remote — at least nine months in the case of pregnancy, and maybe years in the case of AIDS. But, like pregnancy, AIDS once caught, cannot be undone by regret or good deeds.

Those at greatest risk may eventually prove to be in their late teens and early twenties, who are both the most sexually active and who often believe themselves immortal.

From the family planning point of view, the drama of AIDS is forcing public opinion to accept the promotion and distribution of contraceptives much more realistically than the need of family planning alone could ever have achieved. Condoms may have been "superfine" but until recently, one needed a thick skin to promote them. If a girl had an illegitimate child because her boyfriend did not know how to obtain a condom, we could always blame her as a sinner and try to get someone to adopt the child. But the sudden death of tens of thousands of adults of all social ranks cracks the mask of hypocrisy on the face of a society.

The USA is agog because the Surgeon General, Dr. C. Everett Koop, actively promoted condoms in a meeting for students of Liberty College, Virginia, chaired by the Reverend Jerry Falwell. The *Chicken Ranch*, a legal brothel in Nevada, now insists its customers use condoms. On February 14, 1987 — an appropriate date — the *New York Times*, after 15 years of systematic resistance, published its first advertisement for condoms — although the advertiser still had to agree not to mention "contraception." Condoms, which used to get held up for long intervals in the customs of Colombia, Latin American, are now speeding through.

Other barriers will fall. Section 4 (5) of the 1954 Television Act (Britain) explicitly forbade the advertisement of "contraceptives, matrimonial agencies, fortune tellers and undertakers." When the London Rubber Company sponsored a Formula One racing car in the 1970's, the cameras had to pan off it every time it sped past, or they would have broken the law. Today, if condoms are not advertised, undertakers may have to be.

Ted Turner's Cablevision TV station in the USA has taken condom advertisements without blinking, and the big US networks are rethinking their traditional hostility, although they still fear their sponsors may pull out in an act of mass advertising interruptus. With the exception of a few small TV stations, the large networks remain subject to small town criticism, but I predict that these last bastions of public health naivete will fall in the next year.

AIDS treatments are already getting accelerated review by the US Food and Drug Administration, and the epidemic may push that over-conservative organization back into a more realistic attitude toward the risks and benefits of other drugs. Could it be that AIDS will also choke off the avaricious and scientifically illiterate lawyer who has done so much to damage family planning in the USA? Currently, at least one American condom manufacturer is afraid to add a spermicide to its condoms because it cannot get product liability insurance since the Ortho Company lost a $4.8 million case that maintained, contrary to epidemiological evidence, that nonoxynol-9 caused fetal abnormalities.

The National Academy of Sciences and Institute of Medicine in America are calling for an annual budget of $30 million for FY 88 rising to a billion dollars annually in the 1990's for all aspects of AIDS research, education and service. International effort will cost as much or more. The US Agency for International Development has given $2 million to WHO and recognizes more — much more — will be needed. The Agency for International Development spends $17 million a year on providing condoms and only reaches approximately 1% of eligible couples around the world.

Currently, AIDS is moving more rapidly than bureaucracies can react: it takes time for NIH to write a proposal, select competitive bids, choose the best response, and fund the work. WHO can only act if invited by governments, and some Third World governments are still counting cases of AIDS rather than worrying about the spread of the virus, which is the real threat.

The issue that faces us in relation to AIDS is an accelerated version of the problem that has dogged us in relation to too rapid population growth. Human sexual behavior is intrinsically conservative, and the coital expression of sex is regulated by law and restricted by religion. Rapid changes in sexual behavior are difficult to achieve. In the case of the population explosion, vigorous action came one or two generations too late. In the case of AIDS, necessary action which is delayed for a year or two, or possibly only for months, will prove very costly. Elites in both America and Africa have already wasted valuable lead time being too timid about promoting condoms to deter AIDS.

The most aggressive leadership possible is necessary to promote mutually faithful sexual relationships and, where that fails, safer sex practices. Face to face counseling of prostitutes, probably using prostitutes themselves to transmit messages, is urgently needed. There must be a multiplicity of condom outlets; pharmacies, vending machines, mail order, supermarkets, video arcades, hotels, and antenatal and family planning clinics — sadly family planning clinics have often been shy about distributing condoms. Could insurance companies offer discounts to condom users like they do to non-smokers?

In the last analysis, I think birth control has a lot to give and something to benefit by becoming an ally of the new death control.

AIDS does two things: it makes our private, sexual lives public, and it makes the Twentieth Century Adam risk his life for sex in the way

Eve has always done. Unlike most plagues, the elites, or at least elite males, are at a disproportionate risk for getting AIDS. The rich have always gone to prostitutes or played the "sugar daddy." Film stars, priests and politicians are dying, and when a son or daughter goes to university and comes back with AIDS, everyone will take notice.

AIDS is important, but it must not be allowed to push everything else into the background. Every year 400,000 to 500,000 women die from pregnancy, childbirth or abortion. Unlike AIDS victims, pregnant women die mostly in remote areas and nearly all are illiterate and poor. It is a carnage equivalent to crashing a jumbo jet filled with women passengers every five and a half hours, day in and day out throughout the year. Yet, very few people notice. To date the AIDS epidemic in America has killed approximately as many men as women die of childbirth in the Indian subcontinent every three months. Dare we hope that policy makers, professionals and people in general will become more interested in all aspects of preventive medicine because of AIDS?

If ten million people die of AIDS in the 1990's around the world, that will be less than half those who died of influenza a couple of years after the First World War, or somewhat less than twice the number of women condemned to die in childbirth in the same decade. One *decade* of AIDS deaths will only represent about 10% of *one year's* global population growth, or ten months of population growth in the single country of India. Hand guns currently kill about as many Americans as die of AIDS, and smoking will be responsible for ten times as many deaths (350,000) as AIDS this year.

From a scientific point of view, AIDS reminds us of the value of basic research and the utility of epidemiology. The understanding of the AIDS virus has been achieved rapidly and in exquisite detail because fundamental studies had already taken place in this area. Key questions about the natural history of the disease have been and are being unraveled by ingenious and persistent observers in both rich and poor countries. Already, 80,000 tests related to AIDS are conducted each day in the USA.

One of the reasons AIDS has taken off so rapidly is because of exceeding rapid growth of large cities. Recently, Gail Singer interviewed a sample of Californian women under age 25 about their sexual careers. The median age of beginning intercourse was 17 years, but by age 25 one or two women in her sample reported having sex with as many as 500 men. They were not prostitutes, but the remarkable thing is that they had had sexual relations with more partners than there are, or were, adults of the opposite sex in most villages of the Third World or from our agricultural past; and many more than there were in the hunter-gatherer bands that make up 90% of human history.

AIDS, however, is not without precedent. Martin Alonso Pinzon, the captain of the *Pinta* (the first of Columbus's three ships to make landfall in the New World) is said to have died from syphilis shortly after returning home. Fra Ramon, who chronicled Columbus' voyages, mentions that the "sores that we call the French sickness" were described in the folk mythology of the Caribbean islanders. The disease is recorded in parts of Italy from 1494 onwards and was widespread in Europe by 1498. A physician, Ruiz Diaz de Isla, treated some of Columbus's crew, giving an unusually accurate description of syphilis, including the observation that inter-current malaria attack would arrest the progress of the disease — a shrewd observation that was used in therapy until the discovery of penicillin. Whether or not syphilis really was the first export from the New World, it certainly hit Fifteenth Century Europe with exceeding virulence. Victims suffered from pustules that were "dark green, and the sight thereof was more grievous unto the patient than the pain itself; and yet the pain was as though they had lain in the fire."

Just as AIDS has been dubbed the "gay plague," so syphilis, when it first appeared, was described as someone else's problem; the French called it "the disease of Naples," the British the "French pox" and the Japanese the "Chinese infection," and even today, the origin of syphilis can arouse passion among academics. In the same way, we call a contraceptive diaphragm a *Dutch cap* and a condom a *French letter*, while the French call a rubber the *Capot anglais*. But, sexually transmitted diseases have a habit of not remaining someone else's problem, and today the gay plague is turning into a domestic disaster for many heterosexual families.

Whatever its name or origin, syphilis brought about changes in sexual behavior. Calvin was born only seventeen years after Columbus returned and it seems the puritan revolution, at least in part, was propelled by a very real fear of syphilis. Sexual immorality was sternly punished. Certainly, the change in sexual behavior that took place in Sixteenth and Seventeenth Century Europe was profound; illegitimacy fell to low levels, spouses came to depend more on each other than on their kin and the brand of entrepreneurial capitalism that is the basis of so much of western business matured in the sexually more conservative Protestant regions of Western Europe and their North American offshoots.

Our sexual behavior, our social structure, and our communal expectations all interact and the AIDS epidemic is certain to change how we live and, for those who work in family planning, it will bring about formidable changes. When the wages of sin is death and not just a case of the clap, people will become more cautious sexually. AIDS will stretch and perhaps break some health systems. The details of that change may be difficult to predict, but monogamy and chastity now have a powerful new ally. Will family life change now that a recent poll of women in American has shown they fear AIDS more than nuclear war?

How will the church — both fundamentalist and Catholic — accommodate to AIDS? Now that several priests and, one bishop, have died of the disease, will the Vatican become more or less entrenched in its views? Georgetown University Medical School, Washington, a Jesuit foundation, has somehow found ways of counseling AIDS positive patients on "safe sex" practices.

Appropriate and successful health policies will only be possible if individuals of all religious, political, and social backgrounds recognize that responsibility is enhanced by knowledge and choice and that enforced ignorance not only kills the body but paralyzes moral choice.

AIDS — A PUBLIC HEALTH CRISIS

Reprinted with permission
from *Population Reports*
Series L, No. 6, Jul-Aug, 1986
Population Information Program
The Johns Hopkins University

As of August 1986, 71 countries had reported almost 29,000 cases of AIDS. Cases have been reported on all continents, although in many areas the extent is unknown or greatly underreported. Currently, the largest numbers have been reported in the United States, Western Europe, Central Africa, Brazil, and Haiti. Worldwide as many as 5 to 10 million people may be infected with the virus that causes AIDS, known as the human immunodeficiency virus (HIV). Most of these people have no symptoms now but can infect others. Many of these people are expected to develop AIDS eventually. In the US alone, more than 270,000 AIDS cases are expected by 1991.

In North America, Europe, and Brazil, most cases have involved homosexual men or users of intravenous drugs who have shared contaminated needles. In Africa and Haiti, many women are developing AIDS. In these areas sexual intercourse between men and women may be the main route of transmission. The number of children with AIDS is expected to grow, and in some areas AIDS may become a major threat to child survival.

AIDS results from a viral infection that damages the immune system. The damaged immune system cannot protect against certain other infections and cancers, some of which then become the direct causes of death. These illnesses include an otherwise rare form of pneumonia, aggressive Kaposi's sarcoma (a type of cancer), brain infections, persistent diarrhea, and herpes infections. Because of the way that the virus infects cells, developing either a cure or a vaccine is extremely difficult. At best, both are years away.

With no cure or vaccine in sight, the only real hope for controlling AIDS now is education that changes people's behavior. Family planning workers and other health workers must lead, but the mass media, community and national leaders, parents, and teachers also must help. The basic messages are simple, but they must be heard and heeded.

Acquired immune deficiency syndrome — AIDS — is a global epidemic. To date, only 5 years after the syndrome was first described, almost 29,000 cases have been reported in 71 countries around the world, and the World Health Organization (WHO) estimates that the actual number of cases may be as high as 100,000. Although to date most cases have been reported in the US, AIDS appears to be increasing rapidly in some other countries, especially in Africa. In addition to cases of AIDS, 5 to 10 million people may be infected with human immunodeficiency virus, the virus that causes AIDS.

In the US, where AIDS was first reported in 1981, formal nationwide surveillance began in 1982. Between June 1981 and June 1986, 21,517 cases were reported from all 50 states, for a cumulative rate of 9 cases per 100,000 population. Two cities have the highest rates: New York, with 72 cases per 100,000 population, and San Francisco, with 68 per 100,000.

In Europe AIDS is far less common. In the 27 countries reporting to the WHO European Collaborating Center on AIDS, 2,568 cases were identified between 1982 and June 1986, mostly in large cities. As of September, 1985 the rates were highest — between 1.0 and 1.2 per 100,000 population — in Belgium, Denmark, and Switzerland. In Belgium over two-thirds of cases came from Africa for medical treatment.

Among developing areas AIDS appears to be most common in Brazil, Haiti, and Central Africa. Some 739 cases were reported in Brazil by June 1986 and 377 in Haiti by December 1985.

AIDS is rapidly becoming a major public health problem throughout sub-Saharan Africa. Nine African countries have officially reported a total of 378 cases, but WHO estimates that there have been at least 50,000 cases since 1980. The disease may have first appeared in the late 1970's in Zaire, about the same time that it first appeared in the US and Haiti. By 1984, based on hospital admissions and a survey of doctors, researchers estimated an annual incidence of 17 to 18 cases per 100,000 population in Kinshasa, Zaire, and 80 per 100,000 in Kigali, Rwanda. Cases also have been reported in the neighboring countries of Zambia, Tanzania, Kenya, South Africa and Uganda, where AIDS is called "Slim disease" because it causes extreme weight loss. To date, residents of 23 African countries have sought treatment in Europe for AIDS or related conditions.

The reported cases of AIDS are only the tip of the iceberg, for several reasons. First, many cases are not recognized. In the US, for example, 10 percent of AIDS cases may go unreported. Where diagnostic facilities are not available, a majority of cases may be missed. Second, cases of AIDS are reported only when they meet the criteria set up by the US Centers for Disease control. In fact, however, the immune deficiency characteristic of AIDS can lead to many other serious illnesses. These may not be reported or even diagnosed as related to AIDS. Third — and perhaps most important — many people are already infected with the virus that causes AIDS, but symptoms may not appear for several years after infection.

Cases of AIDS in the US and Europe are increasing rapidly. In the US twice as many cases were reported in the second half of 1985 as in the first half of 1984. Some 14,000 to 16,000 new cases are expected in 1986, almost as many as reported from 1981 to 1985. The US Public Health Service estimates that by 1991 more than 270,000 cases will have been reported. In Europe the number of reported new cases increased from an average of 22 per week between March and June 1985 to 31 cases per week between October and December 1985.

It is difficult to gauge just how rapidly AIDS is increasing in places where disease surveillance and diagnostic equipment are inadequate and where persons with AIDS may not seek or have access to medical care. Nonetheless, in Africa reports from hospitals suggest a rapid increase. In Uganda, for example, physicians in Mulago Hospital in Kampala did not see any cases in 1981 diagnosed as AIDS; in 1984 they saw one or two cases per month on average; in 1985, one or two cases per week; and in the first six months of 1986, one or two cases per day. In Zaire, at University Hospital in Kinshasa, cases of cryptococcal meningitis — an infection frequently found in Africans with AIDS — jumped from an average of less than one per year before 1978 to 44 cases over the years between 1978 and 1984 — an average of six per year. At University Teaching Hospital in Lusaka, Zambia, cases of Kaposi's sarcoma — a cancer characteristic of AIDS — rose from about 10 per year before 1983 to 23 in 1983, 37 in 1984, and 25 in just the first four months of 1985. A similar increase has been reported in Kinshasa. Unlike the common, slowly progressing, treatable Kaposi's sarcoma long known in Africa, these cases have taken an aggressive, fatal form similar to Kaposi's sarcoma found in persons with AIDS in the US and Europe.

The epidemiology of AIDS varies markedly in different areas. In North America, Europe, and Latin America, AIDS has occurred primarily in homosexual and bisexual men (that is, men who have sexual relations with both men and women) and intravenous (IV) drug users. In contrast, in Africa and Haiti, women appear to be about as likely as men to be infected and develop AIDS.

In developed countries adults with AIDS have been grouped into 5 categories defined by the US CDC for reporting and surveillance purposes. Because some people in these groups are likely to engage in behavior that may expose them to the virus or because they have received donated blood or blood products, these are identified as high-risk groups. In general, in Europe and the US the distribution among these categories has remained fairly constant since 1981. In Europe, however, the percentage of cases associated with IV drug use has increased sharply sine 1984. Over 90 percent of all US and European cases are men. Most are between the ages of 20 and 49. Children under age 13 make up less than 3 percent of cases. In Africa and Haiti very few people with AIDS report homosexual or bisexual activity. In Africa 35 to 57 percent of reported cases are women. In Haiti, the percentage of cases who are women has increased steadily from 12 percent in 1980-82 to 36 percent in 1985. This and other evidence suggests that heterosexual intercourse is a major means of transmission. At the same time, intramuscular injections are common in these countries and may be an important mode of transmission. All these findings are important to family planning and maternal and child health programs. Because the virus that causes AIDS can be transmitted during pregnancy and childbirth, many infants may develop AIDS. Indeed, up to 14 percent of pregnant women studied in Kampala, Uganda, are infected with the virus.

At present AIDS is a fatal disease. No effective treatment is currently available. Although the interval between diagnosis and death varies widely, in the US about 50 percent of patients die within 18 months of diagnosis; about 80 percent, within 36 months. Some 55 percent of adults and about 61 percent of children diagnosed with AIDS since 1981 have died. Rates are similar in Europe. In Africa and Haiti, survival time after diagnosis is shorter, probably because of later diagnosis and lack of access to care.

In the US, AIDS has become a major cause of death in young men. In New York and San Francisco AIDS is one of the five leading causes of death among men between the ages of 24 and 54. In New York, AIDS has caused almost as much premature mortality in men age 25 to 44 as all forms of cancer.

Infection with human immunodeficiency virus, a newly discovered virus, takes many forms. It ranges from a complete absence of symptoms, to mild illness, to debilitating neurological disorders and fatal disease. AIDS is the end stage of this infection. Many more people are infected with the virus than show any symptoms. This is a cause for major public health concern. How many of these asymptomatic people will develop symptoms and how many will develop AIDS are still uncertain.

In 1986, US CDC classified the clinical features of HIV infection into four broad categories:

I. Initial infection with the virus and development of antibodies

II. Asymptomatic carrier state,

III. Persistent generalized lymphadenopathy,

IV. Other HIV-related diseases including AIDS.

Infection begins when HIV enters the bloodstream and stimulates an immune response and the development of antibodies. The presence of these antibodies (seropositivity) usually indicates that infection has occurred. Most infected people have no symptoms and do not know that they are carrying the virus. Nevertheless, presumably all who are infected, with or without symptoms, can transmit the virus to others.

The majority of people who become infected develop antibodies without any immediate symptoms. A sizable minority experience a short-term illness similar to mononucleosis or, rarely, acute neurological symptoms, such as seizures and temporary motor impairment. This occurs about two to five weeks after initial infection. Antibodies to HIV can usually be detected two to eight weeks after initial infection, although in a small minority six months or more may elapse.

In the second category of HIV infection, the asymptomatic carrier state, infected people have antibodies but no overt signs of disease. Laboratory tests may show a reduced number of T-helper lymphocytes, also called T-4 lymphocytes, specialized white blood cells that help fight infection.

A more severe form of HIV infection occurs when people with antibodies develop symptoms. These symptoms have been variously termed persistent generalized lymphadenopathy, lymphadenopathy syndrome, AIDS prodrome, AIDS-related conditions, lesser AIDS, and AIDS-related complex (ARC). Persistent generalized lymphadenopathy, the third US CDC category, is defined as swollen lymph nodes in two separate sites other than the groin for more than three months. Lymphadenopathy is one of the most common signs of HIV infection, but many persons with lymphadenopathy may not be aware of it.

Persistent generalized lymphadenopathy may occur alone or in combination with night sweats, fever, diarrhea, weight loss, fatigue, and uncommon infections such as oral candidiasis (thrush) and herpes zoster infection (shingles). These symptoms may occur intermittently or persistently, and they vary in severity. They are usually not life-threatening, but diarrhea and weight loss sometimes do cause death.

For some, persistent generalized lymphadenopathy, alone or with other symptoms, is an intermediate stage between initial infection and AIDS. For others, these symptoms appear to be a chronic manifestation of HIV infection. After about two years up to 20 percent of people with these symptoms have developed AIDS. In the longest follow-up to date of people with persistent generalized lymphadenopathy — four and one-half years on average — 12 of 42 men (29 percent) developed AIDS.

AIDS is the end stage of HIV infection. As defined by US CDC, AIDS is characterized by life-threatening opportunistic infections (infections that occur only in people with immune deficiency) and/or cancers that occur in people with otherwise unexplained defects in immunity. These infections occur because people with AIDS have lost most of their natural defenses against certain infections and are unable to fight them off.

AIDS is a syndrome — a complex of diseases and symptoms — resulting from unexplained immune deficiency. In 1982 the US CDC formally established a specific definition of AIDS for surveillance and reporting purposes AIDS was defined as:

(1) the presence of a reliably diagnosed disease, such as *Pneumocystsis carnii* pneumonia or Kaposi's sarcoma, that signals an underlying deficiency in the immune system and

(2) the immune deficiency is not due to drugs, certain types of cancers, congenital disease, or other known causes.

Between 1982 and 1985, HIV was discovered, tests to detect HIV antibodies were developed, and other illnesses associated with the virus were recognized.

Thus in 1985 US CDC expanded its case definition to include:

(3) certain other opportunistic infections and cancers of lymph tissue in people found to harbor HIV or test positive for HIV antibodies.

Since the US CDC definition depends partly on laboratory analyses, WHO is developing a provisional clinical definition for use where laboratory tests are not available.

The spectrum of opportunistic infections and other symptoms in people with AIDS varies in different regions, usually reflecting the infections prevalent in these regions. Some of the differences, however, may be due to lack of diagnostic facilities in some countries to detect certain diseases. In Haiti and Africa the most common opportunistic infections are tuberculosis, cryptococcal meningitis, herpes simplex infection, oral and esophageal candidiasis cryptosporidiosis, central nervous system toxoplasmosis, and skin rashes. Chronic diarrhea and weight loss are very common. In the US, in contrast, 63 percent of people with AIDS are diagnosed with *Pneumocystis carnii* pneumonia. Cryptococcal infections, cryptosporidiosis, and toxoplasmosis have been reported in less than 5 percent.

Kaposi's sarcoma is the most common malignancy in people with AIDS. It has been diagnosed, mostly among homosexual men, in 33 percent of AIDS cases in Europe and 24 percent in the US. In Africans Kaposi's sarcoma is reported in 2 to 20 percent of cases, and in Haitians, in 5 to 12 percent. Other types of cancer, especially Burkitt's lymphoma and non-Hodgkins lymphoma of the central nervous system, also occur in people with AIDS.

Neurological disorders occur in people with HIV infection. These disorders can be severe, including progressive memory loss, dementia, psychiatric symptoms, encephalitis, and meningitis. The virus can infect cells in the brain as well as certain white blood cells and has been isolated from the brain and cerebrospinal fluid of people with AIDS. In US studies 31 to 66 percent of people with AIDS have neurological symptoms.

Most AIDS patients develop multiple opportunistic infections or cancers and die either because (1) the infection cannot be treated effectively, or (2) their weakened immune system impairs resistance to infection and response to therapy. The following are the most common opportunistic infections:

— CRYPTOCOCCAL MENINGITIS, caused by a yeast-like fungus, usually starts with low-grade fever and mild headache. Nausea, vomiting, and blurred vision may follow. Patients become progressively lethargic. If untreated, the disease is fatal. Even with treatment up to one-quarter of patients die of progressive cryptococcal disease.

— CENTRAL NERVOUS SYSTEM TOXOPLASMOSIS, caused by a protozoan, leads to encephalitis (inflammation of the brain). Among the most common early signs are neurologic defects such as seizures and cognitive disorders. Fever, headache, lethargy, and confusion also are common. If untreated, this illness is almost always fatal.

— PNEUMOCYSTIS CARINII PNEUMONIA, caused by a protozoan, occurs almost exclusively in persons with immune deficiency. Symptoms include fever, chills, cough, and shortness of breath. Life-threatening respiratory failure may occur.

— CRYPTOSPORIDIOSIS, another protozoan disease, causes debilitating diarrhea that may last for weeks and even months and is very difficult to treat. Other symptoms include cramps, fever, nausea, and vomiting. Diarrhea can be severe enough to cause dehydration and death unless nutritional supplements are given.

— KAPOSI'S SARCOMA, a cancer of the blood vessels, is the most common cancer in AIDS patients, in whom it is more aggressive than in those who do not have AIDS. Kaposi's sarcoma appears as dark blue or purple raised areas on the skin, often first appearing on the trunk or upper extremities but also on the ears and nose. These skin nodules are not itchy or painful. Although people occasionally service several years, the disease commonly spreads to the internal organs and may eventually cause death. Persons with Kaposi's sarcoma usually die from opportunistic infections.

— TUBERCULOSIS (TB), caused by bacteria, can affect many organs. Disseminated TB is common in AIDS patients. Also, they may develop extremely aggressive tubercular lesions in sites not usually affected by the disease. AIDS patients with tuberculosis usually respond well to treatment.

— HERPES SIMPLEX VIRUSES cause skin lesions in or around the mouth or in the genital and rectal areas, depending on the type of virus. In people without immune deficiency, these lesions are generally mild and temporary, although recurrent. In AIDS cases lesions are more severe and recur more often.

— CANDIDIASIS in the alimentary tract, or thrush, is caused by a yeast. Candidiasis is common and usually benign in infants but is very rare in adults. Two types often occur in AIDS cases. Oral candidiasis, the more common, causes white, usually painless lesions in the mouth. The other type, esophageal candidiasis, may cause pain or difficulty in swallowing. Candidiasis generally responds to treatment, but relapse is common; many patients must be treated for the rest of their lives.

AIDS is less common in children than in adults, but the number of cases in children is expected to rise rapidly. AIDS in children was first diagnosed in 1983 in the US. By July 1986, 321 US children under age 13 with AIDS had been reported. Over 60 percent of these children had died. Disease resulted from infection during pregnancy or child-birth in about three-fourths of these children. Most of the others acquired HIV infection through transfusions. The number of actual cases of AIDS among children in developing countries is unknown. Most countries do not have national reporting yet. Also, diagnosing AIDS in children is difficult because the major symptoms — diarrhea and failure to thrive — are very common and nonspecific.

Little is known about the prevalence of HIV infection among children. In the US, researchers estimate that as many as 1,000 children are infected with the virus but have not developed AIDS. No studies are available, however. In Zaire two studies from Mama Yemo Hospital found that 10 to 12 percent of hospitalized children were infected with HIV in 1984 and 1985 compared with 1 to 2 percent of two healthy control groups.

HIV infection progresses differently in children than in adults. Certain symptoms and illnesses are more common — chronic swelling of the parotid gland, recurrent bacterial infections, central nervous system abnormalities, and lymphoid interstitial pneumonia. Central nervous system abnormalities have been reported in 50 to 80 percent of infected children. In contrast, Kaposi's sarcoma, which is found in over 20 percent of US adults with AIDS, is uncommon in children.

Researchers in New York have reported a distinct syndrome among 20 children infected with HIV in utero. The syndrome involves growth retardation and multiple facial and cranial abnormalities — an abnormally small head, a prominent box-like forehead, and a flattened nasal bridge.

There are no answers yet to some important questions concerning HIV infection in children: (1) What is the likelihood that an infected woman will transmit the virus to her child? (2) What factors increase the risks of transmission from mother to child? (3) Is the virus readily transmitted in breast-milk? (4) Can the prognosis for infected children be improved? (5) Are there risks from immunizing infected children? Answers to these questions are urgently needed to help stem the rising tide of AIDS in the very young.

Overall, how many people infected with HIV will develop AIDS or other symptoms? At this point, it is difficult to say. AIDS is so new that long-term prospective studies are just beginning to yield results. It has been variously estimated that each year 8 to 10 percent of asymptomatic infected persons develop some symptoms and that 2 to 10 percent develop AIDS. One of the longest studies to date followed 57 homosexual men in San Francisco who were known to be infected with HIV, for a median of five years. Among the 57 men, 10, or 18 percent, have developed AIDS, and 27, or 45 percent, have developed other symptoms.

The proportion of infected individuals who develop symptoms or AIDS seems to vary in different groups. For example, after at least three years' follow-up, 34 percent of a group of infected homosexual men in New York had developed AIDS compared with 12 percent of a group of infected hemophiliacs in Pennsylvania. Exposure to as-yet-unidentified risk factors, such as greater dose of the virus, concurrent infections, or drug use, might explain this difference. It is not known exactly when the participants were infected, however. Therefore, the difference may have occurred because the New York group had been infected longer than the Pennsylvania group. The reported incubation period — that is, the time between infection and first symptoms or diagnosis — also varies widely, ranging from 1.5 to 7 years. A mathematical model based on transfusion cases suggests that the incubation period may range from four months to 10 years with a mean of 4.5 years.

Why do some people with HIV infection develop symptoms or AIDS while others do not? Very little is known about the factors that influence progression of HIV-related infection. One hypothesis is that repeated infections and possibly exposure to antigens (infections agents or possibly other foreign substances such as semen or transfused blood) may activate the replication of HIV, leading to various symptoms. Several studies have found that persistent generalized lymphadenopathy or AIDS often occurs in people with current and/or past infection with various other viruses — cytomegalovirus, hepatitis B virus, or Epstein-Barr virus, or with a recent history of sexually transmitted diseases and/or sexual intercourse with many partners without the use of condoms. Not all studies report these findings, however. Another hypothesis is that certain conditions — malaria, certain other parasitic diseases, and malnutrition — may themselves compromise immune function, increasing the chances of immunosuppression with HIV.

Use of certain drugs also may lead to HIV-related illness, but evidence is very preliminary. Several US studies have found that homosexual men with persistent generalized lymphadenopathy or AIDS, especially involving Kaposi's sarcoma, were more likely to have used volatile nitrites (drugs inhaled to enhance sexual pleasure) than healthy men. Others find no such relationship, however.

It has been suspected that pregnancy triggers symptoms in infected women, but the evidence is conflicting. In a US study 6 of 11 asymptomatic women developed AIDS or other symptoms during pregnancy. All of the 11 women were known to have been infected for a least a year because all had previously given birth to a child infected with HIV. Another study in the US, however, reported no progression of illness during pregnancy. A woman with HIV infection needs to use condoms because, if she becomes pregnant, she can pass the virus to the fetus during pregnancy and possibly endanger her own life as well. In addition, using condoms will help to protect her sexual partner.

WHO estimates that five to ten million people worldwide are infected with the virus. Making estimates is difficult because they must be based on small studies of selected populations. In the US possibly one to two million people may be infected. Rates of infection are highest among hemophiliacs, homosexual men, and IV drug users. In Africa also, possibly one to two million people are infected, according to a WHO estimate. High rates are reported in prostitutes and clients of STD clinics, but HIV infection is not confined to any specific group. In studies using two different blood tests to achieve greatest accuracy, from 2 to 14 percent of pregnant women and new mothers in Kenya, Malawi, Uganda, Zaire, and Zambia were infected, as were 6 to 11 percent of male and female blood donors in Uganda and Zaire. in Tanzania, Uganda, and Zambia, infection has been found to be equally common in rural and urban areas. In Latin America 5 to 12 percent of small groups of homosexual men studied in Panama and Peru were infected.

Rates of infection have increased rapidly among some groups in the US, Europe, and Africa. In Nairobi, Kenya, for example, only 4 percent of 58 prostitutes tested positive in 1981 compared with 69 percent of 535 prostitutes tested in 1985. In contrast, a study in Baltimore of homosexual men who initially showed no evidence of HIV infection found, in three successive 6-month periods beginning in April 1984, that 4 percent, 2 percent, and one percent developed antibodies indicating HIV infection. All study participants had been advised about safe sexual practices. The results suggest that educational efforts to change behavior in high-risk groups can have some effect.

Most reported cases of AIDS have been sexually transmitted. Only the most intimate contact, usually involving the transfer of semen or blood from one person to another, can spread the virus. Thus AIDS is not a highly contagious disease. Unlike the virus that causes measles, for example, the virus that causes AIDS is not transmitted through the air. There also is no evidence that it is transmitted through casual contact, by insects, or by food or water. The virus is transmitted:

1. by sexual intercourse,
2. by transfusions of contaminated blood or blood products,
3. by sharing or reusing contaminated needles, and
4. during pregnancy, childbirth, and possibly breastfeeding from woman to child.

Since routes of transmission are limited, a few protective practices — using condoms, limiting the number of sexual partners, sterilizing needles and syringes, and avoiding pregnancy in infected women — can substantially reduce the transmission of the virus. Because the virus may be transmitted by infected people who have no symptoms, the best way to minimize the risk of infection through sexual relations with people who are at high risk is always to use condoms unless partners are known to be free of infection.

Transmission of HIV always involves exposure to body fluids from an infected person. The dose or amount of virus, the route of exposure, and the duration of exposure all may influence the chances of becoming infected. It is not known, however, how much virus over what period of time is needed to cause infection or what other factors affect the chances of infection.

HIV has been isolated from various body fluids. The greatest concentrations have been found in blood, semen, and cerebrospinal fluid. Lower concentrations have been detected infrequently in tears, saliva, breastmilk, colostrum, urine, and cervical and vaginal secretions. HIV also has been isolated in brain tissue, lymph nodes, bone marrow cells, and skin. To date only blood and semen have been conclusively shown to transmit the virus.

Scientists thing that HIV infection is chronic and that infected people will always be carriers. In other words, they are capable of transmitting the virus even though they may have no symptoms of infection.

HIV infection can be transmitted during sexual intercourse between men and between men and women. Some 65 to 75 percent of AIDS cases in the US and Europe have occurred in homosexual and bisexual men. While the number of cases attributable to heterosexual transmission is smaller (at least in the US and Europe), the evidence for heterosexual transmission is convincing. It consists of cases of HIV infection and AIDS in sexual partners of infected persons; in women artificially inseminated from an infected donor; and in female prostitutes.

Certain sexual patterns and practices increase the risk of infection more than others. Relations with multiple sexual partners increases the chances of encountering someone who is infected, especially in an area where HIV infection is very common. Among sexual practices, receptive anal intercourse with an infected partner is especially likely to lead to infection. The mucosa lining the rectum is delicate and tears easily during anal intercourse. This allows infected lymphocytes and virus in semen to enter the tissue and bloodstream of the receptive partner, whether male or female.

The virus is also transmitted during vaginal intercourse. Both male and female partners can be infected in this way. It is not clear whether the risk is the same for both men and women, however. Most sexually transmitted diseases are more readily transmitted from men to women than from women to men. It is also not clear how readily the virus is transmitted during vaginal intercourse or what the chances are of infection associated with a single act of intercourse with an infected person. In both vaginal and anal intercourse, using a condom reduces the chances of transmission.

It is not known whether other sexual practices, such as oral-genital contact or kissing, transmit the virus. Nevertheless, since HIV is found in semen and sometimes in saliva, and since oral-genital contact transmits other infections, most infectious disease experts recommend avoiding these and any other practices that might transfer bodily fluids.

Heterosexual intercourse may be the major route of HIV transmission in developing countries. In central Africa and Haiti, women are as likely as men to be infected, and female prostitutes are thought to be transmitting the virus to their clients. Some 80 percent of African men treated for AIDS in Rwanda and Belgium regularly visited prostitutes, compared with 34 percent of healthy men. Similar results have been reported in Haiti and among Haitian immigrants in the US. Furthermore, both male homosexuality and anal intercourse are said to be rare in Africa. Reliable information on sexual practices is scarce, however.

Heterosexual transmission may be common in some areas for several reasons. Sexually transmitted diseases may facilitate transmission of HIV. Chancroid, herpes, and some other sexually transmitted diseases can cause open genital sores, possibly allowing the virus to enter the bloodstream. Cervical and vaginal infections often produce a copious discharge in the vagina with a high concentration of lymphocytes — and thus also virus — in a woman infected with HIV. Certain sexual practices also may affect the chances of infection. For example, Zairian prostitutes often put objects into their vaginas. This may cause open sores and infection. At the same time, more frequent heterosexual transmission in Africa and Haiti may simply mean that HIV first became established among heterosexual men and women in these areas, in contrast with the US and Europe, where it first became established among homosexual men.

Transfusion of contaminated blood or blood products can transmit HIV. About 2 percent of AIDS cases in the US and about 5 percent in Europe have occurred among hemophiliacs and others receiving contaminated transfusions of blood products. Blood transfusions seem to pose a greater risk to infants than to others. In the US, infants receive less than 2 percent of all transfusions but have accounted for about 10 percent of AIDS cases associated with transfusion. This could be because infants' immune systems are immature, because they receive a larger dose of the virus relative to their body size, or because of a shorter incubation period. Most developed countries are now screening all donated blood. Therefore transfusion-related infections will become extremely rare in these countries. Of course, giving blood poses no risk to the donor as long as a sterile needle is used.

In some African countries blood transfusions may be an important means of HIV transmission. In Zaire, Uganda, and Rwanda, for example, 6 percent or more of samples of donated blood contain antibodies to HIV. In Zaire, studies of adults and children found that those with HIV antibodies were at least twice as likely to have had blood transfusions as those without such antibodies.

Not all blood components transmit the virus. Red blood cells, platelets, plasma, whole blood, and clotting factor concentrate may contain the virus. Other products prepared from blood — albumin, immunoglobulins (gamma globulins), and hepatitis B vaccine — have not been shown to pose any risk. The process of separating and manufacturing these products from whole blood inactivates the virus. HIV antibodies may still be present, and recipients' blood can test positive for six months after they receive the product. This does not indicate infection, however. Heat treatment during the manufacture of Factor VIII concentrate, a blood clotting agent used by hemophiliacs, also inactivates most of the virus, greatly reducing the risk of infection.

HIV is transmitted among intravenous drug users by sharing needles and syringes in which small amounts of contaminated blood are transferred. Intravenous drug use has been linked with 25 percent of AIDS cases in the US and 8 percent in Europe, and these percentages are increasing. Of course, persons infected by contaminated needles can then pass on the infection through sexual intercourse, and vice versa.

If needles used for medical injections are contaminated, they may spread infection. While intravenous drug use is rare in developing countries, many people take antibiotics and other medications by injection for minor and major illnesses. In Zaire, for example, over 80 percent of healthy children and adults had had one or more injections in a 3-year period. Traditional healers as well as trained health workers give these injections, and needles are not always properly sterilized. In fact, outbreaks of infectious diseases such as Ebola hemorrhagic fever have been traced to contaminated needles in clinics. Researchers have suggested that contaminated needles in sexually transmitted disease clinics may be an important means of HIV transmission. At present, there is no direct evidence for this.

It is not clear how important a role medical injections with contaminated needles play in transmitting HIV, in part because injections are so common in developing countries. Two studies in Zaire, one in Rwanda, and one in Haiti have found that people with HIV antibodies or with AIDS had received more injections one to five years before the onset of symptoms than had healthy controls. Other studies in several African countries, however, report no difference in the number of injections.

There has been no demonstrated transmission of HIV as a result of immunization. A Zairian study comparing hospitalized children with HIV antibodies to children without antibodies found no difference in the number of immunizations they had received. Immunization workers are expected to sterilize needles, and immunization involves only a few injections. Also, subdermal or intramuscular injections used for immunization and to treat illness may be less likely to transmit the virus than intravenous injections, especially as practiced by drug users. Less virus may enter the body, and it usually would not enter directly into the bloodstream.

HIV can be transmitted from an infected mother to the fetus during pregnancy or childbirth. The virus has been isolated in breastmilk, and there has been one report of a woman, infected by a postnatal blood transfusion, whose breastfeeding infant became infected.

How often transmission occurs in pregnancy is not certain. Researchers estimate that 20 to 50 percent of infants born to infected mothers also will be infected. Rates are higher among infants of women who previously have given birth to an infected child. Large prospective studies are now underway in the US, Haiti, and Africa addressing this and related questions. Since many women in some countries are becoming infected, AIDS and other HIV-related illness may become a major threat to child survival.

Casual contact or even close family contact has not been shown to spread HIV. To transmit the virus, infected cells or viral particles must pass into the tissue or bloodstream of another person. More than 10 studies involving some 600 family members of people with AIDS in the US, Europe, and Africa show no evidence of transmission of the virus except to sexual partners or to children born to an infected mother. Living in very crowded conditions and sharing bathrooms, kitchens, eating utensils, plates, drinking glasses, and personal items such as combs, towels, and even razors and toothbrushes with infected people before and after they developed AIDS have not led to infection. There also is no evidence that the virus can be spread in food or beverages.

Health workers also face little risk of infection even if they have extensive contact with people with AIDS. Only three to six cases of job-related infection have been reported, and researchers disagree about which of these cases truly resulted from occupational exposure. Among more than 2,000 health care workers tested in the US and Europe, including more than 400 with needlestick or other exposure to patients with HIV infection, no more than four had HIV antibodies and apparently were not infected through intravenous drug use or homosexual intercourse. This amounts to at most 0.25 percent of all these workers and 1.25 percent of those with needlestick injuries. This is considerably lower than the risk of infection with hepatitis B virus. After being stuck with a needle contaminated with hepatitis B, 6 to 30 percent of persons become infected. A deep intramuscular wound with a contaminated needle or accidental self-injection or contaminated blood may be necessary to cause infection with HIV. Even workers bitten repeatedly by an AIDS patient suffering from dementia have not developed HIV antibodies.

In Zaire, 6 percent of almost 2,400 health workers in Kinshasa had HIV antibodies. This rate, however, is the same both in hospital workers who had direct contact with AIDS patients or possibly contaminated instruments and in those who had no such contact. This suggests that few, if any, of these infections involved transmission through professional contact with AIDS patients. Both US CDC and WHO have prepared safety guidelines for health workers.

* * * * * * * * * *

WHO Updates on AIDS Total Reprinted from *CDC AIDS Weekly*
July 6, 1987

The World Health Organization reports there have been 53,121 cases
of AIDS
    The total, as of July 1, 1987, represents an increase of 1,370 cases
since June 1.
    The WHO says that over two-thirds of the cases, or a total of
37,019, have been registered in the United States.

* * * * * * * * * *

West Germany: Police Computer Identifies Those With AIDS
Reprinted from *CDC AIDS Weekly* August 10, 1987

West Germany's interior minister says the police computer system
identifies 343 people infected with the AIDS virus.
    Interior Minister Friedrich Zimmerman says that carriers are identi-
fied for the protection of officers who might come into contact with
them.
    Wilfried Renner, deputy floor leader of the Social Democrats has
called for a special meeting of the parliamentary interior affairs
committee to discuss the police precaution.

* * * * * * * * * *

*AS of January 1, 1982, The Centers for Disease Control in Atlanta
reported 281 cases of AIDS in the United States*

[handwritten note at top: Reagan, American College of Physicians: "When it comes to preventing AIDS, don't medicine & morality teach the same lessons?"]

[handwritten note: A projective, not disruptive term.]

The AIDS Virus
Robert C. Gallo
Reprinted with permission from *Scientific American*
January, 1987

It is a modern plague: the first great pandemic of the second half of the 20th century. The flat, clinical-sounding name given to the disease by epidemiologists — acquired immune deficiency syn- *[handwritten: virology that]* drome — has been shortened to the chilling acronym AIDS. First *[handwritten: created that chill]* described in 1981, AIDS is probably the result of a new infection of human beings that began in central Africa, perhaps as recently as the 1950's. From there it probably spread to the Caribbean and then to the U.S. and Europe. By now as many as two million people in the U.S. may be infected. In the endemic areas of Africa and the Caribbean the situation is much worse. Indeed, in some areas it may be too late to prevent a disturbingly high number of people from dying.

In sharp contrast to the bleak epidemiological picture of AIDS, the *[handwritten: bleak epidemiology]* accumulation of knowledge about its cause has been remarkably *[handwritten: bright virology]* quick. Only three years after the disease was described its cause was *[handwritten: NO!]* conclusively shown to be the third human retrovirus: human T-lymphotropic virus III (HTLV-III), which is also called human immu-nodeficiency virus (HIV). Like other retroviruses, HTLV-III has RNA as its genetic material. When the virus enters its host cell, a viral enzyme called reverse transcriptase exploits the viral RNA as a tem-plate to assemble a corresponding molecule of DNA. The DNA travels to the cell nucleus and inserts itself among the host's chromosomes, where it provides the basis for viral replication.

In the case of HTLV-III the host cell is often a T4 lymphocyte, a white blood cell that has a central role in regulating the immune system. Once it is inside a T4 cell, the virus may remain latent until the lymphocyte is immunologically stimulated by a secondary infec-tion. Then the virus bursts into action, reproducing itself so furiously that the new virus particles escaping from the cell riddle the cellular membrane with holes and the lymphocyte dies. The resulting depletion of T4 cells — the hallmark of AIDS — leaves the patient vulnerable to "opportunistic" infections by agents that would not harm a healthy person.

How HTLV-III manages to replicate in a single burst after lying low, sometimes for years, is one of the most fundamental questions confronting AIDS researchers. Another important question is the full spectrum of diseases with which the virus is associated. Although most of the attention given to the virus has gone to AIDS, HTLV-III is also associated with brain disease and several types of cancer. In spite of such lingering questions, more is known about the AIDS virus than is known about any other retrovirus. The rapidity of that scientific advance was made possible partly by the discovery in 1978 of the first human retrovirus, HTLV-I, which causes leukemia. In its turn the new knowledge is making possible the measures that are desperately needed to treat AIDS and prevent its spread.

The first sign that a new disease was afoot was the appearance of a rare cancer called Kaposi's sarcoma among the "wrong" patients. Kaposi's sarcoma is a tumor of blood-vessel tissue in the skin or internal organs that had been known mainly among older Italian and Jewish men and in Africa. In the late 1970's, however, a more aggressive form of the same cancer began to appear among young white middle-class males, a group in which it had been extremely rare. Many of the new Kaposi's sarcoma patients turned out to have a history of homosexuality, and these young men provided the basis for the first reports of a new syndrome, which came in 1981 from Michael S. Gottlieb of the University of California at Los Angeles School of Medicine, Frederick P. Siegal of the Mount Sinai Medical Center and Henry Masur of New York Hospital. Seen mainly among young homosexual men, the new syndrome included opportunistic infections and a depletion of T4 cells as well as, in some cases, Kaposi's sarcoma. Soon epidemiologists at the U.S. Centers for Disease Control (CDC) noted a dramatic increase in pneumonia caused by *Pneumocystis carinii*, a widespread but generally harmless protozoan. It seemed clear that an infectious form of immune deficiency was on the rise, and the name AIDS was coined to describe it. AIDS was quickly found to be spreading among users of intravenous drugs, recipients of frequent blood transfusions and Haitians. A mysterious and fatal illness, apparently associated with life-style, had appeared.

Hypotheses about the cause of AIDS proliferated rapidly. It was suggested that the disease resulted from exposure to sperm and to amyl nitrate, a stimulant used by some homosexuals. It was even proposed that AIDS had no specific etiologic agent: the patients' immune systems had simply broken down under chronic overexposure to foreign proteins carried by other people's white blood cells or by infectious agents. Yet it seemed more plausible to think of a single *to whom?* cause, and several workers suggested known viruses such as Epstein-Barr virus or cytomegalovirus, which are members of the herpes virus family. Both were long-established viruses, however, whereas AIDS seemed to be a new disease. Moreover, neither virus has an affinity for T cells.

James W. Curran of the CDC and his colleagues, who had been following the nascent epidemic, clearly favored the notion of a new infectious agent. In late 1981, as I listened to Curran outline what was known about the epidemiology of AIDS, I was already in agreement with him. A clue as to what the new agent might be came from the fact that some hemophiliacs had developed AIDS after receiving infusions of a preparation called Factor VIII, prepared from the plasma of many blood donors. In preparing Factor VIII the plasma is passed through filters fine enough to remove fungi and bacteria — but not viruses.

That observation supported those who had argued in favor of a virus. Yet if one could not look to established viruses as the cause, how could the culprit be identified? Any virus that was a candidate would have to fit what was known about the agent, which included the following. It was present in whole blood, plasma and semen as well as in Factor VIII. The epidemiological pattern showed that it could be transmitted by sexual contact, blood and congenital infection. Infection led, directly or indirectly, to the loss of T4 cells.

As it happened, that pattern was familiar to me and my co-workers, because HTLV-I had been isolated in my laboratory in 1978. HTLV-I can be transmitted by blood, intimate contact and congenital infection; it has a strong affinity for T cells. Furthermore, although the chief effect of HTLV-I is leukemia, the virus can also cause a mild immune deficiency in some patients. Accordingly, in the spring of 1982 I proposed that the cause of AIDS was likely to be a new human retrovirus.

To refine and test the retrovirus hypothesis I assembled a small working group of scientists, each chosen for a specific expertise. Along with clinicians, epidemiologists, immunologists, and molecular biologists were investigators experienced in animal retrovirology. One of the retrovirologists, Myron Essex of the Harvard Medical School, had published results lending support to the idea that a human retrovirus might cause AIDS. Essex had shown that a retrovirus called feline leukemia virus (FeLV) can cause either leukemia or immune deficiency in cats. A minor variation in the virus's outer envelope, it was later shown, determines whether infection leads to immune suppression or to cancer.

These suggestive results made it seem even more plausible that a variant of HTLV-I (or its near relative HTLV-II, isolated in 1982) might be the AIDS agent. Essex's group and my own quickly began searching for such a virus. Soon we were joined by a third group, led by Luc Montagnier of the Pasteur Institute, who had been stimulated by the retrovirus hypothesis. All three groups employed the methods that my colleagues and I had developed for isolating HTLV-I: the virus was cultured in T cells stimulated by the growth factor called IL-2 and its presence was detected by sensitive assays for the viral reverse transcriptase.

Those methods quickly produced results. Beginning in late 1982 and continuing throughout 1983 my co-workers and I found preliminary evidence of retroviruses different from HTLV-I or II in tissues from people with AIDS or pre-AIDS conditions. Then in May of 1983 Montagnier and his colleagues Francoise Bare-Sinoussi and Jean-Claude Chermann published the first report of a new retrovirus from a patient with the lymphadenopathy ("swollen glands") typical of some pre-AIDS cases. The French investigators later gave their find the name lymphadenopathy-associated virus (LAV).

The initial report of LAV was intriguing, but it was hardly a conclusive identification of the cause of AIDS. The reason is that the methods then available (reverse-transcriptase assays accompanied by electron microscopy) can show that a retrovirus is present in a tissue sample but cannot specify the precise type of virus. Unique identification is possible only if reagents (such as antibodies) are available that react with the proteins of that virus and no other. Making such reagents requires large quantities of purified viral proteins; to obtain them the virus must be grown in the laboratory.

The new virus (or viruses), however, resisted the early attempts at laboratory culture: when they were put in T cells, the cells died. Hence no specific reagents to the new isolates could be made. We had previously learned how to culture HTLV-I and II, and reagents to those viruses were available. As a result it was possible to show that the viruses present in AIDS patients were not HTLV-I or HTLV-II, but throughout most of 1983 it was not possible to make a positive identification because specific reagents were lacking. Moreover, in the absence of reagents one could not say that any two of the new isolates were the same, which was clearly a requirement for showing that AIDS has a single cause.

The answer to such difficulties was to find a way to grow the virus. In the fall of 1983 my colleague Mike Popovic identified several cell lines that could be infected with the virus but resisted being killed. To obtain them the blood cells of a person with leukemia were separated and allowed to proliferate into clones of genetically identical cells. Many clones were screened, and several were found to have the right combination of qualities; the most productive of them was the clone designated H9. All the resistant lines are made up of leukemic T4 cells that are immortal in culture and therefore an endless source of virus.

Why certain T4 cell lines should resist the cytopathic effects of the virus is a significant question that has not been answered. In the winter of 1983-84, however, my colleagues and I had little time for that puzzle because we were concentrating on growing the virus. By December substantial quantities were being grown, and soon afterward reagent production was under way. With reagents in hand, we could go back and identify the many stored viral isolates. Initial testing showed that 48 isolates from AIDS patients or members of risk groups were of the same type. In contrast, the virus so identified was not found in any members of a control group of 124 healthy heterosexuals.

Continuous production of the virus also yielded enough viral proteins to provide the basis of a blood test. (Although there are several methods of testing blood for the AIDS agent, all of them rely on the reaction between viral proteins and antibodies in the infected persons' blood.) The first blood testing was done by my colleague M. G. Sarnagadharan, working on serum identified only by a code. By means of such "blind" testing Sarnagadharan found virus in the serum of from 88 to 100 percent of AIDS patients (depending on the study), in a high but varying proportion of people in risk groups and in almost no healthy individuals outside the risk groups. The cause of AIDS had been established.

My colleagues and I reported these results in a series of publications in May, 1984. The retrovirus we had identified showed an affinity for T4 cells and also killed those cells. In accord with the prevailing conventions of virus nomenclature, the isolates were given the generic name HTLV-III and individual strains were distinguished by the initials of the patient from which they had come. Later it was shown that LAV is a different strain of the same virus. Later still, the name HIV was coined by a committee set up to resolve the problems caused by the existence of multiple names for the same biologic object.   *vir — the principle causative agent*

Demonstrating the cause of AIDS was a fundamental step. Perhaps equally important from the viewpoint of public health was the fact that growing the virus had provided a basis for a practical blood test. The infected H9 line was given to several biotechnology companies, which used it as a source of viral proteins for a commercial blood test. The commercial test, marketed in 1985, virtually eliminated the risk of contracting AIDS through blood transfusion.

Although only three years have elapsed since the cause of AIDS was identified, much has been learned about how the virus gives rise to disease. When a person is first infected, his (or her) immune system does respond by making antibodies. That response is clearly not adequate, however, and the virus takes hold. In many cases lymphocytes then begin to proliferate abnormally in the lymph nodes. Thereafter the node's intricate structure collapses, and a decline in the number of lymphocytes in the node follows. Soon the number of lymphocytes in the blood also decreases, leaving the patient open to opportunistic infections.

What events at the cellular level underlie this clinical catastrophe? It seems infection may be initiated by free virus or by virus carried in infected cells. Once the virus is inside the body its target consists of cells bearing the T4 molecule in their outer membrane. That molecule defines the category of T4 lymphocytes, but it is also found on cells called monocytes and macrophages, and it appears that T4 carrying monocytes and macrophages are among the first targets of infection by the AIDS virus.

Monocytes and macrophages arise from the same bone-marrow precursors as lymphocytes, but they have different roles in the immune response. Among the roles of the machrophage are interactions with T4 lymphocytes that stimulate the T4 cells to undertake their tasks. Some of the interactions occur in the lymph node, and observations by Peter Biberfeld of the Karolinska Institute in Stockholm and Claudio Baroni of the University of Rome suggest that many T4 cells are infected in the lymph node during contact with a macrophage. After a variable latency the infected lymphocyte may be killed by viral replication.

Clearly the T4 population is reduced by the death of infected cells. The effect is compounded by the fact that the killing halts the normal proliferation of the lymphocytes that accompanies their immune functions. In the interaction with a macrophage the T4 cell not only is primed to respond to a particular protein but also is activated.

Growth factors secreted by the macrophages cause it to begin a process of cell division that ultimately yields a clone of perhaps 1,000 descendants, all programmed to respond to the same antigen (protein). The descendants circulate in the blood and, on encountering the antigen they are programmed for, they induce the maturation of cells called B lymphocytes and T8 cytotoxic cells that attack pathogens directly. In this way the "memory clone" provides part of the basis of lasting immunity.

When a T4 cell infected with the AIDS virus is activated, however, the result is quite different, as Daniel Zagury of the University of Paris has shown in collaboration with me. Instead of yielding 1,000 progeny, the infected T cell proliferates into a stunted clone with perhaps as few as 10 members. When those 10 reach the bloodstream and are stimulated by antigens, they begin producing virus and die. Other suggestions have been made, but I think the direct killing of infected lymphocytes and the abortive expansion of the memory clones are largely responsible for the profound depletion of T4 cells observed in AIDS.

And what underlies these cellular events at the level of molecules? One of the most significant molecules in HTLV-III infection is T4. Indeed, by interacting with the outer envelope of the virus, T4 may provide entry to the cell. The viral envelope consists of a membrane studded with glycoprotein molecules (proteins with attached sugar chains). Each glycoprotein has two subunits, called gp41 and gp120. When HTLV-III makes contact with a cell, gp120 appears to interact with a T4 molecule in the cell's outer membrane. Thereafter the cell's membrane may form a vesicle that draws the virus into the cell. (This process, which is known as receptor-mediated endocytosis, provides entry to the cell for a variety of molecules needed for normal metabolism.)

The by now overwhelming evidence that T4 is involved in infection was gathered in steps. The first step was the clinical observation that the infected cells are T4 lymphocytes. Next, Robin A. Weiss of the Chester Beatty Laboratory in London, Angus Dalgleish of University College Hospital Medical School and David Klatzmann of the Hopital Salpetriere found that antibodies to the T4 molecule, which cover part of its structure, block HTLV-III infection. Then my colleagues and I found infected T4-carrying monocytes and macrophages. Some of the most telling evidence, however, came from Weiss and Richard Axel of the Columbia University College of Physicians and Surgeons, who inserted the T4 gene into cells that do not ordinarily carry the marker and are not infected. Expression of the gene, entailing synthesis of the marker and its insertion into the cell membrane, is sufficient for infection of any human cell.

A similar, if less formidable, combination of evidence implicates T4 in cell death. There too the initial observation was a clinical one: that the T4-lymphocyte population was depleted. In contrast to infection, however, the presence of T4 alone is not sufficient for cell killing. Although monocytes and macrophages can be infected with HTLV-III, they are not easily killed, and the reason may be that they have few T4 molecules on their surface. It seems that although a low level of T4 is sufficient for entry, a higher level may be required for the cytopathic effect. Indeed, as William Haseltine of the Dana Farber Cancer Institute has suggested, the rate of cell killing may be proportional to the concentration of T4 in the surface membrane of the infected cell.

Although no one knows why the death of the T4 cell should depend on the molecule that defines it, some suggestive findings make it possible to formulate a hypothesis. The killing depends not only on the T4 molecule but also on the viral envelope. My colleagues Flossie Wong-Staal and Amanda G. Fisher showed that mutant viruses lacking a piece of the inner end of gp41 have a drastically reduced cytopathic effect. Thus, like entry to the cell, its death may depend on an interaction between the viral envelope and the cell membrane. Perhaps that interaction (which takes place as the virus particle buds from the cell) punches a hole in the membrane. Because the virus buds in a mass of particles, the cell cannot repair the holes as fast as they are made; its contents leak out and it dies.

If that model (for the moment only a model) is correct, attention naturally falls on the question of how the virus is able to raise its rate of replication very rapidly from zero to a level high enough to kill the host cell. That question in turn focuses attention on the viral genome (the full complement of genetic information). The genome's DNA form, transcribed from the viral RNA and integrated into the cell's chromosomes, is called the provirus. The provirus includes the genes for the components of the virus particle, and in order for the virus to replicate, those genes must be expressed. How is gene expression controlled?

The answer (still very much under investigation) appears to lie in a group of regulatory genes whose presence renders the HTLV-III genome more complex than that of any other known retrovirus. The genetic complement of many retroviruses consists chiefly of the three genes that encode the components of the virus particle *env* (which codes for the envelope proteins), *gag* (for the RNA-containing core) and *pol* (for the reverse transcriptase). Those three genes are flanked by stretches of DNA called the long terminal redundancies, or LTR's. The LTR's include DNA sequences that have a role in controlling the expression of the viral genes.

The genome of HTLV-III, however, includes at least four other genes, called *tat*, *trs*, *sor* and 3' *orf*. Rather than encoding viral components, the four additional genes encode small proteins that help to regulate gene expression. The *tat* gene (discovered by Haseltine and his colleague Joseph Sodroski, and independently by Wong-Staal and Suresh Arya in my laboratory) has a dual function. Like its analogues in HTLV-I and II, *tat* appears to regulate the transcription of messenger RNA (mRNA) from the viral genes. In addition the *tat* protein affects events after transcription, perhaps the translation of the viral mRNA into proteins. The *trs* gene (discovered by Haseltine) appears to control the balance among the various forms of viral mRNA. The functions of *sor* and 3' *orf* are unknown.

There are many other unknowns in this complex system, and it is too soon to say confidently how it works. It is not too soon, however, to hazard a general hypothesis, taking as a premise the fact that the virus does not replicate until the T cell is immunologically activated. The LTR's of the AIDS virus share some DNA sequences with the cellular genes that are turned on during immune activation. I think the chemical signals that activate the T4 cell simultaneously activate the viral LTR's. Somehow the small regulatory proteins interact with the provirus to boost synthesis of the viral components very quickly. The components self-assemble and bud from the cell in a pulse that may kill the host.

In summary form that is what is known about how HTLV-III cripples the immune system. Although most of the attention given to the virus has been devoted to that process, it has become increasingly clear that immune deficiency is only one effect of the AIDS agent. The other main type of disease caused by HTLV-III is seen in the central nervous system. HTLV-III was first detected in brain and spinal-cord tissue from AIDS patients by my colleagues George M. Shaw, Beatrice Hahn, Wong-Staal and me in 1984. The infected cells appear to have some of the properties of monocytes and macrophages. Those cells may be able to cross the blood-brain barrier, which separates the central nervous system from the blood supply; perhaps macrophages become infected in the blood and transport the virus from there to the brain.

In the brain and spinal cord the virus appears to have a direct pathogenic effect that is not dependent on the immune deficiency.

The chief pathologies observed in the brain are an abnormal proliferation of the glial cells that surround the neurons and lesions resulting from loss of white matter (which is, along with gray matter, one of the two main types of brain tissue). How the virus causes such anatomical changes is not understood. Nor is it known how the relatively limited range of structural aberrations due to the virus gives rise to a wide range of symptoms including dementia and mimicry of other neurological syndromes such as multiple sclerosis.

Whereas the neurological effects of HTLV-III are distinct from immune deficiency, the third main type of pathology — cancer — has a more ambiguous relation to the crippling of the immune system. People infected with the virus have an increased risk of at least three types of human tumor; Kaposi's sarcoma, carcinomas (including skin cancers often seen in the mouth or rectum of infected homosexuals) and B-cell lymphomas, which are tumors originating in B lymphocytes.

In some instances the tumors appear to be independent of immune deficits, as is suggested by the fact that homosexuals may have an increased risk of developing Kaposi's sarcoma even if they are not infected with AIDS virus. Pathogens other than HTLV-III — perhaps sexually transmitted agents — are likely to be involved in these tumors. Yet infection with HTLV-III greatly increases the risk that Kaposi's sarcoma will develop. Therefore it seems likely that depression of the immune response enables secondary tumor-causing agents to infect and replicate freely. What they are is not known, but one may be human B-lymphotropic virus (HBLV), a new DNA-containing member of the herpes virus family recently isolated by my colleagues Zaki Salahuddin, Dharam Ablashi and Biberfeld and me.

The welter of pathologies caused by HTLV-III seems daunting, but the knowledge already gained about the virus has begun to lay the groundwork for treatment and prevention. The most promising therapies currently under investigation are based on interrupting the reverse transcriptase as it assembles the viral DNA destined to become the provirus. The drugs used for this purpose are chemical analogues of the nucleotides that form the subunits of DNA. When the analogue is supplied to an infected cell, reverse transcriptase will incorporate it into a growing DNA chain. Because the analogue lacks the correct attachment point for the next subunit, however, the chain is terminated. The truncated DNA cannot integrate itself into the chromosomes or provide the basis for viral replication, and so the spread of infection is halted.

Recent tests of azidothymidine, or AZT, have shown that this strategy can reduce mortality among AIDS and pre-AIDS patients as well as moderating their symptoms. AZT was formulated some 20 years ago as an anticancer drug. Although a failure in that role, it was resurrected in 1984 as a possible means of treating AIDS. After initial studies of the interaction of AZT and the viral reverse transcriptase, the drug was brought to the threshold of clinical use by Samuel Broder and Robert Yachoan of the National Cancer Institutes. Recently a multicenter trial was interrupted to begin wide distribution of AZT as a result of the dramatic benefits observed in the tests. It is not known, however, how toxic AZT may prove to be when it is used for a long period.

Perhaps the most important work now being done in the effort to curb AIDS is the development of a vaccine. For a vaccine to be effective it must safely evoke two different types of immunologic response. The B cells must be stimulated to produce neutralizing antibodies, which bind to the virus's envelope and prevent it from entering cells. In addition the cellular system anchored by the T cells must be capable of attacking and destroying cells already infected with the virus. Although, as I have mentioned, people infected with HTLV-III do make antibodies to the virus, the amount of effective, neutralizing antibody is worrisomely low, and of course cellular immunity is subverted by the death of the T4 cells. A successful vaccine must boost both reactions greatly.

That task is made considerably more complex by the virus's great genetic variability. Unlike many viruses, which have only a few strains, HTLV-III comprises a great many variants that form a continuum of related strains. Some pairs of variants differ by as few as 80 nucleotides of the 9,500 making up the viral genome; others differ by more than 1,000 nucleotides. Since the nucleotide sequence of the genome constitutes the genetic code for the viral proteins, such differences translate into variations in protein composition. Differences in proteins may in turn account for variations in biological activity seen among strains of HTLV-III, including preferences for infecting either T4 cells or macrophages.

Intriguingly, Wade P. Parks of the University of Miami (collaborating with Shaw and Hahn in my group) showed that an individual infected with HTLV-III may harbor several strains of the virus, all closely related in their genetic makeup. The fact that all the coexisting strains are closely related suggests that somehow their presence may "vaccinate" the infected person against reinfection by more distantly related strains. This pattern offers hope that a synthetic vaccine may be able to do the same. As yet, however, no manmade vaccine has been able to cope with the profusion of strains. My group and others are working on many approaches to a vaccine, some of which have yielded neutralizing antibodies. Yet so far the vaccines have been type-specific, neutralizing many but not all HTLV-III variants.

The progress made in only three years — identification of the cause of AIDS, formulation of a blood test, the first effective therapy and the beginning of vaccine development — is striking, particularly in view of the fact that AIDS is a viral illness, a type that has generally resisted effective therapy. Yet even if therapy and vaccine are brought into being on the fastest possible schedule, HTLV-III's toll will be heavy: many of the millions already infected will become ill before treatment is available.

The proportion of infected people who do go on to become ill may be considerably higher than what was once thought. Along with Mark Kaplan of North Shore University Hospital on Long Island, Robert R. Redfield of the Walter Reed Army Institute of Research has led the way in developing clinical categories that go beyond classical AIDS to consider HTLV-III infection in its full context. Redfield has developed a six-stage system of classification beginning with a positive blood test and ending with full-blown AIDS. Recently he used that system to follow a group of patients for as long as 36 months and found that about 90 percent of them progressed from the stage in which they began the study to a subsequent stage. Such results suggest that, contrary to what has been suggested, there may not be a large group of infected people who remain without symptoms.

It is difficult to say what the final toll will be. Regardless of its size, however, much of it will be felt in Africa. In some African countries epidemiological results show that a sizable fraction of people in the sexually active age groups are already infected. The high prevalence of infection in Africa is due partly to the fact that universal testing of the blood supply is beyond the economic reach of most African countries. As a result the virus is still being transmitted by contaminated blood. In addition, it appears that the virus has had more time to spread in Africa than it has had in any other part of the world.

Recent results have begun to provide a picture of how the AIDS virus may have come to be. In 1985 Essex and his colleague Phyllis J. Kanki isolated a virus related to HTLV-III in African green monkeys, whose range includes much of equatorial Africa. The monkey virus, which is called simian T-lymphotropic virus III (STLV-III), may well be an ancestor of the AIDS agent. Yet although STLV-III is a closer relative of HTLV-III than any other animal retrovirus is, the relation between them is still not particularly close. Nor is the monkey virus pathogenic in its usual host.

Recently, however, the gap between the simian virus and the human one has begun to be filled by the discovery of a group of intermediate viruses. The first of these, called HTLV-IV, is closely related to STLV-III and is non-pathogenic, but it infects humans. It was isolated by Essex and Kanki in West Africa in 1985. More recently two viruses that are closely related to HTLV-IV but do cause immune deficiency have been discovered in the same region. Called LAV-2 and the SBL virus, they were isolated by the Pasteur group and by a Swedish group respectively. A plausible hypothesis is that STLV-III somehow entered human beings, initiating a series of mutations that yielded the intermediate viruses before terminating in the fierce pathology of HTLV-III.

That those fierce effects are of recent origin is shown by tests done on stored blood serum from many parts of the world. Tests on sera from the 1960's and 1970's detect no antibodies to HTLV-III anywhere except in a small region of central Africa, where the earliest signs of infection have been found in serum samples taken in the 1950's. It appears that after remaining localized for some time, the virus began spreading to the rest of central Africa during the early 1970's. Later in that decade it reached Haiti and may have reached Europe and the Americas from there.

Analysis of the origin and spread of HTLV-III leads to the conclusion that cannot be sufficiently emphasized: AIDS is not a disease of homosexuals or drug addicts or indeed of any particular risk group. The virus is spread by intimate contact, and the form of contact seems to be less important than the contact itself. Rapid spread of the virus depends on the accumulation of a pool of infected people that is large enough for a few exposures to result in infection. The pool need not consist of homosexuals or drug addicts. In Africa the pool is made up of heterosexuals, and Redfield, Kaplan and others have demonstrated heterosexual transmission in the U.S. Until a reliable vaccine is developed, intelligent caution and an understanding of the virus are the best weapons against its spread.

Does this terrible tale have a moral? Yes. In the past two decades one of the fondest boasts of medical science has been the conquest of infectious disease, at least in the wealthy countries of the industrialized world. The advent of retroviruses with the capacity to cause extraordinarily complex and devastating disease has exposed that claim for what it was: hubris. Nature is never truly conquered. The human retroviruses and their intricate interrelation with the human cell are but one example of that fact. Indeed, perhaps conquest is the wrong metaphor to describe our relation to nature, which not only surrounds but in the deepest sense also constitutes our being.

* * * * * * * * * *

World Health Official describes AIDS Threat
Reprinted from *CDC AIDS Weekly* August 10, 1987

The world is facing a precipitous increase in the number of AIDS cases — up to three million new cases by 1991 — irrespective of prevention and control measures, according to the World Health Organization.

Dr. Jonathan Mann, Director of the WHO Special Program on AIDS, told the Third International Conference on AIDS in Washington of "the historical responsibility to take action now against a worldwide epidemic whose ultimate scope and dimensions are as yet unpredictable."

"AIDS has created a worldwide emergency. Global AIDS control will require billions of dollars over the next five years," Mann says. "The disease has assumed pandemic proportions affecting every continent of the world, and further spread of the virus is inevitable. AIDS threatens all countries — there are no geographic 'safe zones' and no racial exemptions."

As of June 1, 1987, 52,535 AIDS cases had been reported to the WHO from 113 countries.

"We are witnessing a rising wave of stigmatization: against Westerners in Asia, against Africans in Europe, of homosexuals, of prostitutes, of hemophiliacs, of recipients of blood transfusions," Mann says.

Beyond the health statistics, the impact of AIDS may be critical to economic and social development, Mann says. "AIDS robs societies of men and women in their most productive years, ages 20 to 49. This has the potential for economic and political destabilization in the severely affected parts of the developing world. Fear and ignorance about AIDS is causing as many tragedies as the disease itself. Today we are seeing a wave of stigmatization as AIDS has become the touchstone for political beliefs and has unveiled thinly disguised prejudices .... Fear about AIDS even threatens free travel between countries."

"A global problem of this magnitude demands a global attack. The challenge to international public health is unprecedented and urgent. The WHO has a constitutional responsibility to direct and coordinate the global struggle against AIDS, " Mann says.

* * * * * * * * * *

AIDS Perceived as Major Health Threat
Reprinted from *CDC AIDS Weekly* August 10, 1987

A survey conducted by the American Broadcasting Company has found that 70 percent of Americans believe that AIDS is the country's greatest health threat.

The June 2 [1987] telephone survey of 509 adults has a margin of error of plus or minus 5 percent. Those surveyed believed that AIDS was a greater threat than cancer, drug addiction and heart disease.

* * * * * * * * * *

Univ. of Calif. Virologist Confident that HIV does Not Cause AIDS
Reprinted from *CDC AIDS Weekly* July 6, 1987

The University of California virologist who wrote that HIV is not the cause of AIDS now says he "wouldn't be afraid to be injected with HIV."

In an interview published in the July 6 issue of the *New York Native*, a weekly newspaper oriented toward the gay community, Peter H. Duesberg said he is becoming more confident that there is no reason to believe that retroviruses are associated with AIDS or cancer.

"The human immunodeficiency virus is consistently latent," Duesberg told *Native* interviewer John Lauritsen. "It infiltrates or infects very low numbers of cells, as few as one in 100,000 . . . and those that are infected don't do anything. The virus just sits there."

Duesberg maintains that the cytopathic activity of HIV is a laboratory artifact and that there is no evidence that cells are killed by HIV in vivo.

"It is very difficult to reconcile the claim that the virus works by killing cells with the fact that it needs mitosis in order to replicate in that cell," he said. "I told [National Cancer Institute researcher Robert] Gallo that I wouldn't be afraid to be injected with HIV. . . . But I said, 'the virus couldn't come from your laboratory; it would have to be cleaner than that.' And, of course, something else could be transmitted, something that could be the real cause of AIDS."

Duesberg also suggests that the fact that an individual is HIV-antibody positive indicates only that that person has an effective immune system.

Calling AZT "a poison," Duesberg told the *Native* that he considers it "highly irresponsible" to treat AIDS patients with the drug. "Even if AZT has a preference for the virus, you will hurt the normal cells no end," he said. "That's guaranteed. That you hurt the virus is rather hypothetical. Certainly by the time a patient has symptoms of the disease, given the long latent period and given the fact that the virus is inactive even in the acute form of the disease, I see no rationale for treating with AZT."

Asked why researchers at the National Institutes of Health and others are so sure that HIV is the sole cause of AIDS, Duesberg suggested that the NIH is a political structure that is under pressure to produce positive results and that depends on favorable publicity.

"The director of the NIH needs someone like Gallo, to say, 'This is my hero,' " he said. "So it becomes an autonomous system which is not necessarily what good science used to be, where you just want to find out what's really going on and challenging in all directions.

Noting that AIDS is a condition, Duesberg suggests that AIDS is not a disease entity and that he finds it difficult to imagine that it is caused by a single pathogen. He acknowledges that he does not know what causes AIDS.

"I doubt that it could be a known virus or bacterium, because the viruses are simply not seen, and most of the known bacteria respond to antibiotics, which I'm sure have been tried and have not been effective," Duesberg said. "So I really wonder what it could be."

While calling Duesberg "an eminent scientist," NCI epidemiologist and section chief William A. Blattner has responded to the virologist's paper, saying that Duesberg is "wrong" and that he lacks a "fundamental understanding of the time-dependent nature of the AIDS epidemic."

The AIDS Virus — Well Known But a Mystery

by Jean L. Marx

Reprinted with permission from *Science,* Vol. 236; 390–92
April 24, 1987

If knowledge is power, then the research community should be gaining a firm ascendancy over the virus that causes AIDS. In the 4 years since that virus, now called human immunodeficiency virus (HIV-1), was discovered, its genome has been cloned and sequenced, and the various genes have been identified, including at least five "accessory" genes that are not found in more ordinary viruses. A great deal has also been learned about the transmission of HIV-1 and the body's responses to it. "Never has so much knowledge been generated in such a short time as in the case of the human retroviruses and AIDS," as Erling Norrby of the Karolinska Institutet in Stockholm, Sweden, put it in his introduction to the session on AIDS research at the seventh annual DNA/Hybridoma Congress.

Much of that knowledge leads to the inexorable conclusion, however, that the AIDS virus has an insidious nature that makes it well equipped to resist immune attack. The virus destroys the immune system instead. The San Francisco meeting, for example, reflected a growing recognition that the virus may spread, both from person to person and also to various types of cells within an individual, by direct cell-to-cell transmission. Moreover, it is apparently able to lurk within some of these cells in latent form. All this means that developing a vaccine to protect against AIDS may be even more difficult than is already thought.

Moreover, despite the large gains in knowledge, many gaps remain. Some of these concern the functions of the HIV-1 accessory genes. Learning how these genes work is important because they provide potential targets for therapeutic drugs. Another unresolved issue concerns the two viral relatives of HIV-1 that were discovered about a year ago. The main question is whether these viruses, which are at least very closely related to one another, are a major cause of AIDS.

Until now, most efforts to develop an AIDS vaccine have focused on the production of antibodies capable of neutralizing the free virus before it infects cells. However, there are indications that the virus may be transmitted not just as the free virus but by direct cell-to-cell contacts. "The most important mode of transmission from person to person is the virus-infected cell," says Jay Levy of the University of California at San Francisco. This would be consistent with the relative difficulty of person-to-person transmission of the AIDS virus.

Infection occurs primarily by sexual contact or direct introduction of contaminated blood into the bloodstream or by transfer from infected mother to child in the womb or during birth, but not by casual contact.

Cell-to-cell contacts may also be instrumental in disseminating the AIDS virus once it is inside the body. Individuals can develop full-blown AIDS, for example, even though they have neutralizing antibodies that might be expected to control the free virus.

Although HIV-1 was originally thought to be specific for infecting a particular type of immune cell — the helper T cell — research over the past year or so has shown that the virus can enter many kinds of cells. A partial listing includes additional types of immune cells, such as macrophages and antibody-producing B cells, the endothelial cells that line blood vessels, and also certain non-neuronal cells. Robert Gallo of the National Cancer Institute and his colleagues have suggested that the macrophage may be the primary culprit in HIV-1 dissemination.

Even though HIV-1 infects many cell types, it preferentially kills helper T cells, the consequent loss of which is the primary cause of the collapse of the immune system in AIDS patients. The susceptibility of helper T cells to killing by HIV-1 has been something of a mystery, especially because virtually all the cells eventually die in AIDS patients even though only a small percentage appear to be infected by the virus. According to William Haseltine of Harvard's Dana Farber Cancer Institute, the susceptibility of the helper cells may be related to the presence on their surfaces of large quantities of an antigen designated CD4.

Investigators have shown that this antigen is the receptor by which the AIDS virus binds to many of the cells it infects, although work by Richard Axel of the College of Physicians and Surgeons of Columbia

University, Robin Weiss of the Chester Beatty Laboratories in London, and their colleagues indicates that the binding is necessary, but not sufficient, for the virus to enter cells. Another, as yet unidentified molecule may be required in addition to CD4. Moreover, according to Levy, the brain cells infected by the AIDS virus show no traces of CD4 antigen production, a finding which suggests the existence of an additional, as yet unidentified receptor.

The complete HIV-1 particle is covered by a membranous envelope containing a complex of two major viral glycoproteins called gp120 and gp41. When the virus attaches to the CD4 antigen on target cells, it apparently does so by means of gp120.

During replication of the virus in infected cells, the glycoproteins are incorporated into the outer cellular membrane and eventually become part of the viral envelope when the particles bud from the cell. Haseltine proposes that the presence of large quantities both of CD4 and envelope glycoproteins on helper cell surfaces can lead to cell death in either of two ways. By binding to CD4 molecules on the same cell, the glycoproteins may cause portions of the membrane to fuse with one another, thereby disrupting the membrane and killing the individual cell.

In addition, the envelope glycoproteins displayed on one cell may bind with CD4 molecules on the surfaces of other, uninfected T cells to form the fused cell complexes called syncytia. "In this way, one infected cell can kill up to 500 uninfected cells," Haseltine says. "It helps to explain how you can get total T-cell ablation when only a few are infected."

In a development consistent with much else in the history of AIDS research, Haseltine's explanation of how HIV-1 kills T cells is not accepted by all researchers. For example, Gallo and his colleagues do not think that syncytia formation contributes to cell death. Flossie Wong-Staal of the Gallo group points out that they have identified an HIV-1 mutant that causes syncytia formation but does not kill cells. The NCI workers suggest than an interaction between the CD4 and gp120 molecules of the same cell leads to the death of that cell. They have evidence suggesting that a portion of the gp41 molecule is also necessary for the lethal interaction.

Even if fusions between infected and uninfected cells do not result in cell death, they may at least contribute to the spread of HIV-1. Macrophages and B cells, for example, carry much smaller numbers of CD4 molecules than helper T cells. Macrophages and B cells can therefore be fusion partners, but are more likely to be infected without being killed as a result. These and the other cells that are infected by HIV-1, but not killed, may serve as reservoirs for maintaining the virus in the body and transmitting it to other cells that might otherwise serve to restore an AIDS patient's immunity.

The importance of cell-to-cell transmission of HIV-1 has implications for vaccine development. "Any strategy for a vaccine against AIDS will have to deal not only with the free virus, but with virus-infected cells," says Dani Bolognese of Duke University Medical Center in Durham, North Carolina. To be effective, a vaccine will have to elicit immune cells capable of recognizing and killing infected cells, in addition to eliciting neutralizing antibodies.

The results regarding the ability of HIV-1 to stimulate cell-mediated immunity are both encouraging and discouraging with regard to potential vaccine development. On the encouraging side, infection with the virus apparently leads to the generation of killer cells. At the meeting, Bernard Moss of the National Institute of Allergy and Infectious Diseases described work in which Bruce Walker and Martin Hirsch of Harvard Medical School found that individuals who have been infected with the AIDS virus produce cells that can attack cells bearing HIV-1 proteins. They do not see the killer cells in persons who have not been infected by HIV-1.

More discouraging, however, is the finding that the killer cells do not necessarily prevent AIDS development. They are found in AIDS patients, as well as in infected individuals who remain healthy.

There are indications that another type of immune cell, which is called the suppressor cell because it acts as negative regulator of immune responses, may help suppress the spread of HIV-1 and perhaps the development of full-blown AIDS. Levy and his colleagues found that they could isolate HIV-1 from blood cells from some healthy, infected individuals and from a patient with a stable case of the AIDS-related cancer Kaposi's sarcoma only when they first removed the suppressor T cells from the samples. "When you have infected people who have gone relatively long times in clinically good health you may have a difficult time in getting the virus out of blood," Levy explains. "The suppressor T cells are keeping the virus in check." They may be doing this by producing an antiviral agent such as an interferon.

The suppressor T cells do not wipe out the virus, however. Once they are removed the virus can be recovered.

Another potential problem with regard to developing a vaccine that elicits cell-mediated immunity is the large number of cell types that can apparently harbor HIV-1 in latent form. Cells that are not making and displaying appreciable amounts of viral proteins might well escape the immune system's killer cells.

This is one of the reasons why researchers are very interested in finding an explanation of how HIV-1 manages to remain latent for long periods of time without either killing the host cells directly or eliciting an immune attack that destroys them. The genes that control the synthesis of the viral proteins provide an obvious place to look for the answer, and the HIV-1 genome comes equipped with a wealth of possibilities in the five accessory genes that are not found in ordinary retroviruses.

Understanding how the genes work may also be important from a therapeutic point of view. The genes are potential targets for therapeutic drugs for AIDS. "While every viral gene is a target for intervention the accessory genes are unique to the AIDS viruses and work late," Wong-Staal notes. The only drug now approved for treating AIDS patients is AZT (3'-azido-3'deoxythymidine), which acts early in the viral life cycle by blocking the reverse transcription of the RNA genome of HIV-1 into DNA. Combining an early-acting drug such as AZT with one that acts to inhibit a late component of the viral life cycle may produce a more effective therapy.

One of the four accessory genes, which is located near the right-hand (3') end of the viral genome and called the 3' open reading frame (3'orf, apparently has a negative effect on HIV-1 replication. When Levy, Cecilia Cheng-Mayer, also of University of San Francisco, and Paul Luciw of the University of California at Davis made deletions in the 3'orf, they found that the replication of the virus increased five- to tenfold. Wong-Staal and her colleagues have made a similar observation. The action of this gene may help to keep HIV-1 replication in check and possibly allow the virus to remain latent.

The other three accessory genes are apparently needed for the production of infectious HIV-1 particles, although just how these genes work seems less clear now than it was a year or two ago. Wong-Staal does not overstate the situation when she says, "There is a lot of confusion about what these genes do." Expression of the gene designated *tat*, for example, increases the synthesis of the viral structural proteins. The normal immune stimulation of HIV-1 infected helper T cells apparently contributes to the death of the cells by setting in motion a train of events that result in *tat* gene activation and increased synthesis of the viral proteins.

Haseltine and Wong-Staal originally proposed that the *tat* gene product works by increasing transcription of the viral genes into messenger RNA, which is the first step in protein synthesis. Then, about a year ago Haseltine and his colleagues concluded that the *tat* product primarily acts after transcription to increase the efficiency with which the viral messenger RNA's are used to direct protein synthesis.

At the meeting, Wong-Staal described her group's latest findings regarding *tat* gene action and concluded that it can increase both transcription and translation, with the amount of *tat* product made determining the balance between the two effects. If just a little of the *tat* protein is produced, the transcriptional effect predominates, whereas higher concentrations stimulate transcription and translation more equally. Haseltine, meanwhile, says that there is currently not enough information to determine whether the *tat* product acts directly on transcription or on post-transcriptional activities.

Haseltine and Wong-Staal also fail to see eye-to-eye on the effects of the third of the HIV-1 accessory genes, which Haseltine calls *art* and Wong-Staal calls *trs*, designations that reflect the researchers' differing views on the gene's mode of action. According to Haseltine, the unspliced messenger RNA for the HIV-1 structural proteins contains a regulatory sequence that would inhibit the synthesis of the proteins if its effects were not counteracted by the *art* gene product. He therefore named the gene *art* for "anti-repression-trans-activator" because it relieves the repressive effects of the inhibitory sequence.

According to Wong-Staal, *trs* gene activity results in decreased transcription of the viral genome, but is also necessary for correct splicing of the messenger RNA's that are formed. An active *trs* (for trans-regulator of splicing) gene is therefore needed for synthesis of the viral proteins, even though it serves at the same time to damp down that synthesis. These ongoing controversies about the mode of action of the HIV-1 accessory genes *tat* and *art-trs* cannot now be resolved.

The fourth accessory gene of HIV-1 is designated *sor* and, according to Wong-Staal, has little effect on the synthesis of the viral proteins, but is necessary for the normal infectivity of HIV-1 viral particles. Finally, Wong-Staal has identified a fifth likely gene in the AIDS virus genome. The function of this "R" gene, as it is called, is currently unknown.

One of the biggest mysteries of current AIDS research concerns the pathogenicity — or lack thereof- of the HIV-1 relatives that were isolated last year by Phyllis Kanki and Myron Essex of the Harvard School of Public Health and their colleagues and by Luc Montagnier of the Pasteur Institute in Paris and his colleagues. The viruses appear to be very much alike. They both resemble simian T-cell lymphotropic virus III (STLV-III) much more closely than HIV-1. STLV-III, which is another AIDS virus relative, is found in wild African Green monkeys, although it does not appear to cause disease in the animals. It does cause an AIDS-like illness in captive macaques, however. Moreover, the human HIV-1 relatives cannot be distinguished immunologically. They also have similar geographical distributions. They have so far been found almost exclusively in the inhabitants of western Africa, or in Europeans who have had sexual contact with western Africans, whereas the African distribution of HIV-1 is mostly confined to the countries of central Africa.

Despite these similarities, the Harvard and French groups report a critical difference between the viruses they have discovered, although the two groups used different approaches to come to their conclusions. The French workers looked for the virus they call HIV-2 in patients who have AIDS but do not show signs of HIV-1 infection. According to Montagnier, he and his colleagues have so far isolated HIV-2 from 30 such patients. Moreover, the virus kills helper T cells that are grown in laboratory dishes. In the view of French workers, the new virus is a significant cause of the immune deficiency.

Meanwhile, Essex and his colleagues have been performing an epidemiological study in which they have looked at the rate of infection with the virus they call HTLV-IV (human T-cell lymphotropic virus IV) in three groups of people in each of six western African countries. The three groups were healthy controls; hospital patients with AIDS-like symptoms; and prostitutes, who constitute a high-risk group for sexually transmitted diseases such as AIDS. In all, nearly 4300 people were included in the study.

The Essex group has not found any correlation between HTLV-IV and AIDS. In each of the six countries there was little difference between the prevalence of HTLV-IV infections in the controls and in the patients with symptoms that might be indicative of AIDS. The prostitutes generally had higher infection rates than the members of either of the other two groups, but did not show signs of disease. Moreover, HTLV-IV, unlike HIV-2, does not kill helper cells grown in culture.

How the divergent conclusions of the French and Harvard groups might be reconciled is currently unclear. One possibility, Montagnier suggests, "is that it is too early to see disease (in the populations studied by Essex). It's just a matter of time." AIDS symptoms usually do not appear until five or more years after HIV-1 infection and HTLV-IV may have entered the populations in question too recently for a significant amount of AIDS to become apparent. Essex discounts this suggestion, however.

He and his colleagues have been doing a prospective study to look for indications of immune deficiencies in a group of prostitutes in the west African nation of Senegal who have been infected with HTLV-IV. During the 18 months the women have been studied, Essex says, they have not shown even subtle signs of immune suppression, which would be detectable in individuals infected with HIV-1 itself for that long.

Essex also notes that HTLV-IV is just as prevalent in Guinea-Bissau as HIV-1 is in the areas of central Africa where AIDS has reached epidemic proportions. Some 10 to 20 years were required for the HIV-1 infection to reach their current prevalence and if HTLV-IV behaves similarly, it should be — but is not — causing detectable AIDS. Essex concedes that HTLV-IV might rarely cause AIDS, but maintains, "It's absolutely clear that infection with this virus is not like infection with HIV-1 in Africa or in homosexuals."

Another mystery concerning the relation between HIV-2 and HTLV-IV recently emerged from work reported by James Mullins and his colleagues at Harvard School of Public Health. These researchers found that the genomes of three HTLV-IV isolates and several STLV-III isolates are nearly identical. This contrasts markedly with the situation regarding HIV-1, the genome of which has been found to vary from isolate to isolate. The same is true with regard to HIV-2. Montagnier's group has compared about ten isolates and, the French researcher says, "Our conclusion is that HIV-2 has the same type of genetic variation as HIV-1." The HIV-2 genome also shows variations compared to those of the STLV-III and HTLV-IV isolates.

The explanation for the apparently much greater stability of the HTLV-IV/STLV-III genome compared to that of the HTLV-1 and HIV-2 genomes is currently unclear. There is a possibility, however, in view of the Essex group's not finding a correlation between HTLV-IV infection and AIDS, that the development of unstable viral strains is related to increased pathogenicity. More work will be needed to resolve these issues. Researchers may have come a great distance in their knowledge of AIDS, but they still have a long way to go.

* * * * * * * * * *

Sweden Closes Gay Saunas Reprinted from *CDC AIDS Weekly* July 6, 1987

The Swedish Parliament has approved a measure that will close sauna and video clubs frequented by homosexuals.

The law, approved by the 349-member Riksdag, took effect July 1, 1987. The measure was approved by 253 members of the parliament. Seventy disapproved.

There have been 113 cases in Sweden, with 63 deaths.

* * * * * * * * * *

It's a Crime   Reprinted from *CDC AIDS Weekly* July 6, 1987

The California Senate has voted to make it a crime for people to donate blood if they know they have been exposed to the AIDS virus or have the disease. State Senator John Seymour of Anaheim says donating AIDS-contaminated blood is a crime equal to murder, saying such a person "just as easily killed a victim as if he had pulled out a gun and shot him."

The measure, approved on a 26 to 2 vote, would make the crime a felony punishable by two, four or six years in prison.

State Senator Milton Marks of San Francisco, one of the measure's opponents, says people with AIDS should be treated medically, not criminally.

* * * * * * * * * *

All AIDS Prisoners to be sent to one facility   Reprinted from *CDC AIDS Weekly* July 6, 1987

All male U.S. prison inmates infected with the AIDS virus are being sent to the U.S. Medical Center for Federal Prisons in Springfield, Missouri, officials say.

The center has 22 inmates with full-blown AIDS cases, and 42 inmates who have tested positive for exposure to the virus but who have no symptoms, according to C. Allan Turner, chief executive officer at the prison.

Maryellen Thoms, a spokeswoman for the U.S. Bureau of Prisons in Washington, says 52 other men in the U.S. prisons are now showing significant symptoms of AIDS and will be transferred to Springfield. "Once testing begins . . . we may find a high number of HIV-positive cases, a number too high for all of them to be placed in Springfield," Thoms says. "Those inmates are under only one limitation — they are not allowed to work in our food-services facility."

* * * * * * * * * *

Increased Resources for Drug Clinics to Combat AIDS Reprinted from *CDC AIDS Weekly* August 1, 1987

New York state and city officials have announced a program to provide AIDS treatment for 3,000 drug users. They say almost half of the city's IV drug users are infected with the AIDS virus.

Deputy Mayor Stanley Brezenoff says the city will turn over a number of city-owned buildings to the state, so that they can be used for drug treatment and methadone clinics.

"There will be no slowing of the transmission of the AIDS virus, of preventing seepage of the virus into the general population, without a meaningful war on drugs," says city Health Commissioner Dr. Stephen Joseph. "The future of the AIDS epidemic in New York and elsewhere in the nation lies in the AIDS-intravenous drug use connection."

Brain Damage by AIDS Under Active Study

Deborah M. Barnes
Reprinted with permission from *Science, Vol. 235; 1574–77*
March 27, 1987

Since 1985, when several groups of investigators reported that the AIDS virus not only enters the cerebrospinal fluid that bathes the brain and spinal cord, but also enters the brain itself, researchers have mounted a massive effort to determine how the AIDS virus so dramatically impairs nervous system function. Within the past year they have documented the neurological symptoms that many AIDS patients develop, ranging from mild confusion and poor coordination to profound dementia and an inability to control movement. Other scientists have identified the cell types — primarily macrophages and monocytes — that contain most of the detectable virus in the brains of AIDS patients. But even with this information in hand, the mechanisms by which the AIDS virus damage the nervous system have remained an enigma.

Now, new information is leading researchers to debate whether AIDS-related neurological damage is caused by direct viral infection of cells in the nervous system — glial cells in particular — or whether the virus mediates its damage indirectly, perhaps by inhibiting the actions of substances that are important for the survival or maintenance of the nervous system. Both ideas have some support, but the new evidence also calls into question the role of the T4 antigen, which on T lymphocytes binds the outer protein of the AIDS virus.

An emerging concept, new in terms of AIDS research but not new to many neuro-scientists and immunologists, is that membrane proteins and responses to secreted factors that are shared by the nervous and immune systems may underlie much of the damage in AIDS.

Perhaps because some of its proteins mimic the structure of naturally occurring substances, the AIDS virus may damage cells of the nervous and immune systems both directly and indirectly.

"Eventually, one-half to two-thirds of the 14,000 living AIDS patients in the United States will develop moderate to severe neurological problems." says Richard Price of the Memorial Sloan-Kettering Cancer Center in New York. Lasts year, Price, Bradford Navia, Carol Petito, and Enn Sook Cho, also of Sloan-Kettering, reported that the evidence of damage to nervous system tissue, even in AIDS patients with severe symptoms, can be surprisingly subtle. Some, but not all, patients show a slight brain shrinkage, enlarged ventricles, abnormally staining white matter, or vacuolar myelopathy, a spinal cord abnormality in which the myelin sheaths surrounding nerve fibers contain abnormal spaces or vacuoles.

At about the same time, Anthony Fauci and Scott Koenig of the National Institute of Allergy and Infectious Disease and their colleagues reported that 95 percent of the detectable virus in the brain occurs in immune system cells, monocytes, or macrophages, some of which fuse to form multinucleate giant cells. Clayton Wiley, of the University of California at San Diego, and Jay Nelson and Michael Oldstone, of Scripps Clinic and Research Foundation in La Jolla, reported that some brain endothelial cells, which line blood capillaries, also contain virus.

To address the issue of how the AIDS virus severely impairs nervous system function, apparently without causing extensive structural damage to brain tissue, scientists are currently pursuing two major research strategies. One is to determine conclusively whether certain cells of the nervous system are susceptible to direct infection by the AIDS virus, and the other is to explore ways in which the virus may damage the nervous system indirectly.

Several laboratories are now pursuing the first research strategy by determining whether neurons or glia grown in tissue culture or those in the brain of an AIDS patient can be infected with the AIDS virus. Jay Levy, Cecilia Cheng-Mayer, James Rutka, Mark Rosenblum, Thomas McHugh, and Daniel Stites of the University of California at San Francisco have preliminary evidence that the AIDS virus will infect two kinds of brain-derived cells *in vitro*. These are glioma cell lines, which are transformed glial cells — non-neuronal cells whose complex functions are not completely understood — and human fetal brain cells that have been subcultured several times.

"Three of the four glioma lines seem to replicate some viral isolates but not others," says Levy. "And the cultures that contain cells which stain positive for GFAP [glial fibrillary acidic protein], a marker for astrocytes, tend to be infected more often." The San Francisco group also finds that the source of a particular viral isolate does not predict the kinds of cells it will infect *in vitro*. Brain isolates infect some, but not all, cultures from brain and peripheral blood, and peripheral blood isolates show a similar heterogeneous pattern of infectivity.

Levy and his co-workers increase their ability to detect viral infection by adding peripheral mononuclear cells to the glioma and brain cell cultures, which Levy notes contain a variety of cell types. But even under enhanced conditions, the AIDS virus reproduces in these brain-derived cells at only 1/1,000 to 1/100,000 its level of replication in T4 lymphocytes.

Despite this low level of infection, however, Levy says that their data "clearly show that the AIDS virus will infect brain astrocytes in addition to infecting brain macrophages and endothelial cells. And cells do not need to have CD4 antigen [also known as the T4 receptor on T lymphocytes to which the AIDS virus binds] to be infectible with the virus." Levy, Nelson, and Wiley also have evidence that spinal cord oligodendrocytes, which make the fatty myelin sheaths that surround nerve cell axons, may also be infectible, possibly accounting for vacuolar myelopathy in some patients.

But David Ho of the UCLA School of Medicine is skeptical about *in vitro* evidence that the AIDS virus infects brain-specific cells directly. "The bulk of the evidence suggests that there is very little direct infection of neural cells," he says. "You can take virus and add it to glial cell cultures, and if you also add T cells you can rescue the virus. But you really don't know that the virus entered the glial cells. It may have only stuck to the surface."

The notion that the AIDS virus actually infects glial cells *in vivo* as well as *in vitro* is strongly supported by new data from Joseph Melnick, Ferenc Gyorkey, and Phyllis Gyorkey of Baylor College of Medicine in Houston. They find that the AIDS virus infects two kinds of glial cells, both oligodendrocytes and astrocytes, in fresh brain biopsy tissue from AIDS patients. The researchers examined tissue from the neocortex of seven patients and found mature virus particles and staining for *cor* protein of the AIDS virus in five of them. They indicate that mature and replicating virions, budding from infected cells, are generally rare, but occur more often in oligodendrocytes than in astrocytes.

"There is now no question that the AIDS virus is harbored in the brain," says Melnick. "What we see in our tiny samples of tissue probably represents what takes place in thousands of places in the brain of an AIDS patient." Melnick describes the Baylor group's recent efforts to find areas of brain cells that contained virus particles as "extremely laborious." He thinks that their ability to examine fresh, rather than postmortem, tissue was a key factor in making electron micrographs that show both intact virus and viral budding from brain glial cells.

Other laboratories are also trying to obtain convincing evidence that the AIDS virus infects brain cells directly *in vitro*, but with ambiguous results. For example, Suzanne Gartner of the National Cancer Institute (NCI) says, "We have not been able to get what I consider a productive infection in primary cultures of brain cells."

Gartner, Mikulas Popovic, Elizabeth Read-Connole, and Robert Gallo, also of NCI, and Werner Mellert of the Institute for Biology Environmental Research Center in Munich, West Germany, are now trying "to see if we can mimic what happens *in vivo*," says Gartner. "In an AIDS patient, the cell type responsible for persistent brain infection is probably the macrophage. Infected macrophages are not like infected T cells; they don't die quickly, so they can continue to produce virus for a long time." To test how infected cells from the immune system might alter normal brain cells, Gartner and her co-workers add already infected T cells of macrophages to cultures of uninfected glioma and human fetal brain cells. "We have some preliminary evidence of infection, but only in a small number of cells," she says.

Their results are very preliminary, but the NCI group is finding that infected macrophages do alter noninfected glioma cells, and they propose two mechanisms by which this might occur. One is that the virus infects brain cells directly. The other is that macrophages, which secrete regulatory molecules under normal circumstances, secrete abnormal factors when they are infected by the AIDS virus. "I think the viral infection is changing the macrophage and then its function is changed," Gartner says.

Not all researchers are convinced that brain macrophages play a primary role in nervous system damage, however. "Everyone is euphoric, thinking that macrophages bring virus into the brain," Price says. "But macrophages could just be an indication of infection. Suppose a very low level of virus infects the brain. Then, the macrophages could come in and pick up virus and amplify the infection. There is no evidence that this happens, but there is also no evidence that macrophages bring virus into the brain either."

Price also questions why it is often difficult to find evidence of viral infection in patients with neurological symptoms. "We find virus in the brain of only about one-third of the demented patients," says Price. "An obvious explanation is that the detection techniques are not sensitive enough. But one of the questions that people have raised is, 'are there some indirect methods by which the virus damages the nervous system?' "

Scientists who pursue this second major research direction envision several possibilities by which damage may occur. First, as Gartner suggests, infected cells may secrete altered factors that can no longer perform some necessary function. Second, infected cells may secrete substances that are actually toxic to some cells. Or then, the AIDS virus may compete for receptor binding sites on cells of the nervous system that would normally be occupied by necessary maintenance or survival factors.

At least two different groups of investigators, Mark Gurney and his colleagues at the University of Chicago and Candace Pert and her co-workers at the National Institute of Mental Health (NIMH), have recently described data that point to the third possibility — specifically, that gp120 (the envelope glycoprotein that surrounds the AIDS virus) may mediate damage indirectly.

Last fall, Gurney, Mark Lee, and Brian Apatoff reported that neuroleukin, a novel factor secreted by stimulated T lymphocytes, promotes the survival of a population of embryonic chick sensory neurons that is insensitive to nerve growth factor. The researchers suggested that, because a region of the neuroleukin protein is partly homologous to gp120 and because neuroleukin can activate B lymphocytes to secrete immunoglobin, there may be a common mechanism by which a product of the AIDS virus both alters immune system function and interferes with neuronal function.

Now, Gurney, Lee, Apatoff, Gregory Spear, and Indre Rackauskas, also of the University of Chicago, in collaboration with Ho have preliminary evidence that fragments of the AIDS virus envelope glycoprotein inhibit the ability of neuroleukin, but not nerve growth factor, to enhance the survival and maintenance of certain nerve cells in vitro. Their new work also shows that brain neurons, specifically septal and hippocampal neurons, respond to neuroleukin, indicating that the trophic factor may work in the central, as well as the peripheral, nervous system.

As yet, however, Gurney and his co-workers have not been able to show that neurons have specific membrane receptors for neuroleukin or to determine whether the AIDS virus envelope glycoprotein competes with neuroleukin for specific binding sites on nerve cells. Additionally, the researchers do not know if adult neurons in the human brain require neuroleukin as a survival factor. But, says Gurney, "with neuroleukin, you have a growth factor that is highly homologous in different species — it affects human B lymphocytes, embryonic mouse brain neurons, and embryonic chick sensory neurons. It may be that a gene product of the AIDS virus, the envelope glycoprotein, is released by infected macrophages in the brain and that it inhibits the function of neuroleukin."

Pert and Joanna Hill, also of NIMH, and William Farrar of the Frederick Cancer Research Facility in Maryland, along with their colleagues also have evidence that the AIDS virus may interfere with the action of a normally occurring substance in the brain. They suggest that a peptide — which Pert and Michael Ruff, of the National Institute of Dental Research, now think is vasoactive intestinal peptide — binds to the T4-like antigen the group has recently identified in brain tissue from rats, squirrel monkeys, and humans. "It could be that parts of the brain — the hippocampus, dentrite gyrus, amygdala, and outer layer of the cerebral cortex in particular — are areas of attachment for the AIDS virus," says Hill. "This could mean that they are sites for infection."

But the accumulating evidence about where and how the AIDS virus affects the brain sometimes points in different directions. For instance, Price's group finds viral antigen staining in AIDS patients' brains, not at the cortical sites that contain T4 receptors, but in the gray matter underlying the cerebral cortex and in the white matter.

Two possible resolutions of this apparent contradiction are that the brain T4 antigen is not a binding site for the AIDS virus or that it is a site that allows binding but not infection. Pert and her colleagues favor the latter explanation and speculate that the AIDS virus may indirectly damage brain neurons important for intellectual function and emotions. "There is a possibility that the T4 antigen is acting as a receptor for an endogenous peptide," Hill says. "But when it is covered up with the AIDS virus, then the endogenous substance may not be able to bind." By this indirect mechanism, the AIDS virus could cause brain damage because it prevents the interaction of brain cells with a substance, perhaps vasoactive intestinal peptide or a related peptide, that is necessary for their survival or function.

Adding to the body of evidence that a T4 receptor is a component of brain tissue, Charles Gerfen and Paul St. John of NIMH have preliminary data suggesting that the T4 receptor "is located on brain neurons and not on glia." They find that staining for the T4 antigen occurs on cells that appear to be neurons in cultures of rat hippocampus. The cells with T4 antigen look like those that "have neuronal morphology and stain positive for neurofilament and tetanus toxin [two markers for nerve cells]," Gerfen says, although he and St. John have not yet demonstrated T4 staining and neuronal markers in the same cells.

Because much research effort is directed toward showing what brain cells have T4 antigen, a critical question is whether the presence of that receptor means that the cell displaying it is susceptible to infection and damage by the AIDS virus. Many researchers think that cells must have the antigen. But, because Levy and his co-workers find that several isolates of the AIDS virus can infect cells lacking detectable levels of T4 antigen, Levy does not think that the T4 receptor "is the sole factor underlying infectivity. Instead," he says, "something about the ability of a viral isolate to replicate makes it different and therefore affects its ability to damage different cells." He proposes that the crucial differences among viral isolates that make them more infectious lie in the core or the 3'*orf* end of the genome, rather than in the envelope glycoprotein, which is known to interact with T4 receptors on lymphocytes.

Farrar suggests that the AIDS virus may infect cells by more than one mechanism and proposes two possible modes of entry. One is the result of binding to the T4 receptor, and the other is "probably not receptor-mediated," he says. "In general, all receptor-mediated processes will occur quickly. But a process that is more amorphous — I like to call it random binding — may occur more slowly. Virus could be incorporated into a cell as a part of the pinocytotic or cell-drinking process, if there is enough of it around." Whether cell types, such as neurons, that actively recycle membrane at their synaptic terminals, take up virus by this method has yet to be determined.

Farrar also thinks that certain products of the AIDS virus genome may, in themselves, be damaging to cells, and he leans toward gp120, the envelope glycoprotein that surrounds the AIDS virus, as the culprit. "We find that purified gp120 by itself has physiological consequences," he says. Although Farrar and Douglas Ferris, also of Frederick, have yet to test the effects of gp120 on neural tissue, his hypothesis adds another possible dimension to the kind of damage the AIDS virus may do to the nervous system — specifically, that direct damage mediated by viral proteins, rather than by the intact virus, might occur.

Still other research points to the idea that much nervous system damage in an AIDS patient is due to infections by different agents, particularly cytomegalovirus (CMV). Because the AIDS virus attacks T4 lymphocytes and suppresses immune system function, many patients with neurological problems are susceptible to multiple brain infections. Wiley proposes that, by infecting the brain of an AIDS patient, CMV can elicit an immune response which then may draw AIDS virus-infected mononuclear cells into the brain.

"Sixty-seven percent of our patients have CMV infections," says Wiley. He and his colleagues are reexamining brain tissue from AIDS patients collected over the past 5 years and find that, for some unexplained reason, an increasing percentage of the brain samples have cytomegalovirus infection and damage. Although CMV brain infections are not common, they arise frequently in AIDS patients, and the DNA herpes-like virus infects both neurons and glia, he says.

Until recently, many researchers were pessimistic that AIDS-related damage to the nervous system could be reversed. But within the past year, Samuel Broder of NCI and his colleagues and Dannie King of Burroughs Wellcome in Research Triangle Park, North Carolina, have reported that 3'-azido-3'deoxythymidine (AZT) appears to slow, or even reverse, some of the neurological symptoms in a subset of AIDS patients.

Broder and his co-workers report that six of seven patients with neurological symptoms who received AZT improved in intellectual or peripheral nerve function. Some improved only temporarily, probably because their doses of AZT had to be lowered, and Broder is cautious about overinterpreting the preliminary results. "These data should not be taken as a final answer, but as an encouragement to do the necessary large-scale studies. Then we may be able to define what kinds of neurological improvements we can expect."

Researchers still do not know precisely how the AIDS virus damages the nervous system, but within the past year they have proposed several hypotheses and are actively testing their ideas. The intact AIDS virus or its protein products may injure the nervous system directly, damage it indirectly, induce nonneural cells to secrete substances that are toxic to neural tissue, or act through a combination of mechanisms. As scientists learn more about how the virus affects cells of the immune system, they may find that many of the same mechanisms are responsible for nervous system damage.

* * * * * * * * * *

Task Force Chairman Proposes Quarantines Reprinted from *CDC AIDS Weekly*, August 3, 1987

The chairman of the Georgia Task Force on AIDS has proposed that the state consider "involuntary commitment" of people infected with the AIDS virus who are "demonstrably dangerous" to others.

The task force has not taken action on the proposal.

"We are still dealing with persons who have not changed their behavior, and we have to have some way of handling them," says Dr. Doug Skelton, dean of Mercer University's School of Medicine. He says male prostitutes are a particular problem group."

"As an example, I would say that verbal threats to continue intravenous needle sharing or unprotected sex with an uniformed partner would constitute dangerous behavior," Skelton says in a letter to task force members.

Skelton has also proposed making it a crime for a person who has tested positive for AIDS antibodies to engage in sexual activity or share needles without informing the other person that he or she is infected.

* * * * * * * * * *

Official Concerned about AIDS in Asia Reprinted from *CDC AIDS Weekly*, August 10, 1987

Dr. Halfdan Mahler, director-general of the World Health Organization, says The spread of AIDS in Asia poses the potential for a "major catastrophe."

Mahler notes that 52,064 AIDS cases have been reported from 116 countries. Only 151 cases have been from Asia, but if you allow AIDS to get into the powder keg of Asia then we really are going to have a problem."

He views India, Bangladesh, Thailand, Indonesia and the Philippines as most at risk. "I fear that once AIDS is getting in there, with their weak health infrastructures . . . you have the potential for a major catastrophe," Mahler said while in Washington, D.C.

Mahler says it is a top priority of WHO to help Asian nations "to build up the proper kind of national strategy for preventing the infiltration of AIDS into their countries.

* * * * * * * * * *

As of July 1, 1982, The Centers for Disease Control reported 685 cases of AIDS in the United States.

II. The Virus And The Community

Shakespeare and AIDS

The Editors

**"Be as a planetary plague, when Jove will
o'er some high-viced city hang his poison
in the sick air.'**

William Shakespeare
Timon of Athens, iv, 3

The influenza epidemic of 1918-19 never really entered the popular imagination even though over 20,000,000 persons died in a brief span of two to three years. There was no DeFoe to count the death carts which rumbled away from the poor tenement areas of the cities in the middle of the night, carrying away individuals, whole families and devastating neighborhoods and villages. There is no great "Influenza novel" or play or work of art to commemorate the death and social disruption of the period. Why?

Maybe it was because of the timing of the epidemic. It happened, after all, at a time when Western Civilization was locked in a promethean struggle of another kind — a clash of ignorant armies marching at one another on distant shores. It happened in a time when politicians were trumpeting the phraseology which would make the world safe for democracy and Johnny would come marching home again soon. However, at a military funeral honoring hundreds of dead doughboys in 1918, those who were carried home in caskets because of the flu were given the same "Died on the field of honor, sir", as those who were mowed down in a hail of bullets in the trenches of Flanders Field.

The Bubonic Plague of the mid-fourteenth century has had much influence on literature and art. It also had at least one contemporary chronicler — Boccaccio — who immortalized not the plague itself as DeFoe and others were to do in future epidemics — but of society's reaction to it. The entire *The Decameron* is set against the background of the plague. The ten young storytellers in the book do what many people would do later — get away while there was still time and try to go someplace where the plague couldn't reach. Given the rudimentary understanding of the time, the characters in *The Decameron* seem to feel, if not to know, that the plague wouldn't strike them if they escaped to the elegant rural villas of their rich families. After all, plagues are something that happen only to the poor and unclean. Money, status and mobility can, and often did, save a great many lives.

Ever since DeFoe's *Journal of the Plague Year* (written about the plague which appeared in London in 1665) published in 1722, there has been a fascination with numbers. DeFoe's protagonist was as much an accountant as he was an observer of more unquantifiable data such as human suffering.

The Black Death of the Fourteenth Century has been attributed with the deaths of from one-quarter to one-third of the entire population of Europe from Scotland to Italy and from Spain to Russia. Depending on whose figures you use as to what the population of this vast region was in the years just preceding the Bubonic Plague epidemic, the real numbers equal from 20,000,000 to 25,000,000 people killed by the flea of *Rattus rattus*. Figures for the Black Death in Asia, the Middle East and North Africa are probably conjectural, however, contemporary reports recount heavy tolls of death in almost every known country during the Fourteenth Century. One thing that is known is that the plague swept out of the steppes of Central Asia, through the Middle East and North Africa before it hit Italy in 1347. Its spread across Europe in the next 5 years is well documented.

Accounts of the Black Death are known for their arithmetic — simple, rather prosaic totaling up of bodies buried in common pits, houses boarded up, villages depopulated and names stricken from the tax rolls.

Alessandro Manzoni wrote what is perhaps the most profoundly moving story about plague and its social consequences. In *The Betrothed*, Manzoni chronicles the day to day impact of the devastating plague of 1628 on the lives of a young couple and their families in a small town in Italy. The plague is not a backdrop in Manzoni. The plague and its consequences are very real. People do drop dead on the streets, bodies do rot and stink in the alleys and churchyards and along the country roads; animals wander aimlessly through the countryside, their keepers having died; and, whole villages disappear from the scene as they are totally depopulated. Some of Manzoni's observations are not too far from some of the analyses of the onslaught of the AIDS epidemic on modern society.

Manzoni writes.... "Anyone in square, or shop, or home who threw out the hint of the danger, anyone who mentioned the word plague, was greeted with either incredulous jeers or angry contempt. The same incredulity, or it would be truer to say, the same blindness and obstinacy, prevailed in the Senate, in the Council of Ten and throughout the whole of the magistrature.... We have already seen how indifferent it [the government] had been at the first announcement of the plague, both about acting and even about keeping itself informed ... the decree about quarantine which was decided on the 30th October, was only drawn up on the 23rd of the following month and was not published until the 29th. The plague had already entered Milan."

Manzoni proceeds to document the origin of the plague according to the popular understanding of its progress: ... "historians say that it was an Italian soldier in the service of Spain; but they do not tally on much of anything else, even on the name ... they differ also as to the day of his entering Milan; ... whatever the date may be, this unfortunate foot-soldier and bearer of misfortune entered the city with a large bundle of clothes bought or stolen from German troops."

From this "patient Zero", Manzoni traces the infection through landlords, a good samaritan who aided the dying soldier and a local friar who ministered to him.

Manzoni tells at length the story of two doctors who had seen the potential devastating nature of the contagion. And, like some of the early sentinels of the AIDS epidemic....."[they], seeing a terrible scourge advancing, labored in every way to prevent it, yet meeting only obstacles where they were looking for help; and finding themselves targets for abuse and being called enemies of their country — *pro patria hostilibus*, says Ripamonti."

When events started overtaking the leadership and bureaucracy of the country....."The [other] doctors who had been opposed to the idea of the contagion, not wanting to admit now what they had derided before, and having to find some generic name for the new disease which had become too common and too obvious to go without one, adopted the name of 'malignant and pestilential fever' — a miserable expedient, in fact a swindle in words, which yet did a great deal of harm; for while it appeared to acknowledge the truth, it had the effect of preventing the people believing what it was most important that they should believe and realize — that the disease was caught by contact. The magistrates, as if waking from a deep sleep, began to pay a little more attention to the warnings and suggestions of the Tribunal of Health, and to see that the orders about segregation and quarantine issued by that Tribunal were carried out."

The Tribunal of Health had funding problems. Even in 1628 it appears that there was not enough money in the public treasury for both guns and public welfare.

The AIDS epidemic has its counters also. The Centers for Disease Control (CDC) publishes a weekly running total of morbidity and mortality of all currently active infectious diseases. AIDS was added in July, 1981 and the tally of dead and dying mounts steadily every Friday. The World Health Organization (WHO) counts the victims internationally and separates them by geographic national boundaries as if such divisions were meant to keep the virus corralled in some mysterious manner. Larry Kramer in his perceptive and touching essay "1,112 and Counting" records not only numbers, but collects tales of woe and personal suffering and individual deaths.

There is also not enough money left in the treasuries of the world to mount effective campaigns against the relentless march of the AIDS virus. So, as money, time, patience and human inventiveness are running out, or at least growing very thin, we can, with Mark Anthony. . . . "Pray to the gods to intermit the plague." (Shakespeare, J. Caesar).

Pneumocystis Pneumonia —
Los Angeles

Reprinted with permission from *Morbidity*
and Mortality Weekly Report
June 5, 1981

*(Editors note: The following is "Document Zero" — the first men-
tion in the medical literature to suggest ... "the possibility of a
cellular-immune dysfunction related to a common exposure".
These patients comprise cases one through five of the AIDS epidemic
in the United States).*

In the period October 1980 — May 1981, 5 young men, all active
homosexuals, were treated for biopsy-confirmed *Pneumocystis
carinii* pneumonia at 3 different hospitals in Los Angeles, California. Two of the patients died. All 5 patients had laboratory-confirmed
previous or current cytomegalovirus (CMV) infection and candidal
mucosal infection. Case reports of these patients follow.

Patient 1: A previously healthy 33-year-old man developed *P.
carinii* pneumonia and oral mucosal candidiasis in March 1981 after a
2-month history of fever associated with elevated liver enzymes,
leukopenia, and CMV viruria. The serum complement-fixation CMV
titer in October 1980 was 256; in May 1981 it was 32. The patient's
condition deteriorated despite courses of treatment with
trimethoprim-sulfamethoxazole (TMP/SMX), pentamidine, and
acyclovir. He died May 3, and postmortem examination showed
residual *P. carinii* and CMV pneumonia, but no evidence of neoplasia.

Patient 2: A previously healthy 30-year-old man developed *P.
carinii* pneumonia in April 1981, after a 5-month history of fever each
day and of elevated liver-function tests, CMV viruria, and documented

seroconversion to CMV, i.e., an acute-phase titer of 16 and a convalescent-phase titer of 28 in anticomplement immunofluorescence tests. Other features of his illness included leukopenia and mucosal candidiasis. His pneumonia responded to a course of intravenous TMP/SMX, but, as of the latest reports, he continues to have a fever each day.

Patient 3: A 30-year-old man was well until January 1981 when he developed esophageal and oral candidiasis that responded to Amphotericin B treatment. He was hospitalized in February 1981 for *P. carinii* pneumonia that responded to oral TMP/SMX. His esophageal candidiasis recurred after the pneumonia was diagnosed, and he was again given Amphotericin B. The CMV complement-fixation titer in March 1981 was 8. Material from an esophageal biopsy was positive for CMV.

Patient 4: A 29-year-old man developed *P. carinii* pneumonia in February 1981. He had had Hodgkins disease 3 years earlier, but had been successfully treated with radiation therapy alone. He did not improve after being given intravenous TMP/SMX and corticosteroids and died in March. Postmortem examination showed no evidence of Hodgkins disease, but *P. carinii* and CMV were found in lung tissue.

Patient 5: A previously healthy 36-year-old man with a clinically diagnosed CMV infection in September 1980 was seen in April 1981 because of a 4-month history of fever, dyspnea, and cough. On admission he was found to have *P. carinii* pneumonia, oral candidiasis, and CMV retinitis. A complement-fixati on CMV titer in April 1981 was 128. The patient has been treated with 2 short courses of TMP/SMX that have been limited because of a sulfa-induced neutropenia. He is being treated for candidiasis with topical nystatin.

The diagnosis of *Pneumocystis* pneumonia was confirmed for all 5 patients antemortem by closed or open lung biopsy. The patients did not know each other and had no known common contacts or knowledge of sexual partners who had had similar illnesses. The 5 did not have comparable histories of sexually transmitted disease. Four had serologic evidence of past hepatitis B infection but had no evidence of current hepatitis B surface antigen. Two of the 5 reported having frequent homosexual contacts with various partners. All 5 reported using inhalant drugs, and 1 reported parenteral drug abuse. Three patients had profoundly depressed numbers of thymus-dependent lymphocyte cells and profoundly depressed *in vitro* proliferative responses to mitogens and antigens. Lymphocyte studies were not performed on the other 2 patients.

(Reported by MS Gottlieb, HM Schanker, PT Fan, A Saxon, JD Weisman, UCLA School of Medicine; I. Pozalski, Cedars-Mt. Sinai Hospital, Los Angeles and Field Services Office of the CDC).

Editorial Note: *Pneumocystis* pneumonia in the United States is almost exclusively limited to severely immunosuppressed patients. The occurrence of pneumocystosis in these 5 previously healthy individuals without a clinically apparent underlying immunodeficiency is unusual. The fact that these patients were all homosexuals suggests an association between some aspect of a homosexual lifestyle or disease acquired through sexual contact and *Pneumocystis* pneumonia in this population. All 5 patients described in this report had laboratory-confirmed CMV disease or virus shedding within 5 months of the diagnosis of *Pneumocystis* pneumonia. CMV infection has been shown to induce transient abnormalities of *in vitro* cellular-immune function in otherwise healthy human hosts. Although all 3 patients tested had abnormal cellular-immune function, no definitive conclusion regarding the role of CMV infection in these 5 cases can be reached because of the lack of published data on cellular-immune function in healthy homosexual males with and without CMV antibody. In 1 report, 7 (3.5%) of 194 patients with pneumocystosis also had CMV infection; 40 (21%) of the same group had at least 1 other major concurrent infection. A high prevalence of CMV infections among homosexual males was recently reported: 179 (94%) of 190 males reported to be exclusively homosexual had serum antibody to CMV, and 14 (7.4%) had CMV viruria; rates for 101 controls of similar age who were reported to be exclusively heterosexual were 54% for seropositivity and zero for viruria. In another study of 64 males, 4 (6.3%) had positive tests for CMV in semen, but none had CMV recovered from urine. Two of the 4 reported recent homosexual contacts. These findings suggest not only that virus shedding may be more readily detected in seminal fluid than in urine, but also that seminal fluid may be an important vehicle of CMV transmission.

All the above observations suggest the possibility of a cellular-immune dysfunction related to a common exposure that predisposes individuals to opportunistic infections such as pneumocystosis and candidiasis. Although the role of CMV infection in the pathogenesis of pneumocystosis remains unknown, the possibility of *P. carinii* infection must be carefully considered in a differential diagnosis for previously healthy homosexual males with dyspnea and pneumonia.

50,265 and STILL Counting
Loren K. Clarke and Malcolm Potts

On March 14th, 1983, Larry Kramer wrote a perceptive and prescient article titled "1,112 and Counting". Kramer was angry and afraid, beginning his piece in the *New York Native*; "If this article doesn't scare the shit out of you, we're in big trouble." His friends were dying and he screamed at the disinterest from Mayor Koch's office, the Centers for Disease Control and the National Institutes of Health. He screamed also at the gay community for attempting to brush off the epidemic — a word rarely applied to AIDS in 1983. Kramer served warning to the political establishment that if something was not done immediately about AIDS in the homosexual community, control of the disease would be lost. He argued that the disease was ignored because it was killing "kinky gays" and not straight wasps.

The tragedy of Kramer's premonition is that he was absolutely right!

Now, on January 4, 1988, we are at 50,265 and STILL counting!

Every Friday as the latest Mortality and Morbidity Weekly Report thuds down on the desks of the nation's hospitals, Cabinet rooms and Board rooms, more and more heads are shaking in disbelief and powerlessness. Scientific understanding has grown, but a therapy is no nearer than when Kramer wrote. The disease is no longer ignored as it was in 1983 but instead it is dividing politicians and almost every other segment of the society into opposing camps.

"We've heard a different theory every week," continued Kramer [there is still no answer]. Five years later a great deal has been discovered about the virus and a lot about its natural history. And tests of extraordinary delicacy are in routine use. But today's facts are much more frightening than yesterday's speculations. In Kramer's worst nightmare, he can hardly have expected that as he wrote about 1,112 AIDS cases, it would soon be shown that a virus was causing the disease and infecting 50 individuals for every one with symptoms of the disease.

The triumph of HIV testing is that it is a safety net for the blood transfusion industry, although it is sad to recall that the blood industry initially resisted the policies that are now in place.

One of the problems of testing is that it has led to uninformed calls for isolation, forced testing and a call for cleansing the society of lepers and whores. Pamphlets circulated at racist rallies in Georgia proclaim "Thank God for AIDS". Preachers of hard line morality demand a strict Biblical law to stem the spread of the infection and have the illusion that a swift cut of the moral scythe will take us back into some disease-free golden age.

Kramer complained of lack of medical interest and delays in publishing research on AIDS. Today, there are specialist journals devoted to the epidemic and the New England Journal of Medicine, which Kramer castigated for its lack of interest, along with its colleagues, is eager to print whatever it can about the disease.

Research money is available at a level that could hardly have been seen five years ago but a therapy is no nearer. Persons with AIDS still stagger from one false promise to another. It's true that sixty otherwise healthy homosexuals with HIV antibodies have been injected with a vaccine based on a protein purified from the coat of the virus, but the burgeoning of scientific knowledge about this miniscule fragment of RNA and its tiny protein coat suggests that it's going to be unusually difficult and enormously time consuming to devise a safe vaccine. The ethics and logistics of trials are formidable.

The advent of AZT has shown that scientific knowledge can be applied to paliative therapies and a host of other chemical entities are under development. It seems that death can be postponed and the quality of life of the individual improved but a cure is as remote as when Kramer wrote in 1983. No guess about the disease in 1983 could have prepared us for the facts we now know that HIV is a slowly progressing virus. An average of more than 9 years between infection and the symptoms of AIDS is extraordinarily frightening. One of the paradoxes of therapies such as AZT is that the better the quality of an individual's life, the more they are likely to infect others unless they change their patterns of behavior.

There is a need today to test AZT, and whatever comes along after it, not only on those with AIDS but on those who have the antibodies and are yet symptomless. Will the side effects be less in an otherwise fit person? Would it be possible to reduce transmission across the placenta if AZT were given to a pregnant woman? But again, this intriguing but frustrating disease is going to be difficult and slow to study. There is no way of randomly assigning death in a clinical trial.

In 1983, Kramer knew it was difficult to change human sexual behavior — "I am sick of guys who moan that giving up careless sex until this blows over is worse than death. How can they value life so little and cocks and asses so much?" There are still those, who in the face of increasingly compelling facts behave with little regard for themselves and sometimes with murderous results for others. At the same time, there is convincing evidence that the gay community has changed its pattern of behavior and no doubt the heterosexual community will as well.

As a new disease, but one that can only be transmitted in "bodily fluids", AIDS inevitably spreads first in those groups who have most sexual partners or use IV drugs most frequently. The logic of the disease is that it will appear first in those minorities whose behavior is furthest removed from the social "norm". As if to further deceive and bewilder policy makers, the disease of AIDS has a deceptively silent beginning. It is spread by fit people who can infect others for years and years before they show signs of the disease themselves. It is easy for politicians to sidestep the issue of AIDS when the real burden of sickness and death from infection acquired today will fall not on the next President of the USA, but on whoever is elected in 1992.

As AIDS begins with people with high risk behaviors, it follows logically that materials designed to educate such groups to change their behavior and to provide them with the means to control the spread of the disease may seem distasteful to the bulk of society. Logic dictates that, if successful, such materials will leave the bulk of society uneasy. Every Madison Avenue executive knows that a successful advertiser must get inside the mind of his audience and design honest, straightforward messages.

In October, 1987, Senator Jesse Helms described his distress at reading a pamphlet put out by the Gay Men's Health Crisis. A politician above everyone else has to have an intuitive capacity for reading the majority's mood and Senator Helms moved legislation to block the use of federal monies for such "blatant" educational materials. In a way, this was a back handed compliment to the pamphlet; by definition if it was to help its target audience, it was almost necessary that it be offensive to the mainstream of society.

For Larry Kramer, in 1983, his first response for gay men to "fight together" for what they thought was their "rights" in a free, democratic society. However, even if the streets were jammed with sign-carrying militants of all persuasions, AIDS is not going to go away merely by throwing epithets or money at it.

Jonathan Mann, director of the World Health Organization's Special Programme on AIDS states in an interview in early January 1988 that, "As of December 1987, there were over 66,000 AIDS cases reported officially to WHO from more than 125 countries. But that number is not accurate because there remain many barriers to the diagnosis, recognition and reporting of diseases in the world. Even in countries like the United States with its very highly developed AIDS surveillance network, an estimated ten percent of the AIDs cases are not reported to the national government. In some countries, particularly in the developing world where the tools to make a firm diagnosis or a disease reporting infrastructure may be lacking, the reported number of cases may represent only a small fraction of the actual total.

Therefore, we estimate that rather than 66,000, between 100,000 and 150,000 cases of AIDS have probably occurred since the beginning of the epidemic. And the number may actually be higher. . . . One of the questions we often ask is how many infected people there really are. The reason we don't know is because we can only know what individual countries can tell us. There is no country in the world today, including the United States, France, Sweden and the United Kingdom, with a really accurate estimate. Nevertheless, despite these difficulties we would broadly estimate that from five to ten million people are infected with the AIDS virus today worldwide. If that is true — and that is an if — then we could predict the number of new AIDS cases that are likely to occur in the next five years. This is because studies in various parts of the world suggest that between 10 percent and 30 percent of HIV-infected people will develop AIDS over a period of five years. If that's true throughout the world, and there are five to ten million people infected today, we could estimate that between *500,000 and three million* new cases of AIDS will emerge over the next five years from people *already* infected with the AIDS virus. If this estimate holds true, there will be anywhere from ten to thirty times more AIDS cases in the next five years than there have been in the last five years. So we are imminently facing a large number of AIDS cases regardless of whether we are stopping the further spread of the virus."

It does not take voodoo mathematics to come to the startling conclusion that what Dr. Mann is implying is that, cumulatively, over the next five years we could witness AIDS cases totalling anywhere from *30 to 90 million*. At a January meeting on the Global Impact of AIDS held in London, speakers were throwing out the possibility of *hundreds of millions* of AIDS cases worldwide by 1992. Perhaps we should have titled this article "One hundred Million and Counting."

Most countries, although significantly, not the United States of America, now have national AIDS committees to coordinate the work of tracking and stemming the infection. Although the US under President Reagan has been tragically slow to set coherant public policy, much of the public response has had to crystalize around the intially unlikely but extraordinarily brave leadership of the Surgeon General — never before has this symbolic and bureaucratically powerless post had so much influence within the community as it has under the patriarcal influence of Dr. C. Everett Koop.

Even though the US has no national AIDS committee, internationally the US became the first government to support the WHO programme and has continually been the largest single donor. In addition, the US Agency for International Development, which has proved unusually innovative and effective in the field of birth control over the last 20 years, has now taken leadership to support AIDS interventions. USAID supports the work of Family Health International, and the Academy for Educational Development in providing resources and technical skills for Third World countries in their battle against the spread of the disease.

But in the United States, where the disease has spread so quickly and dramatically in one, and now another, high-risk behavior group of individuals, the number 50,265 must indeed be regarded as a chilling reminder that the virus is winning! And, after seven years of geometrical growth, just what is the significance of the number 50,265? For one thing it means that there are probably 500,000 to 1.5 million people who have already been exposed to the virus and who are about 50% assured of developing full-blown AIDS. It means that there are anywhere from two to five million individuals who are active in "copulatory networks" in which the virus can jump from individual to individual during the warm and wet activity of human intercourse. It means that the iceberg is larger than the charts of the epidemiologists and mathematicians had imagined. It means that if the society doesn't act soon, the east and west coasts of the United States could be submerged in a flood of AIDS cases which would give a greater credence to the voices in the wilderness and the cry throughout the land could trigger a reign of terror and stigmatization which could develop into a social apartheid — splitting the most advanced industrial democracy in the world into an "Us" and "Them" which could take generations to repair.

(Editor's note) We are taking this opportunity to include the most recent report of AIDS cases in the United States. The following tables are a condensation of the "AIDS Weekly Surveillance Report — United States AIDS Program, Center for Infectious Diseases, Centers for Disease Control, January 4, 1988."

AIDS WEEKLY SURVEILLANCE REPORT — UNITED STATES AIDS PROGRAM, CENTER FOR INFECTIOUS DISEASES, CENTERS FOR DISEASE CONTROL JANUARY 4, 1988

UNITED STATES CASES REPORTED TO CDC

A. TRANSMISSION CATEGORIES

	MALES		FEMALES		TOTAL	
	Cumulative Number	(%)	Cumulative Number	(%)	Cumulative Number	(%)
ADULTS/ADOLESCENTS						
Homosexual/Bisexual Male	32138	(70)			32138	(65)
Intravenous (IV) Drug Abuser	6668	(15)	1843	(50)	8511	(17)
Homosexual Male and IV Drug Abuser	3726	(8)			3726	(8)
Hemophilia/Coagulation Disorder	474	(1)	20	(1)	494	(1)
Heterosexual Cases	913	(2)	1074	(29)	1987	(4)
Transfusion, Blood/Components	749	(2)	395	(11)	1144	(2)
Undetermined	1194	(3)	321	(9)	1515	(3)
SUBTOTAL [% of all cases]	45862	[93]	3653	[7]	49515	[100]
CHILDREN						
Hemophilia/Coagulation Disorder	37	(9)	3	(1)	40	(5)
Parent with/at risk of AIDS	292	(72)	285	(83)	577	(77)
Transfusion, Blood/Components	58	(14)	41	(12)	99	(13)
Undetermined	18	(4)	16	(5)	34	(5)
SUBTOTAL [% of all cases]	405	[54]	345	[46]	750	[100]
TOTAL [% of all cases]	46267	[92]	3998	[8]	50265	[100]

B. TRANSMISSION CATEGORIES BY RACIAL/ETHNIC GROUP

	WHITE, NOT HISPANIC		BLACK, NOT HISPANIC		HISPANIC		OTHER/ UNKNOWN		TOTAL	
ADULTS/ADOLESCENTS	Cumulative Number	(%)	Cumulative Number	(%)	Cumulative Number	(%)	Cumulative Number	(%)	Cumulative Number	(%)
Homosexual/Bisexual Male	23790	(79)	4805	(39)	3223	(48)	320	(69)	32138	(65)
Intravenous (IV) Drug Abuser	1702	(6)	4359	(36)	2407	(36)	43	(9)	8511	(17)
Homosexual Male and IV Drug Abuser	2379	(8)	876	(7)	447	(7)	24	(5)	3726	(8)
Hemophilia/Coagulation Disorder	419	(1)	29	(0)	33	(0)	13	(3)	494	(1)
Heterosexual Cases	323	(1)	1400	(11)	256	(4)	8	(2)	1987	(4)
Transfusion, Blood/Components	867	(3)	168	(1)	78	(1)	31	(7)	1144	(2)
Undetermined	596	(2)	604	(5)	290	(4)	25	(5)	1515	(3)
SUBTOTAL [% of all cases]	30076	[61]	12241	[25]	6734	[14]	464	[1]	49515	[100]
CHILDREN										
Hemophilia/Coagulation Disorder	27	(17)	6	(1)	6	(3)	1	(20)	40	(5)
Parent with/at risk of AIDS	72	(44)	358	(88)	143	(81)	4	(80)	577	(77)
Transfusion, Blood/Components	53	(33)	25	(6)	21	(12)	0		99	(13)
Undetermined	11	(7)	16	(4)	7	(4)	0		34	(5)
SUBTOTAL [% of all cases]	163	[22]	405	[54]	177	[24]	5	[1]	750	[100]
TOTAL [% of all cases]	30239	[60]	12646	[25]	6911	[14]	469	[1]	50265	[100]

C. AIDS CASES BY STATE OF RESIDENCE AND DATE OF REPORT TO CDC

STATE OF RESIDENCE	Year Ending JAN 4, 1987		Year Ending JAN 4, 1988		CUMULATIVE TOTAL SINCE JUNE 1981					
					Adult/Adolescent		Children		Total	
	Number	Percent	Number	Percent	Number	Percent	Number	Percent	Number	Percent
New York	3776	28.8	3963	18.7	12929	26.1	245	32.7	13174	26.2
California	2672	20.3	4825	22.8	11084	22.4	57	7.6	11141	22.2
Florida	943	7.2	1587	7.5	3538	7.1	86	11.5	3624	7.2
Texas	919	7.0	1680	7.9	3435	6.9	30	4.0	3465	6.9
New Jersey	773	5.9	1517	7.2	3141	6.3	99	13.2	3240	6.4
Illinois	363	2.8	631	3.0	1329	2.7	16	2.1	1345	2.7
Pennsylvania	294	2.2	652	3.1	1279	2.6	20	2.7	1299	2.6
Georgia	294	2.2	500	2.4	1064	2.1	14	1.9	1078	2.1
Massachusetts	275	2.1	457	2.2	1020	2.1	18	2.4	1038	2.1
District of Columbia	223	1.7	466	2.2	970	2.0	9	1.2	979	1.9
Maryland	187	1.4	459	2.2	863	1.7	19	2.5	882	1.8
Washington	167	1.3	343	1.6	695	1.4	4	0.5	699	1.4
Louisiana	161	1.2	334	1.6	661	1.3	9	1.2	670	1.3
Ohio	188	1.4	313	1.5	609	1.2	5	0.7	614	1.2
Connecticut	173	1.3	231	1.1	563	1.1	17	2.3	580	1.2
Virginia	156	1.2	231	1.1	553	1.1	9	1.2	562	1.1
Colorado	167	1.3	227	1.1	519	1.0	2	0.3	521	1.0
Puerto Rico	120	0.9	200	0.9	478	1.0	30	4.0	508	1.0
Michigan	145	1.1	213	1.0	454	0.9	9	1.2	463	0.9
Missouri	73	0.6	233	1.1	388	0.8	4	0.5	392	0.8
Arizona	80	0.6	218	1.0	373	0.8	3	0.4	376	0.7
North Carolina	80	0.6	202	1.0	368	0.7	4	0.5	372	0.7
Minnesota	98	0.7	130	0.6	285	0.6	2	0.3	287	0.6
Oregon	65	0.5	160	0.8	278	0.6	1	0.1	279	0.6
Indiana	68	0.5	125	0.6	245	0.5	2	0.3	247	0.5
Alabama	32	0.2	153	0.7	218	0.4	7	0.9	225	0.4
Oklahoma	49	0.4	106	0.5	185	0.4	4	0.5	189	0.4
South Carolina	53	0.4	78	0.4	181	0.4	5	0.7	186	0.4

	No. (%)	No. (%)	No. (%)	No. (%)	No. (%)
Hawaii	55 (0.4)	81 (0.4)	182 (0.4)	1 (0.1)	183 (0.4)
Wisconsin	42 (0.3)	96 (0.5)	173 (0.3)	1 (0.1)	174 (0.3)
Tennessee	74 (0.6)	72 (0.3)	172 (0.3)	1 (0.1)	173 (0.3)
Nevada	38 (0.3)	89 (0.4)	154 (0.3)		154 (0.3)
Rhode Island	30 (0.2)	68 (0.3)	117 (0.2)	3 (0.4)	120 (0.2)
Kentucky	31 (0.2)	47 (0.2)	109 (0.2)		109 (0.2)
Kansas	35 (0.3)	48 (0.2)	102 (0.2)	1 (0.1)	103 (0.2)
Mississippi	28 (0.2)	50 (0.2)	90 (0.2)		90 (0.2)
New Mexico	24 (0.2)	48 (0.2)	90 (0.2)		90 (0.2)
Utah	22 (0.2)	39 (0.2)	87 (0.2)	3 (0.4)	90 (0.2)
Arkansas	28 (0.2)	47 (0.2)	73 (0.1)		87 (0.2)
Delaware	21 (0.2)	36 (0.2)	62 (0.1)	2 (0.3)	75 (0.1)
Iowa	20 (0.2)	27 (0.1)	58 (0.1)	1 (0.1)	63 (0.1)
Maine	20 (0.2)	28 (0.1)	53 (0.1)	2 (0.3)	59 (0.1)
New Hampshire	13 (0.1)	33 (0.2)	44 (0.1)		55 (0.1)
Nebraska	11 (0.1)	23 (0.1)	39 (0.1)		44 (0.1)
West Virginia	8 (0.1)	21 (0.1)	36 (0.1)	2 (0.3)	41 (0.1)
Alaska	14 (0.1)	14 (0.1)	24 (0.0)		36 (0.1)
Vermont	5 (0.0)	15 (0.1)	14 (0.0)		24 (0.0)
Idaho	2 (0.0)	10 (0.0)	13 (0.0)	2 (0.3)	16 (0.0)
Montana	5 (0.0)	7 (0.0)	8 (0.0)		13 (0.0)
Wyoming	4 (0.0)	3 (0.0)	7 (0.0)		8 (0.0)
Virgin Islands	3 (0.0)	2 (0.0)	6 (0.0)		7 (0.0)
North Dakota	3 (0.0)	2 (0.0)	5 (0.0)		6 (0.0)
South Dakota	2 (0.0)	3 (0.0)	4 (0.0)		5 (0.0)
Guam					4 (0.0)
Trust Territory			1 (0.0)		1 (0.0)
TOTAL	13132 (100.0)	21143 (100.0)	49515 (100.0)	750 (100.0)	50265 (100.0)

D. AIDS CASES BY TRANSMISSION CATEGORIES AND DATE OF REPORT TO CDC, TWELVE-MONTH TOTALS

TRANSMISSION CATEGORIES	Year Ending JAN 4, 1987		Year Ending JAN 4, 1988		CUMULATIVE CASES AND DEATHS SINCE JUNE 1981			
	Number	(%)	Number	(%)	Number	(%)	Deaths	(% Cases)
ADULTS/ADOLESCENTS								
Homosexual/Bisexual Male	8465	(65.4)	13305	(63.9)	32138	(64.9)	17645	(63.7)
Intravenous (IV) Drug Abuser	2245	(17.4)	3537	(17.0)	8511	(17.2)	4854	(17.5)
Homosexual Male and IV Drug Abuser	962	(7.4)	1464	(7.0)	3726	(7.5)	2171	(7.8)
Hemophilia/Coagulation Disorder	135	(1.0)	226	(1.1)	494	(1.0)	290	(1.0)
Heterosexual Cases	535	(4.1)	838	(4.0)	1987	(4.0)	1106	(4.0)
Transfusion, Blood/Components	283	(2.2)	616	(3.0)	1144	(2.3)	763	(2.8)
Undetermined	313	(2.4)	828	(4.0)	1515	(3.1)	862	(3.1)
SUBTOTAL	12938	(100.0)	20814	(100.0)	49515	(100.0)	27691	(100.0)
CHILDREN								
Hemophilia/Coagulation Disorder	11	(5.7)	17	(5.2)	40	(5.3)	26	(5.7)
Parent with/at risk of AIDS	155	(79.9)	246	(74.8)	577	(76.9)	347	(75.8)
Transfusion, Blood/Components	24	(12.4)	44	(13.4)	99	(13.2)	67	(14.6)
Undetermined	4	(2.1)	22	(6.7)	34	(4.5)	18	(3.9)
SUBTOTAL	194	(100.0)	329	(100.0)	750	(100.0)	458	(100.0)
TOTAL	13132		21143		50265		28149	

CASES OF AIDS AND CASE-FATALITY RATES BY HALF-YEAR OF DIAGNOSIS, UNITED STATES

	NUMBER OF CASES	NUMBER OF KNOWN DEATHS	CASE-FATALITY RATE
1981 Jan-June	88	82	93%
July-Dec	183	166	91%
1982 Jan-June	365	320	88%
July-Dec	649	566	87%
1983 Jan-June	1225	1091	89%
July-Dec	1599	1369	86%
1984 Jan-June	2471	2012	81%
July-Dec	3229	2603	81%
1985 Jan-June	4445	3440	77%
July-Dec	5664	4077	72%
1986 Jan-June	6994	4335	62%
July-Dec	8094	3750	46%
1987 Jan-June	9170	3095	34%
July-Dec	6014	1179	20%
1988 Jan-Jan	0	0	0
TOTAL	50265	28149	56%

AGE AT DIAGNOSIS BY RACIAL/ETHNIC GROUP

AGE GROUP	WHITE, NOT HISPANIC Cumulative Number (%)		BLACK, NOT HISPANIC Cumulative Number (%)		HISPANIC Cumulative Number (%)		OTHER/ UNKNOWN Cumulative Number (%)		TOTAL Cumulative Number (%)	
Under 5	113	(0)	369	(3)	158	(2)	4	(1)	644	(1)
5 - 12	50	(0)	36	(0)	19	(0)	1	(0)	106	(0)
13 - 19	94	(0)	67	(1)	38	(1)	6	(1)	205	(0)
20 - 29	5774	(19)	3032	(24)	1545	(22)	83	(18)	10434	(21)
30 - 39	13758	(45)	6056	(48)	3279	(47)	210	(45)	23303	(46)
40 - 49	6864	(23)	2171	(17)	1332	(19)	115	(25)	10482	(21)
Over 49	3586	(12)	915	(7)	540	(8)	50	(11)	5091	(10)
TOTAL [% OF ALL CASES]	30239	[60]	12646	[25]	6911	[14]	469	[1]	50265	[100]

REPORTED CASES AND DEATHS BY OPPORTUNISTIC DISEASE CATEGORY

CUMULATIVE CASES/DEATHS

DISEASE CATEGORY REPORTED	Reported Cases Number (% Total)		Known Deaths Number (% Cases)	
Pneumocystis carinii Pneumonia	31733	(63)	17947	(57)
Other Opportunistic Diseases	12947	(26)	7630	(59)
Kaposi's Sarcoma	5585	(11)	2572	(46)
TOTAL	50265	(100)	28149	(56)

Development of the Epidemic
by Michael W. Adler
Reprinted with permission from *British Medical Journal*
April 25, 1987

The first recognized cases of the acquired immune deficiency syndrome (AIDS) occurred in the summer of 1981 in America. Reports began to appear of *Pneumocystis carinii* pneumonia and Kaposi's sarcoma in young men, whom it was subsequently realized were both homosexual and immunocompromised. Even though the condition became known early on as the acquired immune deficiency syndrome, its cause and modes of transmission were not immediately obvious. The virus now known to cause AIDS in a proportion to those infected was discovered in 1983 and given various names. The internationally accepted term is now the human immunodeficiency virus (HIV). More recently a new variant has been isolated, in patients with west African connections — HIV-II/LAV-II.

AIDS was originally defined by the Centers for Disease Control in America as occurring in a person:

(a) with a reliably diagnosed disease that is at least moderately indicative of an underlying cellular immune deficiency — for example, Kaposi's sarcoma in a patient aged less than 60 years or an opportunistic infection.

(b) who has no known underlying cause of cellular immune deficiency or any other cause of reduced resistance reported to be associated with the disease.

This definition was used for surveillance purposes by most other countries. It was subsequently slightly modified in the light of the discovery of the causal agent and the development of laboratory tests to detect antibody and to include additional serious conditions. A further minor modification to take account of the changing clinical pattern will take place later this year.

HIV has been isolated from semen, cervical secretions, lymphocytes, cell free plasma, cerebrospinal fluid, tears, saliva, urine and breast milk. This does not mean, however, that these fluids all transmit infection since the concentration of virus in them varies considerably. Particularly infectious are semen, blood, and possibly cervical secretions. The commonest mode of transmission of the virus throughout the world is by sexual intercourse. Whether this is anal or vaginal is unimportant. Other methods of transmission are through the receipt of infected blood or blood products and donated organs and semen. Transmission also occurs through the sharing or reuse of contaminated needles by injecting drug abusers or for therapeutic procedures and from mother to child. Transmission from mother to child occurs in utero and also possibly at birth. It is still uncertain whether the virus is transmitted through breast milk; only one case has been recorded of possible infection in this way.

There is no well documented evidence that the virus is spread by saliva. It is not spread by casual or social contact. No health care workers have developed AIDS as a result of looking after patients with HIV infection and AIDS. There are, however, four reported cases of documented seroconversion among health care workers after needlestick injuries. Finally, there is no evidence that the virus is spread by mosquitoes, lice, bed bugs, in swimming pools, or by sharing cups, eating and cooking utensils, toilets, and air space with an infected individual. Hence, HIV infection and AIDS are not contagious.

By March 1987, 31,526 adult cases of AIDS had been reported in the USA plus an additional 456 pediatric cases. Most (79 percent) of the cases in children occurred because a parent suffered from AIDS or belonged to a group at increased risk of AIDS; 12 percent occurred as a result of blood transfusions; and 5 percent occurred in children with haemophilia. Information on risk factors in the remaining 4 percent of parents of these children is not complete.

In the United States the rates for cases of AIDS per million of the population show wide geographical variation. New York has a rate of 991 per million, San Francisco 966, Miami 584, Newark 393, and Los Angeles 363 compared with 140 per million for the USA as a whole. In San Francisco and New York AIDS is now the major cause of premature death in young men. Adult cases in Europe totalled 4549 by December 1986 and in the United Kingdom 724 by March 1987. There are at least 25 times more people infected with HIV at any one time than have AIDS. In the UK proportionately more homosexuals have been notified than in America — 89 percent of cases compared with 73 percent. The doubling time of cases in the USA has slowed down since 1981-82. This slowing should not, however, detract from the projected trends. By 1991 there will probably be a cumulative total of 270,000 cases in the USA.

In the USA and UK the first wave of the epidemic occurred in homosexual men, the next and current wave is among intravenous drug abusers, and after this it might affect the heterosexual population. Transmission into the heterosexual population will occur through bisexual men, intravenous drug abusers, and prostitutes. Currently in the United States 7 percent of cases (2369) have occurred among women, and, although the commonest risk factor is intravenous drug abuse (52 percent), the next most common mode of transmission is heterosexual sexual contact (27 percent). In the U.K. 2.6 percent of adult cases (19) have occurred in women. Case reports and epidemiological surveys clearly show that the virus can be transmitted from men to women and from women to men. Studies of heterosexual transmission have shown different rates of transmission, with the female partners of men with AIDS showing the highest rates. Transmission from women with AIDS to their male partners has been reported to be as high as 65 percent. To some extent these varying rates may be due to different study designs.

In Africa strong evidence has accumulated that HIV is spread mainly by heterosexual intercourse. The male to female ratio of cases is virtually 1:1. As well as sexual intercourse, contaminated blood and also possible needles used for therapeutic purposes and vertical transmission are important. It is now recognized that cases of AIDS were first seen in central Africa in the late 1970's. Surveys from some African countries show that the prevalence of infection is high among certain groups — 80-90 percent of prostitutes, 30 percent of their male clients, 30 percent of those attending departments for sexually transmitted diseases, 10 percent of blood donors, and 10 percent of women attending antenatal clinics. Even though the high levels of infection were originally confined to central Africa, the virus and disease are spreading throughout most of that continent.

The advent of an effective antibody test in 1984 has allowed for a clearer understanding of the changing prevalence and natural history of HIV infection. For example, tests on stored samples of serum collected for other reasons from a cohort of homosexual men in San Francisco give an indication of how the epidemic evolved. In 1978, 4 percent were anti-HIV positive; by 1980 the proportion had increased sixfold, to 24 percent. In London and British provincial centers the rate of seropositivity has also increased. These surveys show that the proportion of individuals infected needs to be high before cases of

AIDS start to become apparent. It also underlines the importance of health education campaigns early in the epidemic, when the seroprevalence is low. Once cases start to appear the epidemic drives itself and a much greater effort is required in terms of control and medical care.

The rate of infection has also increased in other groups. In southern Italy the prevalence of HIV antibody among intravenous drug users increased from 6 percent in 1980 to 76 percent in 1985. Similar large increases have been seen in European countries such as Switzerland. In the UK the prevalence varies — from 10 percent in London to 54 percent in Edinburgh. This geographical variation is also seen in the USA, with low rates in San Francisco and New Orleans (less than 5 percent) and high rates in Manhattan and northern New Jersey (greater than 50 percent). Haemophiliacs are the final group with a high rate of infection in the UK (an average national figure of 44 percent). The level of infection in prostitutes tested in the UK and Europe is low, ranging from 0 percent in Italy, France, and England to 6 percent in Greece. Once prostitutes who are also intravenous drug addicts are studied the rate is very much higher — for example, 70 percent in Italy.

AIDS results in a considerable cost not only in human suffering but also to the health service. In New York the estimated lifetime hospital cost of looking after a patient with AIDS is $134,000, whereas in San Francisco it is $25,000 — 32,000. In the UK it is 7,000 — 20,000 pounds. These figures take into account only hospital costs. Other costs include time off work, the effect of the deaths of young people on national productivity, and domiciliary services. AIDS represents the most major public health problem in the world this century. A clear understanding of the epidemiology forms the basis of developing a strategy of control ranging from health education to research.

* * * * * * * * * *

Soldier expelled because of AIDS exposure Reprinted from *CDC AIDS Weekly* August 10, 1987

Israel has expelled eight soldiers from the military because they were found to be carrying AIDS antibodies, according to a military source quoted by United Press International.

"Three soldiers and five reservists were dismissed from the IDF because they are carriers of the AIDS antibody," said the source quoted by the news agency. There are 540,000 soldiers in the Israeli Defense Forces.

The Israeli government says there have been 45 AIDS cases in the country with 33 deaths. Another 239 people have been diagnosed as carrying AIDS antibodies.

Israeli Health Minister Shoshana Arbeli-Almoslino has told the Israeli parliament that officials are considering mandatory testing for some foreigners, military recruits and pregnant women.

Acquired Immunodeficiency Syndrome: Current and Future Trends

by W. Meade Morgan and James W. Curran
Reprinted with permission from *Public Health Reports*
September-October, 1986

The first cases of Acquired immunodeficiency syndrome (AIDS) were reported in 1981 in five young homosexual men from Los Angeles diagnosed with *Pneumocystis carinii* pneumonia. Since that time the number of cases in the United States has continued to increase, resulting in considerable morbidity and mortality. The cost of medical care and social services has been high, and medical practitioners and public health officials have expressed concerns about the adequacy and availability of personnel and facilities to meet future needs. Planning for the future requires accurate projections of the number of persons with AIDS and other medical and social problems related to human T-cell lymphotropic virus/lymphadenopathy-associated virus (HTLV-III/LAV) infection. As a basis for planning, trends among AIDS cases reported to the Centers for Disease Control (CDC) were analyzed, and empirical models were employed to project the number and the distribution of AIDS cases through 1991. In this paper we provide a detailed description of the demographic projections that serve as the basis for the "Public Health Service Plan for the Prevention and Control of AIDS and the AIDS Virus".

Trends in the numbers of AIDS cases in the United States meeting the surveillance definition and reported to the CDC were analyzed for the period beginning June 1981 through May 16, 1986. Surveillance for AIDS is conducted by health departments in every State, district, and U.S. territory. In most areas, surveillance activities are both passive and active. In many areas, public health officials routinely contact hospital personnel to assist in detecting and reporting cases and use record systems such as death certificates, tumor registries, and laboratory data to supplement and validate hospital-based surveillance. Confidential case reports are recorded on a standard form which includes data on patient demographics, opportunistic disease(s), risk factors, and laboratory tests. Information from the forms without personal identifiers is coded and computerized either at CDC or at health departments where it is then transmitted electronically to CDC.

The models used to project the number and the distribution of AIDS cases by patient group, geographic area of residence, gender, race, and age are empirical in the sense that they reflect observed trends in the distribution of reported cases and assume that these trends will continue unchanged over time. The projections involve a two-stage process. First, the cases reported each month are adjusted to obtain estimates of the cases actually diagnosed during that month. Second, a quadratic polynomial is fitted using weighted linear regression to the adjusted case counts as transformed by a modified Box-Cox method, and the resulting model is projected to 1991. The transformation was used to obtain homoscedastic weighted residuals suitable for calculating confidence intervals. The 68 percent (one standard deviation) confidence bounds account for the usual residual variance in the model as well as the statistical error introduced by adjusting the case counts and applying the Box-Cox transformation. The bounds are valid under the assumption that the quadratic polynomial model, as fit under the Box-Cox transformation, will hold throughout the entire period.

To obtain estimates for the number of AIDS-associated deaths, survival times were calculated from surveillance data using the Kaplan-Meier method for life table analysis. The estimated median survival time was 12 months and the cumulative 3-year survival was estimated to be 28 percent. Because of a lack of followup information related to patients' deaths, surveillance data will considerably overestimate true survival rates after the first year. To project AIDS-related mortality reasonably through the third year after diagnosis and beyond, it was assumed that the cumulative survival times follow a negative exponential distribution with 50 percent of patients living at most 1 year and only 12 percent surviving for more than 3 years. The distribution was applied to the upper and lower bounds for projections on the incidence of AIDS to obtain a range for the number of AIDS-related deaths through 1991.

Changes in the distribution of diagnosed cases over time were tested using the chi-square test for linear trends when testing proportions or the Spearman rank correlation when testing continuous variables. To project future trends in the distribution of cases, weighted linear regression on the logits of proportions was used. For each month from January 1983 until April 1986, the logit of the proportion of AIDS cases in each category was calculated ($logit(p)$ $log(p)$ — $log(1-p)$). Weights were taken to be proportional to the inverse of the approximate variance of $logit(p)$, that is $np(1-p)$ where n is the number of AIDS patients diagnosed in the given month and p is the proportion of patients in the particular category. The changes in the logit proportions were assumed to be linear over time. Quadratic effects were rarely statistically significant and were not considered further. Only cases diagnosed after 1982 were used in order to allow times of diagnosis and reporting to have stabilized. The parameter estimates were restricted so that the projected proportions of cases in both 1986 and 1991 would sum to 100 percent. For the 1991 estimates, 68 percent confidence bounds on the resulting proportions were calculated.

Between June 1, 1981, and May 19, 1986, physicians and health departments in the United States reported 20,766 cases of AIDS. Of these, 20,473 (98.6 percent) were diagnosed in adults and 293 (1.4 percent) in children. The number of cases has increased steadily, but the doubling times continue to lengthen, indicating that the rate of increase is not exponential. For example, between July 1981 and February 1982 approximately 1,000 cases of AIDS had been diagnosed and reported. This number increased by 2,000 by July 1983, a 6-month doubling time. More recently the number of cases has increased from 10,000 in May 1985 to 20,000 by April 1986, a doubling time of 11 months. (See Table 1 at the end of this chapter.)

The table depicts the projected incidence of AIDS through 1991. The adjustment for reporting delays indicates that 25,000 cases will be reported that have already been diagnosed through April 1986, although only 20,076 cases had been reported as of that time. It is projected that 115,800 new AIDS cases will be diagnosed in 1986, increasing to 74,000 cases in 1991. The current number of cases is projected to double in 13 to 15 months, while the cumulative case total of 270,000 by the end of 1991 will represent a doubling over a 2-year period from the end of 1989.

The relative distribution of reported adult and pediatric cases has not changed significantly over time (P > .15). It is projected that 1.4 percent of 1986 cases (200) will occur in children under 13 years of age, decreasing slightly to 1.2 percent (1,000) cases in 1991.

Ninety-four percent (18,879) of the total reported adult cases can be placed in patient groups that suggest a possible means of disease acquisition: homosexual or bisexual men with a history of intravenous (IV) drug abuse (8 percent); homosexual or bisexual men who are not known IV drug abusers (65 percent); heterosexual IV drug abusers (17 percent); persons with hemophilia (1 percent); heterosexual sex partners of persons with AIDS, HTLV-III/LAV infection, or persons who are at increased risk for AIDS (1 percent); and recipients of transfused blood or blood components (2 percent). Patients with multiple risk factors are included in the group listed first. The remaining 6 percent of adult cases have not been classified by recognized risk factors although 40 percent of these cases occurred in persons born in Haiti or in central African countries where heterosexual transmission is thought to account for a major share of the cases.

The relative proportion of reported cases among the patient groups with the largest numbers of cases has remained stable over time since 1982, while slight but statistically significant changes have occurred in the smaller patient groups. The most significant change is a decline in the proportion of AIDS patients born outside the United States, in Haiti or central African countries (P < .0001). The number of reported cases among persons born outside the United States has doubled in the past 18 months, compared with a doubling in 11 months for all other AIDS cases in adults. If current trends continue, this group will account for 1.3 percent of cases diagnosed in 1986 and only 0.3 percent of those diagnosed in 1991. The initially higher proportion of AIDS cases among Haitians may have been due to the migration to the United States during the period 1978 to 1981 of persons who were already infected. Two other shifts in the distribution of cases are statistically significant. First, the proportion of diagnosed cases associated with blood transfusions and in hemophilia patients has increased slightly (P> 0.01) even though the proportion remains small (2.4 percent of the total adult cases). No cases of AIDS have been reported in persons who only received transfusions after routine HTLV-III/LAV antibody testing of donors began in the spring of 1985, although one case of a seronegative donor transmitting infection has been reported. These continuing increases represent cases among persons infected prior to April 1985 as well as increased recognition of the disease among transfusion recipients, particularly elderly patients. The empirical model projects that 2.0 percent of adult AIDS cases in 1986 will be in persons whose only risk factor is the receipt of transfused blood or blood components and that this will increase to 2.5 percent in 1991.

The proportion of cases in the heterosexual contact risk group also has increased from 1983 to 1986 (P <.0001) although the total number of cases identified in this group is small (1.5 percent). If current trends continue, the proportion of heterosexual contact cases is projected to be 2.0 percent in 1986, increasing substantially to 5.0 percent in 1991. In addition to those cases reported as a result of heterosexual contacts, it is likely that a major portion of the cases without identified risk factors result from heterosexual transmission of the AIDS virus. An estimated 7 percent of cases diagnosed in 1986 will be among heterosexual contacts, persons born outside of the United States, and persons with no identified risk factor; the majority of cases in these three groups are thought to result from heterosexual transmission. The proportion in these groups is projected to increase to nearly 10 percent in 1991.

The geographic distribution of diagnosed adult AIDS cases has changed markedly from 1983 to 1986. The proportion of cases outside New York City and San Francisco has increased significantly (P>.0001). This proportionate change is most notable in relation to New York City and is primarily due to an increasing proportion of U.S. cases among homosexual men from other areas. The proportion of homosexual cases from outside of New York City and San Francisco has increased from 50 percent of cases diagnosed before 1984 to 65 percent of those diagnosed after 1984. The geographic distribution of cases among heterosexual IV drug users has changed less, with 44 percent of cases diagnosed before 1984 from outside of New York City compared with 47 percent of those diagnosed after 1984. The number of reported AIDS cases doubled in the past 14 months in New York City, in 13 months in San Francisco and in 10 months in the remainder of the United States.

By 1991, only 12 percent of cases are projected to be diagnosed in the New York City and 8 percent in the San Francisco SMSA's, with 80 percent of the cases outside of these areas which had reported more than half of the cases from 1981 to 1983.

The distribution of cases by race in adults did not change significantly from 1983 to 1986, and there has been a marginally significant increase in the proportion of persons with AIDS who are women (P>.02). The mean age among patients diagnosed before 1984 is 36.3

years compared with 37.8 years for those diagnosed after 1984. Nine-ty-three percent of the reported cases are in men; 60 percent are white, 25 percent are black, 14 percent Hispanic; less than 1 percent of adult cases are in persons between 13 and 19 years of age, 21 percent between 20 and 39, 21 percent between 40 and 49, and 9 percent are over 49. The increase in age has occurred primarily among heterosexual IV drug users whose mean age has increased from 34.2 years for those diagnosed before 1984 and 35.1 for those diagnosed after, and among blood transfusion recipients whose mean ages increased from 50.0 to 55.2 years respectively. The increase in age among adults is not significant if either heterosexual IV drug users or transfusion recipients are excluded (P>.15).

Fifty-four percent or 159 pediatric cases have been in children born to a parent with a history of IV drug abuse, an additional 10 percent (28) are among children of parents with AIDS or are at other risk for AIDS, and 13 percent (39) are in children born to Haitian parents. Fifteen percent (44) of pediatric AIDS cases are in children who have received blood transfusions, and 4 percent (12) have he-mophilia. Risk factor information is incomplete or missing for the remaining 4 percent (11 cases).

The distribution of pediatric cases by the patient's age, race and geographic region has not changed significantly from 1983 to 1986. However, the number of cases is relatively small so that there is less ability to detect trends. Forty-nine percent of the cases were diag-nosed in children under 1 year of age; 60 percent of the children are black and 21 percent are Hispanic; 38 percent have been reported from New York City, 14 percent from New Jersey and 14 percent from Florida. The distribution of pediatric cases by geographic area is similar to that of cases in women who use IV drugs or are born outside of the United States.

AIDS will become an even more serious public health problem in the United States during the next 5 years with a concurrent need for medical and social services for AIDS patients. The empirical model projects that 74,000 patients will be diagnosed in 1991 alone. An estimated 70,000 patients diagnosed during previous years will also require care during 1991.

These projections are conservative since they are based only upon cases reported to CDC. A review of death certificates over a 3-month period in four different metropolitan areas in the United States sug-gested that an additional 10 percent of diagnosed cases of AIDS are not reported to the CDC. At least an additional 10 percent of patients may be seriously ill with other Group IV HTLV-III/LAV infections which do not fit current surveillance criteria (such as severe constitutional disease or "wasting syndrome" without a specific opportunistic infection or tumor). Thus the figures we present may underestimate by 20 percent or more the future morbidity and mortality due to HTLV-III/LAV infection.

Because of the lengthy period between infection with HTLV-III/LAV and the diagnosis of AIDS, most of the cases projected to occur in the next 5 years will be among persons already infected. Thus the majority of cases in 1991 will be in homosexual and bisexual men. Cases in "other heterosexual men and women" are projected to increase to more than 7,000 (nearly 10 percent). Most of these will occur among those already infected. Future trends in the geographic distribution of cases also reflect the current distribution of AIDS virus infection.

The empirical models do not consider the availability of therapy, vaccine, preventable cofactors or the effectiveness of primary prevention efforts. If effective therapeutic regimens soon become widely available, the course of disease could be altered for those already infected. However, effective primary prevention of future HTLV-III/LAV infections through vaccines, counseling and testing, and education will have little impact on the number of cases occurring before 1990 due to the long incubation period and the large number of persons already infected. In some areas, prevention efforts have already been successfully implemented so that the empirical model may overestimate future cases, that is, among persons with hemophilia and recipients of transfusions.

Epidemiologic models for projecting the future incidence of AIDS will require additional information on the incidence, prevalence, and natural history of HTLV-III/LAV infection and on the effectiveness of efforts to prevent virus transmission. Our current understanding of the severity of AIDS and projections for the future underscore the need for continued commitment to research for a vaccine and therapy. Primary prevention and education activities must be widely implemented now throughout the United States to curtail the further spread of infection and future AIDS cases.

* * * * * * * * * *

Mayor closes pool because it was used by AIDS patient
Reprinted from *CDC AIDS Weekly* July 10, 1987

City officials in Williamson, West Virginia, have reopened a swimming pool that had been closed for cleaning after the city's mayor found out that someone carrying the AIDS virus had used the pool.

Mayor Sam Kapourales says he told pool officials to tell swimmers to leave because a pump had malfunctioned. Pool officials say that attendance was down after the pool's reopening. The pool was cleaned with 12 to 16 times the usual amount of chlorine and other chemicals. State health officials say the AIDS virus cannot be spread in swimming pools.

"They can accuse me of overreacting all they want, but there are different reports and new findings every day concerning the AIDS virus," says Kapourales. "There are too many unknowns."

"Parents can use their own judgement whether or not they want their kids to swim there, but as far as I know it is safe. That is what the health department told us," Kapourales says.

Some residents of the town have urged the mayor to close the pool for the rest of the season.

Kapourales says he instructed the head lifeguard to tell the AIDS patient not to enter the pool because of a "state law that bars persons with infectious or communicable disease, or open sores."

By mid-1983, there were 2,450 reported AIDS cases in the United States.

Table 1. Incidence of AIDS and associated mortality, United States, May 19, 1986

Year	Number of cases diagnosed during year	Projected cases		Number of deaths during year	Projected deaths	
		Lower bounds	Upper (68 percent) bounds		Lower range	Upper range
1981 and before	321	. . .	. . .	146	. . .	. . .
1982.	1,002	. . .	. . .	382	. . .	. . .
1983.	2,736	. . .	. . .	1,225	. . .	. . .
1984.	5,456	. . .	. . .	2,829	. . .	. . .
1985[1].	8,775	. . .	. . .	5,178	. . .	. . .
Projected						
1986.	15,800	14,800	16,400	9,000	8,700	9,200
1987.	23,000	21,000	25,000	14,000	13,000	15,000
1988.	33,000	27,000	36,000	21,000	18,000	23,000
1989.	45,000	33,000	51,000	30,000	24,000	33,000
1990.	58,000	40,000	69,000	41,000	31,000	47,000
1991.	74,000	46,000	92,000	54,000	37,000	64,000

[1]The numbers of diagnoses and deaths for 1985 are underestimated since reporting for this year is not yet complete.

AIDS: Has the Problem Been Adequately Assessed?

Victor De Gruttola, Kenneth Mayer and William Bennett
Reprinted with permission from *Reviews of Infectious Diseases*
March-April, 1986

The initial perception that acquired immunodeficiency syndrome would be a disease confined to certain social groups is now changing. However, the potential magnitude of the epidemic is not yet known. Success in identifying the causal agent (the virus termed LAV or HTLV-III) and in unraveling the biology of the syndrome has been encouraging, but it gives no grounds for complacency. As the following analysis indicates, the available epidemiologic data, though limited, are consistent with projections that the virus is capable of spreading to a very large proportion of sexually active individuals — well beyond the groups that have hitherto been identified as "high-risk". A greater prevalence of virus in the sexually active population will make control of blood and blood products that much more difficult and thus will also favor increased rates of infection outside the existing reservoir. It is not yet known whether the risk of developing AIDS among those infected either through sexual contact or through exposure to contaminated blood products will be as great in the future as it has been for the cohorts that have already been studied.

It seems probable that gay men infected early in the epidemic had unusually frequent exposure to a variety of sexually transmitted diseases and, as a result, the onset of disease in them may have been hastened. Route of entry may also have affected the interval of time from exposure to onset of disease in a way that will not be characteristic of individuals infected later in the epidemic. Although results from longitudinal studies of the natural history of AIDS will not be available for many years, sources of data currently available permit analysis of the effect that cofactors or route of entry have on the time to onset of disease. Such analyses are not straightforward, however, and will require development of nonstandard statistical methods. Pending the results of such analyses, there is no reason to believe cofactors that are rare among Americans are required for the development of AIDS. Therefore, unless a major effort is made, and rapidly, to obtain better data about transmission of the virus and to use these data to intercept transmission, an epidemic that is already tragic may reach devastating proportions.

To date, the most comprehensive campaign by public health officials to limit spread of the disease has been directed toward the control of blood and blood products by discouraging high-risk donors, by testing donated blood for the presence of HTLV-III, and by heat-treating cryopreciptated factor VIII. However, transmission by blood and blood products has so far played a relatively small part in the spread of the virus. Efforts to influence patterns of needle sharing by users of illicit drugs may have some effect, and serious consideration should be given to making disposable needles readily available to addicts in jurisdictions where sale is currently restricted. In Canada, where needles are sold without prescription, only one person whose sole exposure was through intravenous drug use had appeared among the country's 196 cases of AIDS by March 1985 (0.5 percent as opposed to approximately 17 percent in the U.S.). However, sexual contact, which ultimately links most subgroups of the population in a common pool, is the major avenue of transmission and the one where effective prevention could make the greatest difference. Unfortunately, sexual behavior is a topic that people find difficult to think about and deal with.

Early surveillance suggested that three interrelated patterns of behavior were implicated as major risk factors: male homosexuality, multiple partners, and receptive anal intercourse. The odds of an AIDS patient having all these factors was very much higher than the odds in the unaffected population, and case control studies of homosexual men have by now confirmed the importance of the latter two behavior patterns, and not homosexuality *per se*, as being the source of risk. The high odds ratios found in the first studies have made it tempting to assume that altering these behaviors would, at least in principle, be the most effective way to limit spread of the epidemic. Unfortunately, however, the cumulative risk of developing AIDS over extended periods is not necessarily reduced to low level even if individuals can be persuaded to reduce the number of partners or to avoid just those sexual practices initially identified as hazardous.

At the beginning of an epidemic, a high odds ratio associated with any given behavior implies only that the disease may be more efficiently transmitted through that behavior than others. As the epidemic progresses, however, and virtually all of those in the category of highest risk have become infected then less efficient means of transmission begin to account for an increasingly large proportion of the total number of cases. Consider the case in which investigators at an early phase of the epidemic find an odds ratio ("risk ratio") of approximately 10 to 1. If the organism is persistent, eventually every member of the lower-risk group could develop the disease. Thus, a high odds ratio associated with any given sexual practice when HTLV-III first entered the population of the United States does not imply that avoiding such a practice will be sufficient to reduce risk of developing AIDS to a "safe" level as the epidemic matures.

To be sure, an infectious disease may remain confined to a subgroup of the whole population as a result of differences in sexual practice. For example, if the infectious period of a given disease is considerably shorter than the average interval between each new sexual contact in one social group but not in another, then sexual transmission of the disease will tend to damp out in the first group but persist in the second. On the other hand, if a chronic infectious carrier state characterizes a disease, it will be subject to transmission even by infrequent contacts and inefficient practices. The infectious period for HTLV-III may be lifelong; reversions from the retroviral infection to a virus-free state appear to be very rare, if they occur at all. Current research suggests that the virus is being sexually transmitted from females to males, both in the United States and in Africa. In Africa, the rates of heterosexual transmission appear to be great enough to do so in other ecologic and cultural settings remains to be established.

If the average annual number of sexual partners drawn from a vulnerable population is reduced, the arrival of maximum risk will be postponed but the ultimate level it reaches will not be lowered. Consider, for example, an early stage of the epidemic, when the prevalence of infectious carriers is 2 percent of a given population. If one person selects two partners from that population and another selects 30, the first would be less than one-tenth as likely to encounter the virus: his probability is 4 percent compared with 44 percent. But if, at a later time, the prevalence has increased to 40 percent, the first individual now has a risk almost two-thirds that of the second: 64

percent compared with nearly 100 percent. In such a setting reducing one's number of new sexual partners to any number greater than zero may be insufficient to substantially reduce the risk of infection in the long run. This appears to be the situation currently facing the homosexual population. Seroprevalence of HTLV-III in samples of homosexual males from major urban areas in the United States and Europe has been rising steadily over the past few years and has now reached a level as high as 73 percent in one San Francisco cohort. The proportion of seropositive individuals who are also infectious is not known. On the whole, though, it appears that the risk associated with any sexual encounter in this population is already substantial.

Thus, sexually active individuals (that is, those having sexual relations outside an established monogamous relationship) cannot achieve a large reduction in their risk of exposure by reducing their number of sexual contacts unless exposure to multiple partners makes an independent contribution to the risk of developing clinical disease (because of some as-yet-unidentified biologic effect of exposure to a variety of partners.) It has been speculated that there might be such a relationship, perhaps in connection with exposure to multiple sperm antigens, but there are indications from the epidemiologic data that multiple partners are not a precondition of susceptibility to AIDS; that is, some individuals with few partners or in serially monogamous relationships have developed antibodies to HTLV-III or AIDS.

Surveys conducted in New York and San Francisco early in the epidemic did find an association between multiple partners and risk of AIDS, as would be expected if the virus was still relatively uncommon even in high-risk populations. More recent surveys of asymptomatic gay men in Boston, northeastern Ohio, and Denmark have not found any clear-cut association between presence of antibody to HTLV-III and total reported number of partners. In Boston, the number of sexual partners from high-risk areas as well as specific sexual practices, rather than total number of partners, is found to be associated with presence of antibody. In Denmark, seropositivity is most strongly associated with sexual exposure to men from the United States. Increased frequency of receptive anal intercourse is also independently associated with seropositivity, but number of homosexual partners is not. These findings imply that the greater risk associated with multiple sexual partners is a result of increased probability of exposure, rather than increased susceptibility to infection once exposed. Although sample sizes have been too small to support a firm conclusion, the conservative assumption must be that all those who are sexually active and engaging in practices associated with some detectable level of risk may become exposed to HTLV-III.

It is already clear that enormous numbers of people have been exposed to HTLV-III and that even more will be exposed in the near future. What proportion of them will develop the disease? Landesman et al. have reported that between 4 percent and 19 percent of subjects infected with the virus have developed AIDS during one to four years of follow-up, and an additional 25 percent have developed symptoms suggestive of AIDS-related illness. These estimates should be regarded as indicating a lower bound unless cofactors that increase the risk of developing AIDS were more prevalent among those infected with HTLV-III early in the epidemic than among those who are being infected now or who will be in the future. Data from various cities have given an annual incidence of AIDS in seropositive homosexual men as ranging from 2-10 percent. These rates reflect not only the underlying biology of the disease but also when, where, and how the infected people were identified.

It is becoming apparent from several lines of evidence that the period of latency from exposure to illness may be five years or longer, and so far there is no reason to reject the assumption that risk of developing the clinical syndrome continues for many years after exposure; it may even increase for some years. Estimates that the typical latency period is one to two years (derived from data on recipients of blood transfusions) were biased because cases of AIDS that developed rapidly were oversampled. A model-based approach designed to correct for this bias produced an estimate of 57 months; the reliability of this estimate remains to be established.

Other currently available sources of data can provide a basis for estimating the period that elapses between the moment of infection with HTLV-III and onset of disease. The effect that route of entry as well as biologic and behavioral cofactors have on this period could also be inferred from existing data sets. Because the data have been generated by unusual sampling schemes, nonstandard statistical methods are required for their analysis. Development of appropriate statistical techniques, however, would permit estimates to be obtained from the following sources: (1) blood donors believed to be infected with HTLV-III at the time of donation; (2) recipients of contaminated blood; (3) cohorts of hemophiliacs for whom time of AIDS diagnosis is known and time of infection may be estimated, and (4) cohorts of homosexual men followed in clinical trials for hepatitis vaccine. Although the experience of individuals identified in each of these ways may not be directly applicable to other populations, appropriate analytic methods could correct for some of the biases. Then, the severity of other biases (for which adjustments are not possible) might be estimated by comparing the results from all of the different sources.

The ways in which route of entry and frequency of exposure to HTLV-III affect time to onset of disease are not easily established, but obtaining an estimate is crucial to developing reliable projections and ultimately, to providing effective counseling for affected individuals. Recipients of contaminated blood transfusions are believed in most cases to have had a single exposure to the virus, whereas men who have acquired AIDS through sexual contact may have had many. The experience of these two groups might appear all but impossible to compare, if only because time to onset of disease is accurately known only for recipients of contaminated blood who have developed AIDS. An indirect analysis might, however, yield this valuable information. It is possible to obtain distributions of times to onset that are conditional on the development of disease within a given period. Such distributions could be developed for both the cohort of people with transfusion-derived disease and for the cohort of 6,875 men followed in the hepatitis trial in San Francisco who have acquired the disease sexually. Comparing the results of these analyses for the two different groups would give some indication of the differences in their risk of developing AIDS once infection with HTLV-III had been established. Stratification of these analyses by age, sexual behavior, prior health status, and chronologic time could indicate the effect of cofactors on risk of developing disease.

Even without sophisticated modeling, however, the data from the cohort of gay men in San Francisco are consistent with a long latency. Although prevalence of the virus in this cohort was already at 24 percent in 1980 and is now, at 73 percent, much nearer to saturation, the annual incidence of AIDS is still approximately doubling, as it has been since 1981. By the end of 1984, 166 of these men were known to have developed AIDS. An additional 96 cases were reported in the first eight months of 1985.

If the average latency period is several years, as some investigators have suggested, then most of the recently diagnosed cases of AIDS have resulted from exposures occurring when HTLV-III infection was still rare. The implications of this projection, if it receives support from further investigation, are extremely grave.

The ultimate magnitude of the national epidemic could also be estimated by comparing the growth rates in cities of high prevalence (chiefly New York and San Francisco) with rates in areas of lower prevalence. Sooner or later, as most of the vulnerable population in any given area becomes exposed, growth rates will have to slow down. Projections are difficult to make in the absence of a good estimate for the prevalence of HTLV-III infection and the average length of the latency period, but examination of data currently available suggests some alarming trends.

The rate of increase in the number of reported cases of AIDS from the first 39 weeks of 1984 to the first 39 weeks of 1985 for a few selected geographic regions is as follows: the United States as a whole, 1.86; New York City, 1.56; San Francisco 1.61; California (including San Francisco), 2.02; New England, 2.02; District of Columbia, 1.75; Pennsylvania, 1.77; West-South-Central 1.85. Growth in New York and San Francisco now appears to be slightly below the national average. This change could indicate either that alarmed inhabitants of these cities have shifted to safer sexual practices or that a high proportion of the susceptible population has already developed AIDS. The latter explanation is the more optimistic, because it would indicate that the incidence is reaching some kind of maximum in areas of high prevalence. That explanation is only plausible if new cases of AIDS are more likely to develop in recently infected people than among those who have been infected for longer. Even if slowing of the rate was the result of a saturation of the susceptible population, however, this saturation may only apply to the pool of highest-risk individuals. Individuals at lower risk will develop disease at a slower rate; the crest of the epidemic for them will occur later.

The former explanation, that of behavioral change, does not necessarily promise any lasting amelioration of the epidemic's course. Change in sexual behavior, especially if it affects frequency but not type of act, is likely only to slow the rate of increase, not to lower the maximum number of people who will ultimately be exposed. Thus, there are many reasons for suspecting that the modestly slower growth rate in New York and San Francisco as compared with other regions of the United States does not imply that the crest of the epidemic will soon arrive; the lower rates of growth may even be partly artifact. Small changes in how the growth rates are established (for example, calculating the rate of increase using the first 22 weeks instead of the first 39) brings the rate in San Francisco above the national average. This instability in the comparative growth rates is more likely to reflect reporting practices (for example, submitting case reports in batches) than underlying trends in the epidemic. Moreover no such slowing has been observed in California (not even among the hepatitis B cohort, which is nearly "saturated" by the virus), and many areas that still have a lower prevalence (such as the District of Columbia and Pennsylvania) show a growth rate that is not very different from that in New York and San Francisco.

Apparent rates of growth have probably also been affected by rapid changes in diagnostic criteria. There is good reason to believe that diagnosis has generally become more accurate because the proportion of AIDS patients with Kaposi's sarcoma (a distinctive entity) has been diminishing in relation to other manifestations of the syndrome. This trend suggests that early in the course of the disease, many patients with opportunistic infections may not have been identified as AIDS patients. (Alternatively, patients with Kaposi's sarcoma alone may come to be differentially underreported if they are diagnosed and managed as private outpatients). During the period of increasingly accurate diagnosis, the apparent growth rate of the epidemic would have been accelerated by diagnostic improvement alone, whereas now, in regions of diagnostic sophistication, it would be expected to diminish — as is currently observed to be the case in New York and San Francisco. On the whole, reported regional growth rates do not give much encouragement to the hope that the epidemic is reaching some kind of maximum as a result of saturating the potentially vulnerable population.

Current efforts to model the epidemic may be able to give firmer predictions, but modeling is made difficult by the large number of parameters that affect the rate of growth of the epidemic. Even without sophisticated models, however, we are inclined to predict that, in the country as a whole, the prevalence is likely to double many more times before it reaches a plateau.

This inference can be drawn from the mere fact that growth is not much slower in areas where the disease has been longest established, is currently most prevalent, and is most accurately diagnosed, as compared with areas where it has been recently introduced. Two conditions could mitigate this prediction. The first would be observed if latency is short enough that the effect of safer practices can be reflected in a reduced incidence of AIDS within several years. The second would be that cofactors required for the development of disease are less prevalent in populations that currently have a low incidence of AIDS.

Given that HTLV-III is becoming rapidly more prevalent and that an appallingly high fraction of exposed people may develop AIDS and the related debilitating syndromes, it becomes imperative to identify measures that may reduce the risk of transmission, pending emergence of definitive means of prevention or cure. Efforts are already being made to diminish the risk of medically transfusing the virus. As we have observed, the strikingly high fraction of cases in the United States attributable to intravenous drug abuse might be lowered if sterile needles were made available over the counter in areas where they are currently available only by prescription. But numerically the greatest yield appears likely to come from shift to safe, or safer, sexual practices.

The history of sexually transmitted diseases is not encouraging in this regard; high-risk behavior persisted among both heterosexually and homosexually active people even in the era when syphilis was pandemic and more likely to be lethal than now. Nonetheless, there currently appear to be major changes in behavior in response to the epidemic. Preliminary analysis of a seroepidemiologic study in Boston indicates that the number of men who have decreased their frequency of high-risk sexual practices is more than twice that of those who have increased these behaviors over the last five years. From this survey, it also appears that subjects who have recently decreased the practice of receptive anal intercourse or have never engaged in this practice still have lower rates of infection than those who have continued it.

Neither sexual activity nor the AIDS epidemic is going to disappear. Well-designed, detailed, and impartial study of sexual behavior in relation to disease transmission is, therefore, an imperative need. But waiting for definitive research results to undertake a public-health campaign is not a feasible option.

If the foregoing arguments about the nature and spread of HTLV-III prove valid, to isolate "promiscuity" as the most important risk factor would be an inadequate approach. Specific protective behaviors during sexual contact are likely to yield a greater margin of safety.

The realization is growing that AIDS will not remain confined to the social groups initially identified as high-risk. It would be unrealistic to respond to this awareness simply by adding new categories (such as prostitutes and their clients) to the list of high-risk groups and assuming that the disease will not affect "ordinary people" — however such people may be defined. As a sexually transmitted disease, AIDS has the potential to affect a very large and diverse population.

Despite considerable ignorance about which sexual practices are and which are not likely to transmit the virus, the potential magnitude of the problem is such that recommendations for protective behavior must be made. Either of two perspectives may be adopted in proposing preventive measures. The sexually active individual presumably wishes not only to reduce but virtually to eliminate his or her risk of exposure to the virus. Once prevalence is relatively high, a person is unlikely to derive much benefit from reducing the number of his or her sexual contacts; even a 10-fold reduction in the cumulative number of partners, everything else being equal, would not clearly reduce the cumulative risk of infection. Without further research, a reasonable level of safety can only be attributed to sexual practices that do not involve exposure to saliva, semen or blood — in essence, mutual masturbation or intercourse with a condom (and the efficacy of the latter is at least open to question, given the current state of knowledge about the efficacy of condoms in actual use). For the individual, compliance with such a restrictive regimen may be highly unappealing, but a candid assessment of the current state of knowledge leaves little alternative.

On the other hand, spread of HTLV-III in the population as a whole may well be retarded by changes in behavior that fall short of absolute safety for the individual. Reduction in numbers of partners and shift to practices that reduce, without eliminating, the risk of transmission will slow the rate at which the virus enters new pools of sexually interacting individuals and increases its prevalence once it is established. The time at which virtual saturation of the susceptible population occurs (a matter of four or five years in one high-risk group of homosexual men in San Francisco) might be considerably delayed for pools in which the incidence of infection is still low.

Can HTLV-III become as prevalent among heterosexually active individuals as it currently is among some groups of homosexually active men? If there are important cofactors affecting homosexual men that are not present among heterosexuals, the answer may be no. Observations made in Central Africa indicate that the virus can be transmitted from women to men as well as from men to women, although it is not yet clear whether conditions there affect susceptibility to the disease. The fact that the male-to-female ratio of prevalence of disease is much closer to 1.0 in Zaire than in the United States does not imply that the virus is as easily transmitted from women to men as vice versa, although the association of the virus in men with sexual contact with prostitutes does imply that it is transmitted that way. Otherwise, all the indications are that the virus is capable of following the same general course among sexually active heterosexuals as it has already among homosexual men, although growth will undoubtedly be slower.

The perception of AIDS as a disease that would remain confined to high-risk and socially stigmatized groups may have retarded efforts at research and education. This consequence would have been unfortunate in any case. It represents, however, a kind of complacency that simply cannot be supported by the currently available evidence, incomplete as it is. Urgently needed is research to specifically analyze the relation of sexual practices to the transmission of HTLV-III in both high-risk and exceptional cases; to explore the efficacy of condoms, virucidal agents, and other methods that may interrupt transfer of the virus; and to develop educational methods or other interventions that will promote reduction of high-risk behavior while affirming the validity of the sexual identity of individuals at risk. But even without more sophisticated information, programs to inform sexually active individuals of the risk they face and of the plausible means to avert it have a vital role to play in diminishing the impact of this national tragedy.

* * * * * * * * * *

Majority support AIDS testing of all
Reprinted from *CDC AIDS Weekly* August 3, 1987

A Gallup Poll (1987) indicates that 52 percent of those surveyed favor AIDS tests of all Americans.

The survey found that 90 percent believed there should be tests for immigrants seeking residence in the United States; 88 percent supported AIDS tests of Federal prisoners. Eighty percent believe that people seeking marriage licenses should be tested. The testing of visitors from foreign countries was supported by 66 percent of respondents.

College graduates were opposed to testing of all Americans, by a margin of 58 to 39 percent. Those who had not completed high school supported such widespread testing, by a 64 to 34 percent margin. The survey also found that 43 percent of those responding said they avoided associating with people they thought might have AIDS.

Public Knowledge about AIDS Increasing

by M. J. Campbell and W. E. Waters
Reprinted with permission from *British Medical Journal*
April 4, 1987

We have previously shown that in Southampton the public is reasonable well informed about the basic facts of the acquired immune deficiency syndrome but that the newspaper advertising campaign conducted by the Department of Health and Social Security in the spring of 1986 had had little effect on knowledge. These findings attracted some attention, and in the week of their publication in October 1986, the government set up a special committee chaired by Lord Whitelaw to investigate methods of transmitting information about AIDS. This drew the attention of the media, and there have since been innumerable references to AIDS in newspaper articles and television programmes as well as several further newspaper advertisements. In January 1987, the government announced that it would start a television advertising campaign and simultaneously deliver information leaflets to all households. As the television campaign was based on the assumption that the level of knowledge about AIDS was still insufficient we decided to monitor the level of knowledge before the campaign to see whether the increased attention by the media had increased public knowledge and to give a baseline from which to judge the campaign.

Three hundred questionnaires about AIDS, together with covering letters and stamped addressed envelopes, were posted in Southampton in early December 1986. The recipients were chosen by a 1 in 500 systematic sample from the Southampton electoral roll. The method of sampling and certain key questions were identical with those used in the previous two surveys in February and June 1986.

The initial response rate was 61 percent. Reminders were sent in January, and these brought the eventual response rate to 69 percent, but as the distribution of reminders overlapped with the distribution of the leaflet and the start of the television campaigns we could not use the later replies in the analysis.

In the table the answers to question 1 were judged to be correct if the respondent mentioned immune deficiency. In question 9 the ranges given were 0-99, 100-499, 500-999, 1000-1999, and >2,000; the answer was judged to be correct if the 500-999 ranged was ticked (in contrast with the June survey, when the 100-499 range was correct). Questions 1-8 (answered explicitly in the newspaper campaign) were scored 1 for a correct answer, 0 for don't know or missing answer, and -1 for an incorrect answer.

The mean score was 5.67 (changed from June 1986 $+0.52$, $z = 2.31$, $p = 0.02$, 95 percent confidence interval 0.07 to 0.97). Though the response rates were not identical, the results seem to indicate a small overall increase in knowledge about AIDS.

The table shows some interesting changes from the June survey. It is encouraging that the message that AIDS is a virus for which there is no cure or vaccine has sunk home. More people now realise that the infection cannot readily be caught by sharing washing, eating, or drinking utensil, but public uncertainty about whether it can be caught from blood or blood products and whether donated blood is tested for AIDS seems to be greater. There was a 34 percent increase in the number of people who believe that the statement "Women are at much less risk of catching AIDS" is false, and the recent publicity states that all promiscuous people are at risk, though most cases to date are still in homosexual men.

Additional questions ascertained that 94 percent of the respondents thought that the government should advertise the facts about AIDS on television, 62 percent thought that television advertisements should contain explicit language, 55 percent thought that television advertisements should contain explicit diagrams, and 89 percent thought that education about AIDS and how to avoid it should be given in schools. About 10 percent thought that doctors, dentists, and nurses were at high risk of catching AIDS, but 9 percent failed to recognise that drug abusers who share injection equipment were at high risk and 20 percent failed to recognize that the sexual partners of drug abusers were at high risk. None of the official literature actually describes the symptoms of AIDS, and this was reflected by the fact that 44 percent of the respondents could not name a single sign or symptom.

Our results suggest that, even before the government's leaflet and television campaigns, the publicity surrounding AIDS had increased the public level of knowledge about the disease. In view of the danger of social isolation of AIDS sufferers it is encouraging that 76 percent now believe that the infection is not readily caught by sharing washing, eating or drinking utensils. A Market of Opinion Research International poll, conducted at about the same time as our survey but comprising face to face interviews with 1093 adults aged 18-54, also found that people were becoming more knowledgeable about AIDS. In the MORI poll the one question on which answers of young single adults differed from those of the total sample was on the possibility of catching AIDS from saliva; half of the total population believed that this was not possible compared with 72 percent of young single adults. This is one subject on which there has been some controversy.

Our questionnaires were returned by only two-thirds of the sample population, but they allowed us to monitor changes in knowledge. In view of the recent survey that showed that possibly seven million people in Britain have difficulty in reading a simple fire warning there may still be many who are impervious to written advice. The form of the television advertisement also needs to be considered. One respondent whose first language was not English, who was later interviewed after the first television advertisement, thought that AIDS was associated with the use of pneumatic drills! Even before the television advertisements, however, the intense media coverage of AIDS seems to have resulted in an increase in the level of public knowledge. Our findings suggest that there is much support for further health education.

* * * * * * * * * *

High mortality rate noted in pediatric AIDS cases Reprinted from *CDC AIDS Weekly* August 10, 1987

Twenty-four of 30 children treated for AIDS at a hospital in Montreal since 1981 have died of the disease.

Dr. Normand Lapointe, head of immunology at Ste. Justine Hospital, says half of the children died within 14 months of diagnosis.

Speaking to a national conference of pediatricians, Lapointe said a study of 60 children infected with the virus found that 30 had the disease.

He says the study indicates that about half of pregnant women who have the virus will pass it on to their offspring.

* * * * * * * * * *

High rate of infection noted in blacks and Hispanics Reprinted from *CDC AIDS Weekly* August 10, 1987

Two surveys released by the San Francisco Department of Public Health show significant levels of AIDS infection in black and Hispanic communities in the city."One study says that about 36 percent of the blacks and 13 percent of Hispanics in San Francisco were at high risk of infection with the AIDS virus because of drug use or sexual habits. "This shows a very significant problem," says Dr. David Werdegar, public health director. "We consider it a major priority. In each group, there is lack of information and a high risk."

Fairbank, Berman and Maullin conducted the study of 400 black adults and 404 Hispanic adults.

The researchers found that seven percent of blacks said they were IV drug users, and half said they shared needles. Almost 15 percent said they were either bisexual or homosexual. Seven percent of Hispanics reported being homosexual or bisexual. Two percent were drug users who said they shared needles. Eighteen percent had multiple sex partners.

* * * * * * * * * *

Former medical official urges tests for all with jail threat Reprinted from *CDC AIDS Weekly* August 3, 1987

The former president of the Georgia Medical Association says all Georgians over the age of 10 should be tested for AIDS, and those who refuse should be jailed.

"It's my recommendation we handle this just like any other sexual disease for which tests are required," says Dr. John Watson Jr., immediate past president of the group. "Somewhere down the road, I guess there's got to be a catch-all where if a person is supposed to be tested and is not, then he's going to be incarcerated."

Watson, a Columbus radiologist, says he was expressing his own opinion, not that of the association.

Speaking to the Georgia House Subcommittee on General Health, which was holding a hearing in Columbus on AIDS issues, Watson contended that all Georgians over 10 should be tested twice a year, and test result cards should be issued so that medical workers can know if a patient has AIDS.

On January 1, 1984, the Centers for Disease Control reported 3,741 cases of AIDS in the United States.

AIDS — The Government Spells Out the Facts

Reprinted with permission from *Punch*
November 26, 1986

A stark message to each and every one of us in our homes. Please read this leaflet with the utmost care. Thank you for not smoking.

WARNING: THIS DOCUMENT CONTAINS CERTAIN WORDS

IS THERE SERIOUS CAUSE FOR CONCERN?

Naturally your Government is concerned. Of course we as a Government are concerned and it is right that we should be concerned. We shall never turn our backs on that concern, for this is a matter which concerns some people more than others, if for example they have come into contact with strangers, or have been taking stimulants, or share a toothbrush, and so on and so forth. Now some people have said that we don't seem concerned. But let us just look at the facts. This Government has shown more, much more, concern than any previous Government towards this menace in our midst. That is our style. We are concerned and we shall continue to be concerned. That is our policy. And we shall stick to that policy, as stick to it we must and stick to it we shall.

We have not flinched from the facts. To take just one example, we have not hesitated to tell people straight that it is probably all right, on the whole, to shake hands with other people, or to be in the same room as strangers. "But, and this is an important but, if they are in any doubt whatsoever, they should rinse any affected parts in proprietary household bleach or pop along to the local Advisory Centre for Gay Haemophiliac Drug Abusers".

This is the sort of positive advice on which we all can act.

IS THERE ANYTHING TO BE DONE?

What we must do, and do quickly, is to tackle the problem we as a nation are facing. Each and every one of us must tackle it with resolution, with determination, with guts. We shall need to have strength. We shall need to have unity. We shall need to pay attention to personal hygiene and to steer clear of this and that and we shall need to deploy our resources, substantial resources, there must be no mistake about that.

Very well. We have those resources. The economy is much stronger today than when we faced up to the plague. Today our attitude is quite different. We have created a fresh climate of optimism where once there was only despair. We have provided a whole range of new opportunities where once there was only decline and decay. People have learnt to stand on their own two feet and not to cling on to others. It cannot be over-emphasised how important that is.

To take just one example, the British condom industry is today the envy of the world, yet until recently people said there was no call for it. We have proven those people wrong. Condom production has more than doubled in recent months — yes, doubled! That is the measure of our recovery and there must be no turning back now, we must take the next step forward.

IS THERE A WAY FORWARD?

There is always a way forward. Firstly we have to take those condoms and be sure they are put where they are most needed. And, you know, it is not just condoms. We have to look at a whole range of resources if we are to achieve a really long-lasting result which we as a nation must have if we are to face up to this very difficult situation, because there are no magic cures, no easy panaceas.

CAN YOU CATCH IT OFF PEOPLE IN THE STREET?

There is absolutely no earthly reason why ordinary, decent, honest, hard-working, God-fearing people need have any real concern provided they do not go about doing things which no ordinary, decent, honest, hard-working, Godfearing person would do willy-nilly.

This may perhaps seem harsh but the plain fact of the matter is that for far too long, far too many people have been going about doing things willy-nilly and the time has come to call a halt, or at the very least be more careful. Many people are now saying that they have had enough. And they are right to say when enough is enough. To have any more could put YOU at risk. We have said and we will go on saying that it is no good at all looking at this problem in isolation. We have to look at the person next to us at home or in the street or in the car or in bed or wherever it may be and we have to ask ourselves: is that person one of us, or one of them?

IS IT TRUE WHAT THEY SAY ABOUT US ALL DROPPING DEAD?

In a democracy there will always be arguments and it is right that there should be arguments because that is the strength and the essence of our freedom. People should be free to say what they feel and to express those very real concerns which affect us all as we go about our daily lives.

Often we have to find a way to face up to sometimes difficult decisions and, let's face it, they are difficult decisions, they are matters of judgment and of sound common sense. If, for example, at a dinner party you are offered a four-letter word you may have to find a way politely to refuse, but without causing offence or embarrassment to your host, who probably means well.

No, we must say firmly, that isn't the way. It really isn't, you know.

HOW CAN I MAKE MY HOME MORE SECURE?

Wherever you live, you are part of a community at risk from AIDS. It may be large or small, in a town or in the country, but the residents of any community possess a very detailed knowledge of their neighbourhood which even the local GP or "bobby on the beat" may find hard to achieve.

A policeman or GP may not recognise someone in your garden as a stranger or AIDS carrier, but a neighbour might. It is this kind of awareness and willingness to help that is the basis of Neighbourhood AIDS Watch.

By being a good neighbor and keeping an eye out for anything suspicious, you can help prevent the spread of AIDS. These are some of the things you should report:

— Strangers with shifty-looking eyes or funny walks.
— People hanging about in pairs.
— Anyone loitering suspiciously near an opium den.
— Someone you don't know in your local gay singles bar.
— anyone who asks to borrow your toothbrush or "vibrator".

If you see anything you believe is suspicious around your neighbour's house, paint a black cross on the front door and inform the authorities.

Thank you for your prurience.

NOW WASH YOUR HANDS!

III. Where is AIDS Going?

The Editors

For every person with AIDS there are approximately 50 individuals infected with HIV. The future course of the pandemic will be determined by the proportion of individuals who eventually develop ARC or AIDS, the rapidity with which society changes its behavior and its practices and the rate of heterosexual transmission — a variable which is still hard to predict in many places.

Once the symptoms of AIDS appear — such as weight loss, opportunistic infections and Kaposi's sarcoma, then without exception the person with AIDS is under sentence of death. Men, on average, live a little over one year from the onset of symptoms, and women an even shorter interval. Infants succumb to AIDS more rapidly than adults.

AIDS-related complex (ARC) is a condition with enlarged lymph glands — and some symptomatic details — which commonly progress to full blown AIDS, but it is not quite as clear as with AIDS, how long an individual with ARC may survive.

The best estimate for the mean incubation period of AIDS is approximately 8 years after infection. It is this long, silent interval of infection which makes the disease so dangerous. Throughout the whole of this period, the individual has HIV in his or her body fluids and has the potential of infecting others. This prolonged, infectious viremia, makes AIDS a unique disease. It may well be that individuals vary in their infectiousness, perhaps becoming more likely to infect others the longer they have their disease. It is this last aspect of AIDS which is still poorly understood.

A remarkable and profound difference exists between AIDS in Africa and AIDS in America, at least at the present time. AIDS in Africa is manifestly spread by heterosexual intercourse and has already devastated whole urban populations. Among the street children of one large African city, driven there by war and famine, 8 out of 100 children tested under the age of 13, carried the virus.

In North America and Europe, the overwhelming majority of persons with AIDS have been infected through homosexual intercourse, or IV drug abuse and heterosexual HIV transmission is still at a low level. Seven percent of cases in the US are in women who have acquired the disease from their partners, but in nearly all cases the men involved were bisexual or IV drug users.

Perhaps the most remarkable contrast of all is that in Africa up to 80 percent of prostitutes in some cities are HIV positive and in all cases seem to have acquired the disease from sexual intercourse, whereas in the US, although increasing numbers of prostitutes are HIV positive, many of them have gotten their disease from IV drug use. Even more significant, in New York, it is estimated that out of approximately 10,000 AIDS cases, only 20 can be traced to infection acquired from prostitutes, whereas in Nairobi, one informed guess is that from one-half to three-quarters of all AIDS cases have been spread by relations with prostitutes.

What is the cause of these profound differences? A pessimistic explanation is merely that the longer an individual has HIV infection, the more likely he or she is to spread the disease and therefore it is only a matter of time before the industrialized nations have the same pattern of disease as Africa. The alternative explanation is that there are factors in Africa that are accelerating the transmission of the disease which may not exist in other countries. One that has been suggested and is biologically plausible is that the presence of another sexually transmitted disease, such as gonorrhea or herpes may multiply the risk of transmission. If a man has a bacterial infection in his reproductive tract, more white cells carrying HIV may enter the semen. If either sex has an additional venereal disease then it may make it more easy to acquire HIV infection. In particular, genital ulcers may make it easier for the fragile HIV virus to get across from one partner to the other.

One thing is known for certain about the next Administration of the United States — the next president will see more people die of AIDS than were killed in World War I, World War II and in Vietnam! Yet it is even now foreseeable that his administration will continue to stumble towards the declaration of a clear national policy on AIDS. AIDS will also probably be a burning issue during the 1988 campaign and politicians would do well to listen to the scientific community and the growing groundswell of frustration and fear among the American voting public. We can only hope that the voices of the public health establishment will be listened to more carefully than the strident voices of those who would form public policy on the basis of Biblical writ.

AIDS is the only totally new disease in the history of the modern world. It did not arise spontaneously or fall off a tree, but probably jumped to humans from some other primate. The epidemic is at any point in time a deep and silent enemy — it is spread by seemingly healthy people who can infect others for years and years before signs of the disease itself appear. The average time from infection to symptom is now calculated to be as long as eight years. We are looking at the epidemic today through the small end of the telescope, that is we are seeing cases of AIDS appearing which were contracted five to eight years ago. The cases of AIDS now being acquired will not appear in the CDC Mortality Register until close to the year 2000.

What we need to understand is the way in which society copes with high risk groups today will determine whether the rest of the population is exposed to the risk of AIDS tomorrow. If AIDS is to be contained we must pay attention to the current groups in which the disease is manifesting itself and provide realistic information and services of the type they need.

It is at this point that society's response to the AIDS epidemic and our future plans become confused, uninformed and finally counterproductive. We are like a person whose neighbor has a fire in their kitchen when asked for a fire extinguisher gets a lecture on fire-proof house construction.

Nationally and internationally, money is beginning to be put into AIDS programs, but the harsh reality is that the money is being spent on counting the dying and cleaning up the blood supply. Little or none of it is being put into any real effort to slow the spread of the disease in high-risk groups.

We may not like our neighbor's religion, color or the garbage they put in the yard, but if their house burns down, so may ours.

a. Transmission

The Case against Casual Contagion

by Merle A. Sande
Reprinted with permission from *New England
Journal of Medicine, Vol. 314; 380-82.*
Copyright 1987 Massachusetts Medical Society
February 6, 1986

The epidemic of acquired immunodeficiency syndrome has become an epidemic of fear. Although our understanding of the disease has been progressing rapidly, the new knowledge has often produced more public concern than relief. The identification of the etiologic agent as a virus — although of critical scientific importance — did little to quell the fears of either the medical community or the general population. Instead, people reacted to the fact that AIDS is caused by a virus with a hysteria reminiscent of another viral infection — the polio epidemic of the early 1950's.

As each new observation was announced, concern intensified. Isolation of the virus from semen explained the rapid spread of the disease in the sexually active male homosexual population but also aroused the fear of potential spread in the heterosexual population. The recognition of an asymptomatic-carrier state amplified the fear of sexual contagion in our society, and that fear was further intensified by reports of widespread transmission of the AIDS virus by heterosexual activity in Africa. The recognition that contaminated blood and blood products were the vectors for transmission of the virus to transfusion recipients and patients with hemophilia and that intravenous drug users acquired the infection by sharing needles raised the possibility that health care workers could be at similar risk from occupational exposure. Probably the most sensational information, and perhaps the most misleading, was that the virus had been isolated from saliva and then from tears. This suggested to the public that the disease might be spread by food handlers, by kissing or shaking hands, or even by contact with fomites. The media did little to dispel these notions; on the contrary, the public was led to believe that AIDS was a highly contagious disease.

The belief that the AIDS virus can be transmitted by casual contact has produced numerous political, legal, and ethical dilemmas. Responses have been varied, including calls for quarantine, mass screening of all potentially infected persons, expulsion from military service of all antibody-positive personnel, and exclusion of infected children from schools. In some cases refusal to care for AIDS patients has been condoned.

Throughout the epidemic, the Centers for Disease Control has had a critical role in countering such reactions. Rational guidelines (based on the best available data on the modes of transmission) for preventing the transmission of the AIDS virus were developed and widely publicized early in the course of the epidemic. However, the response of public officials has been erratic, and the public remains confused.

Where are we now, five years after the epidemic became evident? First of all, although the epidemic is still increasing at an alarming rate nationwide, there is some indication that the rate of increase is slowing in certain areas, such as New York City, and in San Francisco the number of new cases has actually been constant for the past year. This observation may reflect a slowing of the rate of viral acquisition. According to one recent epidemiologic survey in San Francisco, only 5 percent of seronegative homosexual men acquired evidence of infection between 1984 and 1985.

Secondly, and surprisingly, the disease has remained confined largely to the high-risk groups (homosexual men, intravenous drug users, patients with hemophilia and persons who received transfusions before blood screening was introduced, and the offspring and sexual partners of members of these groups), and the distribution of cases among these groups has been remarkably constant throughout the epidemic. In only 5 percent of cases is the mode of transmission unknown. Thus, there is no evidence that the disease is spreading to other populations.

Thirdly, certain factors have been shown to potentiate the transmission of the AIDS virus in the high-risk groups. Very early in the epidemic, studies from the CDC demonstrated that the risk of spread in the homosexual male population correlated with the number of sexual partners. This behavior accounted for the rapid dissemination of the disease throughout the country. Rectal receptive intercourse and the exchange of blood through the sharing of needles are activities that promote viral transmission. These activities may allow fluids containing infected cells to enter the circulation of the uninfected recipient.

In addition, intrauterine spread or vertical transmission of the disease from mother to fetus is an established mode of transmission. The chance that an infected mother will transmit the virus to her unborn offspring may be as high as 50 percent. Unfortunately, clinical AIDS is much more likely to develop in an infected infant than in an infected adult. The virus has been isolated from breast milk, and breast feeding could represent another mode of transmission.

Furthermore, there seems to be no doubt that the disease can be spread by heterosexual sex. Although heterosexual transmission has been postulated as the predominant mode of transmission in equatorial Africa, studies conclusively documenting this remain to be published. That the virus can be transmitted from men to women during vaginal intercourse is supported by the fact that female prostitutes in Africa appear to be at extremely high risk of infection. According to the CDC, the total number of such cases in the United States in which heterosexual transmission has been implicated remains low — only 180 so far — and the disease in 152 of these cases was transmitted from a man to a woman. On the other hand, examples of sexual transmission from a woman to a man are more difficult to document; only 28 cases have been reported in the United States.

It is possible that the difference between the two sexes in the rate of transmission is due to the fact that there are more male intravenous drug users and bisexuals capable of transmitting the disease to women than there are infected women capable of transmitting the virus to men. Although it would appear that the potential for the future spread of this disease in the heterosexual community remains a serious problem, we still do not know the relative risk of spread of the virus through vaginal intercourse and are even less secure in our knowledge about transmission from women to men. To date there is no evidence that the disease is spread by oral intercourse or by kissing.

Finally, remarkably consistent current data indicate that occupational exposure to patients infected with the AIDS virus does not pose a serious risk to health care workers. Over 1750 health care workers with intense exposure to patients with AIDS have been studied for evidence of antibody to the AIDS virus. Of the coworkers not otherwise members of high-risk groups (e.g., homosexual men or intravenous drug abusers), less than 0.1 percent were found to be antibody positive. In our institution (San Francisco General Hospital), more than 300 health care workers with intense and sustained exposure to patients with AIDS for nearly four years have been studied; all are antibody negative, with the exception of 14 of 50 homosexual male hospital workers.

Can the disease be contracted by an accidental needle stick with a needle contaminated by blood from a patient with AIDS? Probably yes, but with an extremely low frequency (less than 0.5 percent). Only one documented case, in a British nurse who acquired the virus after actually receiving a microinjection of blood after an arterial puncture, has been reported. Three additional cases of possible needle-stick transmission in the United States have been suggested but not proved. One worker was not available for follow-up, and the other two denied high-risk activity; it is possible that in each of these three cases, acquisition of the virus could have been through one of the more well-described routes. In addition, over 660 subjects (including one who acquired hepatitis B) with needle sticks from infected needles have been studied and found not to have seroconverted. The low frequency of transmission of the AIDS virus by accidental needle stick as compared with that of hepatitis B, in which 20 to 30 percent of those so exposed acquire the virus, may be due to the large differences in the concentrations of infections particles in the blood (up to 10/13 viral particles per mililiter for hepatitis B, as compared with 10/4 for AIDS). One can therefore conclude that caring for AIDS patients, even when there is intensive exposure to contaminated secretions, is not a high-risk activity. Infection-control committees should therefore implement policies to minimize accidental needle sticks and develop infection-control procedures based on the current CDC recommendations.

Friedland offers strong supporting evidence that the AIDS virus is not transmitted by casual contact, even within a family unit in which there is intimate contact with infected persons. Of 101 subjects tested who were living in a household with a documented carrier of the AIDS virus, none acquired the virus, and it seems clear that the one antibody-positive subject was infected by vertical transmission in utero or at the time of birth. The implications of this study are strengthened by the fact that the infection-control procedures followed by many health care workers were obviously not employed in the families studied. The duration of exposure reported was certainly sufficient, and the interactions numerous enough, to provide every opportunity for the virus to be spread within the family if such transmission was likely. Other, smaller family studies have produced results consistent with those of Friedland. Only 1 of 35 household members associated with 14 seropositive Danish patients with hemophilia had serum antibody to the AIDS virus. This person had engaged in vaginal, oral and anal intercourse with one of the infected patients with hemophilia. The failure of the virus to spread in the secretion-rich environment of the family may in part be explained by the very low isolation rate recently reported in samples of saliva. Ho and his colleagues could isolate HTLV-III from only 1 of 83 saliva samples cultured from antibody-positive subjects, although the virus was detected in 28 of the 50 blood samples tested from the same population. Others have confirmed these studies.

The picture is therefore clear. The AIDS virus is spread sexually, by the injection of contaminated blood, and vertically from mother to fetus. Other modes of transmission are extremely rare. Persons at high risk of acquiring the virus are men who are homosexually and bisexually active, intravenous drug abusers, persons receiving infected blood products intravenously, and children born of infected mothers. At intermediate risk are persons, especially women, who engage in heterosexual sex with members of high-risk groups Groups whose members are highly unlikely to acquire the virus (i.e., virtually no-risk groups) include health care workers caring for AIDS patients and anyone who has casual contact with persons infected with the AIDS virus, including food handlers, schoolchildren, co-workers, and family members. On the basis of these facts, the keys to preventing transmission of the virus are (1) the screening of all donated blood and (2) education and other attempts to modify risky sexual behavior and intravenous drug abuse.

It is now time for members of the medical profession, armed with this knowledge, to take a more active and influential role in quelling the hysteria over the casual transmission of AIDS. We need to support public and medical officials who oppose universal screening, quarantine, the exclusion of students from classrooms, and the removal of employees, including health care workers, from the work place. The evidence presented by Friedland is a powerful argument with which to counter the public's fear of casual contagion and should be used to thwart attempts to discriminate against persons in the so-called high-risk groups.

Update: Acquired Immunodeficiency Syndrome in the San Francisco Cohort Study, 1978-1985

Reprinted with permission for *MMWR*
September 27, 1985

Between 1978 and 1980, a cohort of approximately 6,875 homosexual and bisexual men who had sought evaluation for sexually transmitted diseases at the San Francisco City Clinic was enrolled in a series of studies of the prevalence, incidence, and prevention of hepatitis B virus infections. In 1981, six of the first 10 men reported with acquired immunodeficiency syndrome in San Francisco were discovered to be members of the City Clinic cohort. Subsequently, the Department of Public Health and CDC began a study of cohort members for AIDS and for infections with human T-lymphotropic virus type III/lymphadenopathy-associated virus (HTLV-III/LAV), the cause of AIDS.

In a representative sample of cohort members, prevalence of antibody to HTLV-III/LAV measured by an enzyme immunosorbent assay, increased from 4.5 percent in 1978 to 67.3 percent in 1984. From January through August 1985, HTLV-III/LAV antibody prevalence further increased to 73.1. The number of AIDS cases reported among cohort members increased from 166 in 1984 to 262 in August, 1985.

Thirty-one members of the sample who consented to have their earliest specimens tested had antibody to HTLV-III/LAV at the time they enrolled in studies between 1978-1980. By December 1984, two (6.4 percent) had developed AIDS, and eight (25.8 percent) had AIDS-related conditions, as defined by CDC. Symptomatic infections with HTLV-III/LAV thus had occurred in 10 (32.2 percent) of the 31 men after a follow-up period averaging 61 months. No further cases of AIDS have been reported in the 29 men through the first 8 months of 1985.

Sixty members of the cohort who were seronegative in 1984 were tested again in 1985. An average of 14 months after their last specimens were collected, nine (15.0 percent) were found to have developed antibodies to HTLV-III/LAV. Five of the nine had reduced their numbers of sexual partners since their last visit; two had not changed; and two had increased their numbers slightly. Each man who seroconverted had engaged in sexual activities that resulted in the exchange of semen and other body fluids. Two seroconverters who reported sexual exposures with only one steady partner since their last negative test had engaged in receptive anal intercourse with ejaculation by their respective partners.

Men who remained seronegative were not shown to differ significantly in sexual practices from those who seroconverted, but the number of seroconverters available for comparison is small.

EDITORIAL NOTE: The cumulative incidence of AIDS in City Clinic cohort members is now 3,825 per 100,000, the highest of any reported population. Almost three-quarters of cohort members have serologic evidence of HTLV-III/LAV infections. The long-term prognoses for these men is unknown. The fact that two-thirds of men infected for over 5 years have not developed AIDS or AIDS-related illness is an encouraging indication that infection with this virus is not necessarily followed by rapid development of symptoms and death.

Studies from New York City, San Francisco, and elsewhere suggest that many gay men have changed their sexual lifestyles. Between 1980 and 1983, rates of rectal and pharyngeal gonorrhea in men in Manhattan decreased 59 percent. Surveys of self-reported behavior of gay men in San Francisco have shown decreases in both the average number of sexual partners and sexual practices known to transmit HTLV-III/LAV infection. However, as the prevalence of HTLV-III/LAV infection in a population increases, substantial changes in both the numbers of sexual partners and types of sexual practices will be necessary to reduce the risk that susceptible gay men may become infected.

Epidemiology of AIDS in Women in the United States 1981 through 1986

by Mary Guinan and Ann Hardy

Reprinted with permission from *JAMA*, Vol. 257; No. 15; 2039-42. April 17, 1987

A lthough women with acquired immunodeficiency syndrome constituted less than 7 percent of all AIDS cases as of November 1986, the occurrence of AIDS in women is of special interest for several reasons. Women with AIDS or with human immunodeficiency virus (HIV) infection are the major source of infection of infants with AIDS, and the second most common route of transmission of AIDS to women is through heterosexual intercourse. Trends in AIDS in women may help to determine future trends for pediatric cases and may be a good surrogate for monitoring heterosexual transmission of infection.

We reviewed all cases of AIDS in women reported to the Centers for Disease Control, Atlanta, as of November 7, 1986. Only those that fulfilled the surveillance case definition were included in our analysis. Cases of AIDS in women were placed in only one transmission category in a hierarchical fashion, using the following order: (1) intravenous drug use, (2) coagulation disorder, (3) heterosexual contacts with a person at risk for AIDS, (4) transfusion with blood or blood products, and (5) undetermined.

For analytic purposes, we divided the heterosexual contact group into (1) those patients who had heterosexual contact with a person at risk for AIDS, and (2) those patients whose AIDS was presumed to be acquired by heterosexual transmission, i.e., those born in countries where heterosexual transmission is thought to play a major role (i.e.,

Haiti and countries in Central Africa). Adult patients were those 13 years of age and older. Pediatric patients were those 12 years of age and younger.

We analyzed the data by year of report. Reporting of AIDS cases was initiated in the late spring of 1981; therefore, data are incomplete for that year. Although cases reported in 1981 were used in the descriptive analyses, trend analyses were performed only on cases reported in 1982 and thereafter. Since the homosexual/bisexual male risk group has no equivalent female risk group, we excluded homosexual/bisexual men when comparing cases of AIDS in men and women in other transmission categories.

As of November 27, 1986, a total of 27,140 cases of AIDS in adults had been reported, 1,819 (6.7 percent) of whom were women. Between 1982 and 1986, the proportion of adult women with AIDS did not change significantly. Women with AIDS were significantly younger than non-homosexual/bisexual men with AIDS. A larger proportion of women compared with men with AIDS were in the 20- to 29-year age group (32 vs. 20 percent, $P<.001$), and a lower proportion were in the 40- to 49-year age group (11 v. 18 percent, $P<.01$). The vast majority of women with AIDS were of reproductive age, with 79 percent between ages 13 and 39 years. Over half of the women with AIDS were black. We found no significant differences between heterosexual men and women with aids in race or disease category.

Forty-three states have reported cases of AIDS in women, with 15 states, Puerto Rico, and the District of Columbia reporting ten or more cases. The geographic distribution of AIDS in women was similar to that in men. New York had the highest number of both men (7727) and women (855) with AIDS. Although California accounted for the second largest number of men with AIDS (6068), this state had only the fourth largest number of women with AIDS (106). New Jersey and Florida had the second and third highest numbers of women with AIDS (245 and 188). The highest proportion of women with AIDS were in New Jersey and Connecticut (both with 16 percent), Puerto Rico (12 percent), Florida and Rhode Island (11 percent) and New York (10 percent).

The major transmission category for women with AIDS (52 percent) was intravenous drug use, and the second largest category was heterosexual contact with a person at risk for AIDS (21 percent). Men with AIDS outnumbered women with AIDS in all risk categories except heterosexual contact with a person at risk for AIDS. Only 1 percent of non-homosexual/bisexual men with AIDS are in this group, compared with 21 percent of women with AIDS ($P<.0001$). Of the

456 total reported adults with AIDS whose only risk factor is hetero-sexual contact with a person at risk for AIDS, 381 (84 percent) were women.

Heterosexual contact with an intravenous drug user accounted for 67 percent of women with AIDS in this category, whereas 16 percent of contacts were bisexual men, 1 percent were men with hemophilia, and 167 percent were men with other or unreported risk factors.

Excluding homosexual/bisexual men, the overall ratio of men with AIDS to women with AIDS was 3:1. The ratio was highest for hemo-philiac/coagulation disorder cases (33:1). For cases in the categories of intravenous drug use, transfusion, born in a country with hetero-sexual transmission, and undetermined categories, the ratios ranged from 2:1 to 4:1, whereas for cases in the category of heterosexual contact with a person at risk for AIDS, the ratio was 0.2:1.

The proportion of women with AIDS in the intravenous drug use group decreased between 1983 and 1986 (P<.01). In comparison, the proportion of men with AIDS in the homosexual/bisexual and intravenous drug user categories has remained remarkably stable between 1982 and 1986. A downward trend was noted in the propor-tion of both men and women with AIDS in the category born in a country with heterosexual transmission. The proportion of women with AIDS in the heterosexual contact category increased from 12 percent to 26 percent between 1982 and 1986 (P<.0001). The proportion of women with AIDS in the undetermined transmission category remained stable.

Between 1982 and 1986, the increase in the number of women with AIDS in the intravenous drug user, heterosexual contact, and unknown risk groups was paralleled in the increase in pediatric pa-tients whose mothers were in these risk groups. The only discordant group in which the temporal trends for women and children with AIDS were not similar were those born in a country with heterosexual transmission. For all other categories, trends in women with AIDS are good predictors of trends in children with AIDS whose mothers are in these risk groups.

Reported cases of AIDS in women increased in parallel with cases in men from 1981 through 1986. Over 70 percent of women with AIDS were of black or Hispanic origin, and over 80 percent were of childbearing age. Intravenous drug use was the major risk factor for women with AIDS, and the second most common risk factor was heterosexual contact with a person at risk for AIDS. Heterosexual contact is the only transmission category where women with AIDS outnumber men with AIDS. Moreover, the proportion of women with

AIDS in this category has increased annually between 1982 and 1986. In the United States, at the present time, a heterosexual woman is at greater risk for acquiring AIDS through sexual intercourse than is a heterosexual man.

The larger number of heterosexually acquired AIDS cases among women is likely the result of two factors: (1) a greater proportion of men are infected, and therefore a woman is more likely than a man to encounter an infected partner: and (2) the efficiency of transmission of HIV from man to woman may be greater than from woman to man.

Receptive anal intercourse has been associated with an increased risk for AIDS and for HIV antibody in homosexual men, but apparently not in heterosexual women. We did not have sexual practice data and therefore could not assess this risk in our study. However, the low frequency of anal intercourse reported in other studies of infected women suggests that sexual acquisition in women occurs most commonly through other types of intercourse.

Human immunodeficiency virus has been transmitted to women during artificial insemination when infected semen was injected directly into the uterus through a catheter. Therefore, transmission of the virus presumably can occur during penile-vaginal intercourse. It is unknown whether the risk of HIV infection is the same if the portal of entry of the virus is the vagina or rectum. Direct viral access to the blood occurs when skin or mucous membranes are not intact. Breakdown of cells of these surfaces during intercourse may be more likely during anorectal intercourse. However, if HIV can pass through intact mucous membranes, the risk of transmission through the vagina or rectum may not be different.

One reason for the high rate of women with AIDS who have no identified risk may be that some women were unaware of their exposure to a person in the high-risk group. The two groups most likely to infect women during heterosexual intercourse are men who are intravenous drug users and bisexual men. It may be difficult to assess these risk factors in prospective sex partners. Casual partners, especially, may not reveal that they are members of a high-risk group for AIDS. Therefore, women engaging in casual sex in the United States should be aware of their risk for HIV infection, especially in geographic areas (e.g., New York City and San Francisco) where infection rates are high for men in known risk groups.

Because women may transmit HIV infection to their newborns, it is important to screen and counsel high-risk women concerning their risks. If present trends continue, the number of children with AIDS born to mothers whose risk is either undetermined or associated with heterosexual contact with a person at risk for AIDS will increase. Women in these groups may be unaware of their risk and would not request counseling or HIV testing before they became pregnant. Therefore, primary prevention of HIV infection in women is necessary to prevent the majority of cases of AIDS in children that would result from these maternal risk groups. Counseling has been initiated for intravenous drug users in some areas.

It is difficult to identify and target a large proportion of women who are at risk of acquiring infection through heterosexual intercourse. Therefore, from a public health point of view, it is important to educate all women about their risk of sexually acquired AIDS and to encourage risk-reducing behavior, including celibacy and having only one lifetime sexual partner. Sexually active women who have more than one lifetime sexual partner and those who are sexual partners of HIV infected men or men in high-risk categories may reduce their risk by insisting that their partners always use condoms during intercourse.

Positive HTLV-III/LAV Antibody Results for Sexually Active Female Members of Social/Sexual Clubs — Minnesota

Reprinted with permission from *MMWR*
November 14, 1987

In June 1986, two sexually active women in Minnesota were found to have antibody to human T-lymphotropic virus type III lymphadenopathy-associated virus (HTLV-III/LAV). Both belonged to social/sexual clubs whose stated purpose was to provide their members (primarily couples) with opportunities for social and sexual contacts. Each of the two seropositive women reported having sexual contact with a number of other persons from these clubs, including two men who were bisexual.

Infection was detected in these two women during a serologic screening program conducted by the St. Paul Division of Public Health, in consultation with the Minnesota Department of Health. This screening was undertaken because members of these clubs were known to have been involved in outbreaks of other sexually transmitted diseases (including syphilis and gonorrhea). From a total of 285 members (143 women and 142 men) of two of these social/sexual clubs in the Minneapolis-St. Paul area, 134 volunteers were tested with an enzyme-linked immunosorbent assay (ELISA) for antibody to HTLV-III/LAV in June and July 1986. Any ELISA-positive specimens were also tested with the Western blot assay. All 75 men tested had negative ELISA results for antibody to HTLV-III/LAV. Two of 59 women tested had positive antibody test results for HTLV-III/LAV with both ELISA and Western blot. Antibody results for these women were again positive with ELISA and Western blot when repeated 6 weeks later. The seroprevalence rate of 3 percent among female club members tested is significantly higher than the seroprevalence rate of zero (none of 56,000) among female blood donors in Minnesota.

The two seropositive women had belonged to two different social/sexual clubs for approximately 2 years. Both denied intravenous drug use, a history of blood transfusions, or receipt of clotting factor concentrates. One woman was 31 years old, married, and had sexual relations only with other club members; her husband (also a member) had negative test results for HTLV-III/LAV antibody. The other woman was 25 years old, unmarried, and occasionally had sexual relations with men outside the club.

Each of these two women reported having had sexual contact with more than 25 other club members, including five men with whom they had both had sexual intercourse. Two of these five men could be located for testing and had negative results for HTLV-III/LAV antibody. Two of the other three men whose serologic status could not be determined were reported to be bisexual men with whom both women had had repeated vaginal and anal intercourse.

An additional bisexual man who was a former member of one of these clubs is known to have developed acquired immunodeficiency syndrome. He had no history of sexual contact with either of the seropositive women or with either of the two bisexual men who had sexual contact with these women.

To date, 55 of the 134 club members tested for antibody to HTLV-III/LAV (including the two seropositive women) have participated in follow-up interviews and have received counseling about their sexual practices and attitudes. Four (15 percent) of 27 men reported homosexual contact with other club members as well as with men who were not members of either of the two clubs. When asked whether they perceived themselves as being at increased risk of having AIDS, 40 members (73 percent) replied that they did not. One man reported that he "usually" used condoms while having sexual intercourse. When asked whether they would continue to participate in the activities promoted by social/sexual clubs if they knew such activities were associated with a high risk of having AIDS, 54/55 (98 percent) answered that they would not.

When it was known that one member of each of the two clubs was positive for HTLV-III/LAV antibody, both clubs disbanded. In an effort to minimize the transmission of HTLV-III/LAV, educational programs for sexually active adults (including former club members) are currently being implemented in the Minneapolis-St. Paul area. Follow-up studies of former club members are planned to assess whether other changes in sexual behavior are occurring.

* * * * * * * * * *

By June, 1984, AIDS cases in the United States had passed the 5,000 mark.

b. Modeling the Epidemic and Predictions
The March of AIDS

by Reiner Klingholz
Reprinted from *World Press Review (Die Zeit)*
February, 1987

AIDS has the world surrounded. By mid-November, 78 coun- tries had reported a combined total of 35,883 cases to the World Health Organization. The US accounts for three- quarters of all the cases in these statistics. Japan reports only 21 cases.

Many lands, such as East Germany, the Maldives and Nigeria, with a population of 100 million, say they have no AIDS cases. Islamic na- tions deny the malady's existence within their borders. A Soviet spokesman describes AIDS as a Western disease, and in Sri Lanka an official says he believes that it is only found among Tamil terrorists.

No one believes such politically colored reports. Even correct statistics can reflect only the tip of the iceberg. In no country are all actual cases of the disorder recognized and reported. In many parts of the Third World even the expertise needed to diagnose AIDS does not exist.

WHO has sounded its disaster alarm. "I cannot imagine any health problem in this century being worse," says Halfdan Mahler, the head of WHO. "All of us underestimated it." WHO epidemiologists in Gene- va have gathered together the fragmentary information from around the globe and made a prognosis: in 1990 the organization foresees costs in the area of $1.5 billion to control this worldwide epidemic. As many as 50 to 100 million people may be infected by then.

In Africa, the continent in which the AIDS virus is most widespread, the virus is spreading far faster than in the industrial West. Over the next decade, the virus will reach as much as 70 percent of the population in some areas. "Entire regions," says one expert, "will be depopulated."

While it is no longer certain that the AIDS virus got its start in Africa, many researchers, such as Reinhard Kurth, a virologist at the Paul Ehrlich Institute in Frankfurt, still believe in an African origin. He believes that the malady has long existed as a "village disease" in isolated areas. It was only after the great migration from rural areas that the virus reached urban areas and found ideal conditions for its spread.

It is only in the last few years that the epidemic has overrun Central and East AFrica. In 1984, for the first time, AIDS patients were filling the hospitals of Zaire, Rwanda, Zambia, Kenya, Uganda and Tanzania. Today epidemiologists are finding the virus in the lands of the Sahara as well as in South Africa. Apparently, only some isolated groups, such as the pygmies, who still live as hunters and gatherers, are spared.

In Uganda, where AIDS is known as "slim disease" because of its victims' wasted bodies, it was not until 1982 that enough people died of it for others to take notice. "It was a typical smugglers' disease," says Jack Jagwe of the Ministry of Health in Kampala. "The people were always traveling, and carried the virus from one brothel or bar to the next."

When doctors carried out the first thorough investigation in Uganda's Rakai district this year, they came to a horrifying conclusion: In 14 percent of all blood samples, there was evidence of the AIDS virus. Worse, three-fourths of the sex partners of those who tested positively were infected. Similar results have emerged from the entire Central African AIDS belt.

"Six percent of all blood samples tested in Zaire are positive," reports Peter Piot, a Belgian expert on tropical diseases. "In Kigali, the capital of Rwanda, it is 18 percent." Another study shows that a third of all the sexually active men between 30 and 35 in Lusaka, the capital of Zambia, have the virus in their bodies.

Because homosexuality is relatively rare in Africa, AIDS there is transmitted overwhelmingly by heterosexual contact. Men and women are equally affected by the epidemic. An exception is South Africa: There, homosexuals have been infected from contact with Americans, while infections among heterosexuals — both blacks and whites — have obviously crossed the border from Zaire. Since many African women of childbearing age carry the virus, more and more babies are being born with AIDS. Thirteen percent of the newborns in a Kinshasa clinic come into the world doomed.

A study at Nairobi's Kenyatta Hospital shows just how fast a virus can spread in a society where sexual partners change frequently. Within six years, 60 percent of all prostitutes examined were carriers. In the slums of Nairobi today, there is almost no prostitute who is not affected by the virus. The women, most of whom were forced by poverty to leave their native villages, have about 1,000 customers a year. After spending a while in the slums, the women return to their families on the land. They bring the deadly plague with them.

The firestorm of disease also has been fed by other infections, such as malaria, yellow fever, tuberculosis and leprosy, and by undernourishment and pregnancy. All of these burdens weaken the immune system and make it easier for the virus to establish itself.

African blood transfusions carry a high risk of infection. The expensive AIDS-antibody tests for blood are used almost nowhere, so most blood banks are contaminated. Anyone in Rwanda, Uganda or Zaire who receives a transfusion runs an 8 to 18 percent chance of acquiring AIDS.

"We urgently need foreign help," says Jagwe of Uganda. "Instituting blood testing would cost more than our entire national health budget." The US spent $60 million on such testing last year. For the Third World, such testing might be even more expensive: While such a test in West Germany costs about two dollars, American firms operating in developing countries charge five to eight dollars for it.

Demographers looking at a continent threatened with overpopulation must now take some new factors into account. The disease is most heavily affecting the group made up of sexually active men and women between 15 and 35 — the very economically productive generation on which these poor nations are pinning their hopes. And tourism — for many African lands one of the most important sources of hard currency — could be destroyed. Later, foreign firms may resist investing in lands where an increasing share of the work force is dying off. "By the time that half a region's population is sick and unable to work, if not even sooner," says Gerhard Hunsman, an AIDS expert in Gottingen, Germany, "its entire infrastructure will collapse. The area will cease to be inhabitable."

Even if an effective vaccine against AIDS becomes available in a few years, no one in Africa will be able to afford it. In the same region where mankind took its first steps more than four million years ago — in Ethiopia, Kenya, Uganda, Zaire and Tanzania — Homo sapiens is now in danger of being wiped out.

The Dynamics of the AIDS Epidemic

Roy M. Anderson and Robert M. May
Printed with special permission from the authors
December 1, 1987

The molecular structure and much of the functioning of the HIV virus that causes AIDS have been elucidated in a remarkably short time. In contrast, we still have at best vague estimates for many of the basic quantities that are needed to make predictions about the probable future course of the epidemic.

Taking these basic epidemiological parameters one by one, we first observe that there is considerable uncertainty about the magnitude of the probability that HIV infection will be transmitted from an infected individual to a susceptible partner, over the duration of a given sexual relationship (homosexual or heterosexual). The probabilities both of acquiring and of transmitting infection depend also on the rate at which a given individual acquires new sexual partners; surprisingly little information has been gathered about the distribution functions characterizing the varying degrees of sexual activity among groups of homosexuals, bisexuals and heterosexuals in developed countries, much less in developing ones. Turning from these transmission probabilities and contact rates — which can be altered by social changes, such as adopting "safe sex" practices or reducing numbers of partners — we note there is much uncertainty about the duration of infectiousness among those infected with HIV virus, and also about the fraction of those infected who will eventually develop full-blown AIDS disease, and die soon after. Earlier estimates were that maybe 20-30% of those infected would eventually develop AIDS, typically after about 5 years; this estimate is the basis of the widely quoted CDC projections about AIDS in the USA, discussed further below. The more recent National Academy of Sciences/Institute of Medicine Report estimates this fraction at something more like 25-50% or more. Some recent evidence points to 75% or more of all infectees developing AIDS up to 8 years or more after initial HIV infection; these high estimates come from studies of individuals infected by blood transfusions (which give a chance to pin-point the date of infection), and such infections could conceivably be atypical, and more likely to cause AIDS. Not only is the fraction likely to proceed from HIV infection to AIDS disease and death uncertain, but the duration of infectiousness in HIV infectees is unknown. It could, at worst, be that those who do not develop AIDS disease remain asymptomatic transmitters — "Typhoid Mary's" — of HIV virus the rest of their sexually active lives. The above catalogue is cast in terms of sexual transmission of HIV infection, largely because to date, homosexual transmission accounts for 70-80% of all AIDS cases in the USA, and an even larger fraction in Europe, while heterosexual transmission seems to predominate in Africa. Cases resulting from needle-sharing among drug users, from vertical transmission from infected mothers to offspring, or from blood transfusions represent a significant minority of the total of all cases, and many of the population-level ideas developed below apply to these non-sexual roots of transmission. In what follows, we will, however, confine attention to sexual transmission.

To some extent, the much faster rate of acquiring knowledge about molecular and immunmological aspects of the biology of the HIV virus than about epidemiological aspects derives from the large numbers of appropriately-trained people and well-equipped laboratories that could rapidly turn attention to the former aspects of the problem. Probably more important, however, is the fact that the virus itself can be studied in the laboratory, and significant things learned about it in weeks or months. In contrast, direct assessment of many of the population-level characteristics of the virus-host association involve epidemiological studies of large numbers of people over long spans of time. It is, for example, ultimately difficult to be sure whether there will be individuals who are infected with HIV, and who remain infectious for 20-30 years or more without exhibiting AIDS or other symptoms, until we have followed a cohort of such infectees for such a period!

In the face of these uncertainties, most projections about future levels of HIV infection or AIDS-related deaths are based on using refined statistical techniques to extrapolate from past and current trends. Such extrapolations are likely to be reasonably reliable for predictions about the immediate future. But, as we shall see below, many population-level aspects of the transmission dynamics are likely to change (in non-linear ways) as the epidemic progresses, such that projections derived essentially from curve-fitting to current trends are not reliable for the long run (which for AIDS may mean beyond a few years). This point is not as widely understood as it might be, partly because figures like the widely-cited CDC estimate of "179,000 deaths" from AIDS in the USA by 1991 convey a misleading sense of accuracy. In fact, as the CDC report itself makes clear, even the first digit is uncertain here, and the actual number may lie anywhere from one hundred thousand to several hundred thousands, depending on what assumptions are made about durations of infectiousness, fractions infected with HIV who develop AIDS, rate of spread by heterosexual transmission, or rates and magnitudes of changes in sexual habits.

The present article focuses on things that can be learned from mathematical models for population-level aspects of the processes whereby HIV infection is transmitted. We show how such models can be used to make indirect assessments of some important combinations of the epidemiological parameters, whose lack of amenability to direct measurement has just been discussed. It will also be seen that these models overturn some incorrect impressions that might seem "intuitively obvious".

In what follows, the distinction between HIV infection and AIDS disease needs continually to be kept in mind. Data about number of cases of AIDS are much more abundant than about number of cases of HIV infection, because the constellation of opportunistic infections characterizing AIDS, and usually leading to death within a year, lend themselves to diagnosis (although not all cases are reported as such; even in developed countries, compassion for families arguably results in some AIDS deaths being attributed to other causes). HIV infection by itself presents little in the way of clear-cut symptoms, and such information as we have from the early 1980s and before comes from detection of HIV antibodies in blood sera that were serendipitously collected and stored for other purposes (such as a study of hepatitis B virus among homosexual males in San Francisco in the late 1970s and early 1980s). Thus by the end of 1986 diagnosed cases of AIDS had been reported in 74 countries, with more than 25,000 cases in the USA, nearly 3,000 cases in other countries in the New World, and more than 3,000 cases in Europe. Estimates of the number of HIV infections in the USA, on the other hand, are necessarily much less precise, and range from under one million to as many as two million or more. Up to this time, most of these cases in developed countries are attributed to homosexual/bisexual males. In Africa, where transmission appears to be primarily heterosexual, the fraction seropositive among healthy populations (not AIDS cases) ranges from 0.7% for blood donors in Zaire, to as high as 18% for blood donors in Kigali, Rwanda. A study of some 600 seronegative men and women working in a general hospital in Kinshasa from 1984 to 1985 found the annual incidence of HIV antibodies was around 0.8%, a figure which Quinn thought might be representative of the annual incidence of new HIV infections in Central and East Africa. Throughout Africa, reported cases of AIDS now number several thousand, and many more seem likely to exist unrecorded; Quinn et al. estimate the current annual rate of appearance of cases of AIDS in Central Africa to be around 0.5 to 1.0 per 1,000 adults.

In the relatively early stages of the epidemic, the rate at which new infections are produced by a given infected individual depends on the probability of transmission for the type of relationship between infector and infectee that is in question (homosexual males, intravenous drug users, etc.), and on the effective average number of such contacts with susceptible individuals, per unit time. In this early phase of the epidemic, the number of HIV infections grows exponentially, doubling at a roughly constant rate. Earlier summaries that serological evidence from the USA and from EEC countries suggests that the number of HIV infections doubles roughly every 8-12 months in the early stages of the epidemic, corresponding to the product of the probability of transmission and contacts with susceptible individuals having a value of around 1 per year. Although neither the average transmission probability among homosexual males, nor the effective average rate of acquiring new partners is well know, this population-level estimate of the product is consistent with independent rough assessments that the average rate of acquiring new partners may be around 10 per year (for homosexual males in large cities in developed countries) and the probability of transmission is around 0.1.

These calculations recognize that the chance of a given individual acquiring infection is likely to depend approximately linearly on the number of new sexual partners acquired per unit time, and on the probability that any one partner is infectious; the latter probability, in turn, has the feature that more promiscuous individuals are both more likely to be acquired as partners and are more likely to be infected and infectious. That is, individuals who are highly sexually active are both more likely to acquire infection and more likely to transmit it. The upshot is that the "effective average" rate of acquiring new partners is not simply the mean of the distribution in such rates, but rather is the average of the number-of-partners-squared, divided by the mean. This apparently recondite mathematical point derives basically from the disproportionate part played by highly promiscuous individuals in the early stages of the epidemic, and estimating the rate of acquiring new partners as simply the average number of partners can lead to significant underestimates. As an illustrative but otherwise hypothetical example, consider a population of homosexual males among whom 50% are relatively monogamous, acquiring new sexual partners at the rate of roughly 1 per year, while the remaining 50% have around 19 new partners annually. The mean number of new partners is then 10 per year, but the epidemiologically-relevant quantity is the mean-square to mean ratio which is significantly larger.

This initial phase of exponential growth slows down once a substantial fraction of the most sexually active individuals are infected, essentially because many newly acquired partners among this initially disproportionately important category of individuals are already infected. The number of HIV infections in the population as a whole continues to rise, but now more nearly linearly (that is, doubling times lengthen rather than remaining constant as for exponential growth) as infection continues to spread to less promiscuous individuals from the now almost saturated "core group". Thus the shape of the curve of rising levels of seropositivity for HIV differs from the simpler curves characteristic of childhood infections, such as measles, which continue to rise roughly exponentially until around half the at-risk population is infected; the spread of measles is a more homogeneous process than is HIV among groups characterized by great variability in degrees of sexual activity. Such changes in the underlying dynamical processes make for serious complications in projections based on curve-fitting.

If a fixed fraction of those infected with HIV went on to develop AIDS after an incubation period of constant length, with the remaining fraction never developing AIDS, then the curve for the rise in AIDS cases over time would have the same shape as the seropositivity-versus-time curve, displaced in time by the length of the incubation period. In reality, the incubation period is not of constant duration, but rather there is a distribution of durations of incubation periods, the exact nature of which remains uncertain. Current evidence suggests some infectees may develop AIDS within a year or so, but that 4-6 years may be more typical, and the possibility that a substantial fraction of infectees may develop AIDS after significantly longer incubation periods cannot be ruled out. Thus the patterns of rise in total number of AIDS cases over time depends both on the rise in HIV infection (which in turn depends on transmission processes, as just discussed) and on the distribution of incubation times. This means that observed doubling times for diagnosed AIDS cases cannot be used to make direct estimates of the combination of transmission parameters in the way that doubling times for seropositivity levels can, which is a pity because data on AIDS cases are much more abundant and reliable than are data on seropositivity levels. It seems probable, however, that the distribution in incubation periods is of secondary importance in determining the basic patterns of increase in numbers of AIDS cases, and that these data yield estimates of the combination of transmission parameters in broad agreement with those obtained more directly from changes in seropositivity levels over time.

As the epidemic progresses, not only is the pool of susceptibles gradually used up, but also infectious individuals are removed. For HIV, such removal can derive from the debilitation and eventual death consequent upon full-blown AIDS, and it might also derive — although very little is known about this — from the infectiousness of asymptomatic carriers of HIV infection declining over time. A basic quantity characterizing any infectious disease is its "basic reproductive rate", defined as the number of infections produced, on average, by an infected individual in a wholly susceptible population; the infection will tend to invade a susceptible population and cause an epidemic if this reproductive rate exceeds unity, and not otherwise. For HIV, the basic reproductive rate among homosexual males is the product of the transmission probability times effective average number of partners, and the average duration of infectiousness. Unfortunately, the average duration of infectiveness is not known. Again, population-level models enable us to make an indirect inference about the magnitude of the basic reproductive rate.

In simple mathematical models for epidemics such as measles in populations that are to a reasonable approximation "homogeneously mixed", the total number ever infected during the course of the epidemic depends only on the above-defined basic reproductive rate of the infection. But we have just seen that substantial heterogeneity in levels of sexual activity within a population can significantly affect the dynamics of the HIV epidemic, and one consequence is that the fraction ever infected depends both on the basic reproductive rate for HIV and on the actual distribution in rates of acquiring new sexual partners. Among homosexual males in large cities in the USA, seropositivity levels are already around 50% or more; that is, around half the homosexual population of San Francisco, New York, and probably Los Angeles is already infected with HIV. The fraction eventually infected will, of course, thus be at least 50%. Were we dealing with a classic epidemic in a homogeneously mixed population, this would merely tell us that the basic reproductive rate probably exceeded 1.4 (before changes in behavior began to affect the dynamics of the epidemic, as its nature became better understood in the mid-1980s); since we know the basic reproductive rate necessarily exceeds unity for the epidemic to be possible, this estimate of a lower limit of 1.4 is not very helpful. But, given the levels of variability in rates of acquiring new sexual partners that have been reported for homosexual males in large cities, we find that seropositivity levels of 50% cannot be attained unless the basic reproductive rate exceeded 5 or more in the early stages of the epidemic. Given that the basic reproductive rate is the product of one per new partner per year and the average duration of infectiousness, this may characteristically be around 5 years or more. Such an estimate is consistent with HIV infectees remaining infectious throughout the incubation period, currently estimated as around 5 years; the estimate is, however, also consistent with the proportion of HIV infectees who develop AIDS being infectious for less than the incubation period, while a remaining proportion who do not develop AIDS remain infectious for much longer times (possibly for the remainder of their sexually active lives).

In the absence of a vaccine against HIV infection or any effective treatment for AIDS disease, the only way to halt the spread of the disease is to reduce HIV transmission, which ultimately means reducing the basic reproductive rate by persuading people to change their habits. The larger the initial value of the basic reproductive rate, the more difficult this task. The estimate that the original value of the basic reproductive rate probably exceeded 5 is thus not encouraging. It suggests that HIV among homosexual males in large cities is more "intrinsically spreadable" than smallpox (where basic reproductive rate is 2 — 4), possibly comparable with polio (approximately 5), although possibly below measles (approximately 15); remember that 5 is a lower limit, and the basic reproductive rate could be significantly higher for HIV.

The above remarks have concentrated on transmission of HIV among homosexual males in developed countries, where this category accounts for three-quarters or more of all AIDS cases so far. HIV infection from blood transfusions, or by vertical transmission from mothers to fetuses, could not by themselves perpetuate an epidemic; such infections represent a small fraction of AIDS cases but should not discount their significance in terms of numbers of afflicted individuals. Shared needles among drug users is a transmission process that almost certainly sustains its own epidemic among that population, and most of the ideas developed above apply, *mutatis mutandis*, to those circumstances; fewer data are available for these groups than for homosexual males. Setting aside transmission associated with blood transfusions, with needle-sharing itself, or with drug-using male partners, most cases of AIDS among females in developed countries currently appear to derive from HIV transmission from bisexual male partners who are infected. The transmission dynamics of such infections depends essentially on the spread of infection among bisexual males, which, in the absence of detailed information, may be taken to be as for homosexual males. This suggests the incidence of AIDS among such female partners of bisexual males should double at roughly the same rate as for the male homosexual population, which is indeed what the data seem to show.

Given that HIV infection is already established — albeit at low levels as yet — among heterosexuals in developed countries, what is the chance of an epidemic sustaining itself and spreading by purely heterosexual transmission? The accumulating evidence leaves no doubt that this is predominately how AIDS has spread and is spreading in Africa. Data from the distribution by age and sex of the first 500 cases of AIDS diagnosed in Kinshasa (Naipaul's city in *The Bend in the River*) in the last half of 1985 show that there are roughly equal numbers of cases among males and females (45% to 55%), and the age distributions correlate with probable levels of sexual activity (differently for males and females, as discussed below). The relatively low levels among those under 20 years of age seems to us to rule out any significant transmission from needle-sharing in public health programs or from insect vectors. Tests for HIV antibodies in blood sera stored from earlier studies (often for different purposes) show seropositivity levels among female prostitutes rising from 4% in 1980-81 to around 51% in 1983-84 and 59% in 1985-86, and from 1% to 14% and 18% at the corresponding times for males attending a clinic for sexually transmitted diseases in Nairobi. Recent seroprevalance levels among high-risk groups, such as female prostitutes, in Africa, have been reported to range from 27% to 88%, depending on socioeconomic status and geographic location. In a general survey of pregnant women in Nairobi, seropositivity levels rose from 0% in 1980-81 to 2% in 1985-86; and a similar survey of pregnant women in Kinshasa shows seropositivity levels rising from 0.2% in 1970 to 3% in 1980-81 and 8% in 1985-86.

Further evidence for heterosexual transmission as the dominant mode in Africa comes from a study of 2,400 AIDS cases diagnosed in adults in Europe up to 31 March 1986: for the 2,235 cases thought to originate in Europe or elsewhere other than Africa and the Caribbean, 92% fell in the risk-categories usual for adults in developed countries (homosexual/bisexual males, intravenous drug users, blood transfusions), with a male:female ratio of 16:1; for the cases thought to originate in Africa (177 cases) or the Caribbean (61 cases), only 10% fell in these categories, and the male:female ratio was 1.6:1 (undoubtedly biased by the fact that more males than females travel to Europe from Africa and the Caribbean).

The kinds of mathematical analysis sketched earlier apply also to heterosexual transmission of HIV infection, except now we must deal with two reciprocating populations: males transmitting infection to females, and females transmitting infection to males. We need to consider separately the probability that an infected female will transmit infection to a susceptible male, and that an infected male will infect a female. It seems likely that the male-to-female transmission probability may be higher — possibly substantially higher — than the female-to-male transmission probability. For gonorrhea, which is admittedly a weak analogy, male-to-female is roughly twice female to male. Both transmission probabilities may, moreover, typically be higher in Africa than in developed countries owing to the widespread incidence of gonorrhea, genital ulcers, syphilis and other sexually transmitted diseases that often disrupt the integrity of the genital epithelia and thereby facilitate transmission of HIV during vaginal intercourse. In studies among prostitutes in Nairobi, HIV seropositivity was significantly correlated with the presence of other sexually transmitted diseases, and in another study in Zambia, seropositivity in men was also correlated with the presence of genital ulcers; these may, of course, be correlations without causation.

Less obviously, we also need to know the two separate distributions in the rates of acquiring new sexual partners by males and by females. As before, the quantities that influence the dynamics of transmission are not simply the mean numbers of new sexual partners per unit time, but rather the ratio of mean-square to mean numbers for females acquiring male partners and for males acquiring female partners. Although the mean rate at which males acquire new female sexual partners must obviously be identical with the mean rate at which females acquire male partners, these factors will not be identical if the variability in levels of sexual activity among males differs significantly from that among females. As an illustrative example, which may be broadly representative of the situation in some parts of Africa, consider heterosexual transmission of HIV within a population in which all males are moderately promiscuous, all having around 4 new (female) sexual partners per year, while the female population is more heterogeneous in its sexual habits with 90% having 1 new (male) partner per year and the other 10% having on average 31 new partners annually. Both male and female populations have the same average number of 4 new sexual partners per year, as they clearly must. For males, the epidemiologically-relevant quantity is also 4 per year. But for females, the ratio of mean-square to mean number of partners is approximately 24 per year.

As in the somewhat simpler studies for transmission among homosexuals, the models for heterosexual transmission suggest that in the earlier stages of the epidemic — before any subgroup becomes saturated with infection — the incidence of HIV infection among males and among females grows roughly exponentially at the same rate in both populations. The doubling rate now corresponds to a doubling time significantly shorter than the average duration of infectiousness. In developing countries, we would expect to find the female-to-male transmission probability and probably also the male-to-female transmission probability less than the probability of transmission among homosexuals. We would also expect the appropriately-averaged rates of acquiring new sexual partners by women and by men to be less than the rate of acquiring new partners for homosexuals in large cities in the developed world in the early 1980s. Overall, therefore, we would expect the doubling rate to be smaller — and the doubling time to be longer — for heterosexual transmission than for homosexual transmission of HIV in developed countries. Whether or not a self-sustaining epidemic can be generated by purely heterosexual transmission in developed countries depends on the magnitude of the basic reproductive rate for such transmission. Such an epidemic is likely to take off if the basic reproductive rate exceeds unity, and not otherwise. At present, uncertainties surround each one of the 5 quantities entering into this expression for the basic reproductive rate (especially the female-to-male transmission probability), nor is there enough data to attempt the kind of indirect inference of the basic reproductive rate from population-level considerations, as we did for homosexual transmission in developed countries. We believe that reasonable estimates span a range of basic reproductive rate-values from just below unity to significantly above unity.

In the early, exponentially growing stages of such an epidemic of heterosexually-transmitted HIV infection, we expect the ratio of sero-positivity levels among males to that among females to be roughly constant. This result is in direct contradiction to the expectation — explicitly or implicitly stated in essentially all writing on the subject — that the ratio of HIV infections, and thence of AIDS cases, among males and females should be roughly equal if infection is transmitted heterosexually. Indeed, given the expectation that the male-to-female transmission probability may be significantly larger than the female-to-male probability, we could regard the 1:1 sex ratio among cases more as a problem to be explained than as a confirmation of hetero-sexual transmission.

If we were heedless of variability in degrees of sexual activity among male and female populations, the rates of acquiring new part-ners would be identical for female and male. Although the numerical illustration given above makes no claim to be other than qualitative, it may well describe roughly the kind of situation pertaining in much of Africa, where the majority of females have relatively monogamous marriages or "union libres" (persistent cohabitation without formal marriage), but where many of the male partners in such relationships are less monogamous, with the books kept in balance by a cadre of young female prostitutes. Such differences in the distributions of degrees of sexual activity among males and females probably leads to ratios of acquiring new partners significantly above unity which counterbalances the above-noted expectation that probability of transmission is likely to be significantly below unity. By the time one takes the square root of the product of these counterbalancing ratios, it would not be surprising to have a number around unity; we believe this is probably the real — and more complicated — explanation for the ratio of male to female cases of AIDS in Africa being around unity.

With the above assumptions about qualitative differences in male and female patterns of sexual activity in Africa, a more detailed analy-sis of the dynamics of heterosexual transmission leads us to expect the "core group" of female prostitutes relatively rapidly to attain high levels of seropositivity, accompanied by moderate levels among males and lower levels among the female population more generally. This accords with the observations about seropositivity levels in Africa among female prostitutes, men attending clinics, and pregnant women, that were discussed above. The theoretical analysis also matches where the average age of female AIDS patients is significantly below that for males (30 years versus 37 years); in this study, females with AIDS were more likely than males to be unmarried (61% versus

36%). Another study, in Kigali in Rwanda, identified 43% of female AIDS patients as prostitutes.

More generally, a growing amount of data confirms the correlation between rates of acquiring new sexual partners and the probability of acquiring HIV infection or AIDS disease, both for heterosexual transmission in Africa and homosexual transmission in the developed world. Reviewing data from Africa, Quinn et al. report that "case-control studies have shown that AIDS patients have a significantly higher number of heterosexual partners than controls (mean of 32 versus 3) . . . and that the risk of seropositivity increases significantly with the number of different sexual partners per year." There is also a similar correlation between HIV seropositivity levels and numbers of sexual partners among homosexuals in San Francisco.

Bearing all this in mind, our guess is that, in developed countries, HIV could well spread by purely heterosexual transmission within relatively promiscuous subgroups. The long-term possibility of a much more generally disseminated epidemic seems to us to depend crucially on whether a significant fraction of HIV infectees remain asymptomatic carriers (never developing AIDS) essentially for the remainder of their sexually active lives. If this is so, then quite modest levels of promiscuity could result in HIV infection spreading slowly, over decades, among a population who would not think of themselves as promiscuous. In our earlier language, such long duration of infectiousness among a significant fraction of infectees corresponds to the basic reproductive rate for heterosexually-transmitted HIV being very large.

This brings us to a final important point to do with predicting AIDS cases. It might at first seem that the larger the fraction of HIV infectees who go on to develop AIDS and die, the larger the eventual number of deaths from the epidemic. This is not necessarily so. Contrast the following two possibilities, neither of which can be ruled out by currently available data: in Case A, 30% of those infected develop AIDS, remaining infectious typically for 5 years and then dying, while the remaining 70% of those infected remain asymptomatic yet infectious for 30 years; in Case B, 100% of those infected develop AIDS, remaining infectious typically for 8 years and then dying. Notice immediately that the characteristic duration of infectiousness is larger in Case A ($0.3 \times 5 + 0.7 \times 30$ 22.5 years) than in Case B (8 years); this means the basic reproductive rate for HIV infection is almost three times greater under assumption A than under B. The total number of deaths caused by AIDS in either case depends on the fraction ever infected with HIV and on the fraction of those infected who develop AIDS. For Case A, with its substantially larger basic reproductive rate, a larger fraction of the population will acquire HIV infection, but a smaller proportion (30% of these will die. In contrast, in Case B a smaller fraction will be infected, but all who are, will die. We simply cannot say whether Case A or Case B will result in a larger total number of deaths, until we have made a detailed analysis of the nonlinear way the differences in the basic reproductive rates are likely to affect the numbers ever infected. The results of such a calculation are sensitive to the amount of variability in degrees of sexual activity; the greater this variability, the more likely that Case A will lead to more deaths than Case B, in defiance of simple intuition.

For homosexually-transmitted HIV infection in developed countries, our preliminary calculations suggest that the total number of AIDS deaths increases as the fraction of HIV infectees going on to develop full-blown AIDS increases up to around 50% or so, but that total deaths remain roughly constant, or can even decrease, as they increases toward 100%. As emphasized at the outset, current evidence cannot rule out values as low as 20-30% or as high as 100%. Given this uncertainty, it is well to recognize that projected total deaths do not simply rise as estimates rise, but rather that nonlinearities in the transmission processes can produce counter-intuitive outcomes not easily foreseen by curve-fitting.

Uncertainties about the future of the relation between HIV infection and human hosts are matched by uncertainties about the past. The virus does seem to be the latest example of Pliny's *ex Africa aliquid semper novi*, with the earliest serological evidence for HIV found in samples collected in Kinshasa in 1959. Other stored sera from West and East Africa in the 1960s and 1970s have also indicated seropositivity, with seropositivity in 10 of 144 children from Burkina Faso in 1963, and in 50 of 75 children from Uganda in 1972-73. Questions have, however, been raised about the validity of these results (based on enzyme-linked immunosorbent assays and Western blot tests) from stored specimens in areas where malaria is endemic.

Watching Southern evangelists on television in the USA, it is clear that many regard the virus as a divinely-created agent of retribution. A more prosaic, but ultimately almost equally speculative, explanation is that HIV may have arisen by mutating and making the jump from other primates to humans, following a route broadly analogous to that whereby smallpox, measles, and other viruses probably entered the human population from domestic animals some 10,000 years ago. For these more familiar childhood infections, human aggregates of several hundred thousands are needed before the viruses can maintain themselves and spread. So too, it may have required the relatively recent patterns of population growth, urbanization, and possibly greater promiscuity associated partly with the consequent breakdown of older cultures in Africa, to have created conditions for HIV to establish itself there as a heterosexually-transmitted infection. By the same token, the basic reproductive rate for HIV in developing countries was presumably largest among homosexual males in large cities, whence its appearance there in the USA in the late 1970s and somewhat later in Europe.

Whatever the past history, hopes of halting the spread of HIV infection among heterosexuals and homosexuals over the next few years, and thus of reducing AIDS deaths over the next decade and more, rest on persuading people to change their sexual habits. The collection of injunctions summarized as "safe sex", among which use of condoms is probably the single most important, can reduce transmission probabilities. Reductions in the rates at which new sexual partners are acquired lowers the rate at which new infections are produced (partly by reducing the rates at which infectious individuals, who are usually asymptomatic, spread infection and partly by reducing the effective number of susceptibles who are at risk). Our estimate of the basic reproductive rate of HIV infections among homosexuals in developed countries unfortunately suggests that changes must be fairly substantial if this epidemic is to be halted; the basic reproductive rate for heterosexually-transmitted HIV in developed countries may, however, be significantly lower and thus more amenable to being reduced below unity by such cultural changes. The kinds of constructively aggressive programs of public education currently being launched in Britain — although not on anything like the same scale in the USA — face the difficulty that they aim to change behavior in sensitive areas, particularly among young people just entering the sexual arena. Mechanisms of denial are strong, and it seems easy for people genuinely to believe one thing, yet do another.

Cluster of Cases of the Acquired Immune Deficiency Syndrome — Patients Linked by Sexual Contact

David Auerbach, William Darrow, Harold Jaffe
and James Curran

Reprinted with permission from *The American
Journal of Medicine*
March, 1984

Acquired immune deficiency syndrome (AIDS) was first suggested in June 1981 by a report of Los Angeles of *Pneumocystis carinii* pneumonia in five previously healthy homosexual men. Subsequently, Kaposi's sarcoma and a variety of opportunistic infections other than *P. carinii* pneumonia, such as chronic, progressive herpes simplex virus infection, central nervous system toxoplasmosis, cryptococcal meningitis, and disseminated cytomegalovirus infection were also found to be manifestations of AIDS. The abnormality in cellular immune function has been indicated by cutaneous anergy, lymphopenia, and T-cell deficiency.

If AIDS is caused by an infectious agent, evidence of person-to-person spread might be expected. None of the five homosexual men first reported from Los Angeles with *P. carinii* pneumonia gave histories of sexual contact with other patients. In a subsequent series of 41 cases of Kaposi's sarcoma reported from New York City, four homosexually active men were reported to have had "transient, intimate sexual contact with other men in this Kaposi's sarcoma group". In March 1982, several persons in southern California informally reported to public health officials that some men in whom AIDS was later diagnosed had attended the same social gatherings and may have had sexual contracts with one another. Consequently, an investigation was initiated to assess the social and sexual relationships among homosexual men in whom AIDS had been diagnosed.

Of the 19 patients with Kaposi's sarcoma or *P. carinii* pneumonia reported from southern California, eight were alive and 11 had died at the time this investigation was initiated. Interviews were conducted with the eight living patients and with the close companions of seven of the dead patients. Names of sexual contacts were obtained during 13 of the interviews. Nine of the 13 patients were found to have had sexual exposure with other AIDS patients within five years of the onset of symptoms. Four of these nine had had sexual exposures with more than one other patient. The observation that nine of 15 patients who were interviewed named at least one other reported patient as his sexual partner was not expected and seemed highly unusual.

AIDS developed in four men in southern California after they had sexual contact with a non-Californian, Patient 0 (Figure 1). In Patient 0, lymphadenopathy developed in December 1979, and Kaposi's sarcoma was diagnosed in May 1980. He estimated that he had had approximately 250 different male sexual partners each year from 1979 through 1981 and was able to name 72 of his 750 partners for this three-year period. Eight of these 72 named partners were AIDS patients: four from southern California and four from New York City.

Because Patient 0 appeared to link AIDS patients from southern California and New York City, we extended our investigation beyond the Los Angeles-Orange County metropolitan area. Ultimately, we were able to link 40 AIDS patients by sexual contact to at least one other reported patient. Of the 40 linked patients, 22 resided in New York City, nine resided in Los Angeles or contiguous Orange County, and another nine were living in eight other cities in North America when their illnesses were diagnosed. Twenty-four of these men had Kaposi's sarcoma, six had *P. carinii* pneumonia, eight had both Kaposi's sarcoma and *P. carinii* pneumonia, one had disseminated cytomegalovirus infection, and one had central nervous system toxoplasmosis. Thirty-six of these men were white (not Hispanic), three were Hispanic (two originally from Puerto Rico and one originally from Mexico), and one was black. Their median age was 36 years.

These 40 patients were compared with the 208 other homosexual male patients with AIDS who were reported to the Centers for Disease Control as of April 12, 1982, but not named as sexual partners of patients included in the cluster. The 40 linked patients (16.1 percent of the total reported) were significantly more likely to be white and to have only Kaposi's sarcoma than the 208 other patients. However, the two groups were not significantly different with respect to all other variables available from surveillance reports.

The 29 patients who were linked and interviewed (72.5 percent of 40 patients) and the 49 nonlinked patients who were interviewed (23.6 percent of 208 patients) were compared with respect to selected behavioral characteristics. The 29 linked patients were significantly more likely than the 49 nonlinked patients to have met sexual partners in bathhouses, have been frequent users of inhaled amyl or butyl nitrite, and have participated in the sexual practice of "fisting" (manual-rectal intercourse). Patients in both groups tended to have large numbers of sexual partners. Use of recreational drugs other than nitrite inhalants and participation in sexual activities other than "fisting" were not significantly different for the two groups.

To estimate a possible latency period for AIDS among members of the cluster, we looked at the 20 patients who apparently had had sexual exposures with only one other reported patient. Nine of these 20 reported having had sexual relations with their partners for a period lasting no longer than 30 days. Of the nine, three showed symptoms before or at about the same time as their partners, and six noted symptoms after their partners became ill. In these six patients, symptoms were first noticed a mean of 10.5 months (range 7 — 14 months) after having had sexual contact with one of four partners who also was a reported patient.

The four partners may have been sources of AIDS. Three of the possible sources of AIDS were asymptomatic at the time of sexual exposure. The fourth possible source was Patient 0. Lymphadenopathy had already developed in Patient 0 when he had sexual contact with two men in whom AIDS subsequently developed, and he had skin lesions of Kaposi's sarcoma at the time of sexual contact with a third.

Although the cause of AIDS is unknown, it may be caused by an infectious agent that is transmissible from person to person in a manner analogous to hepatitis B virus infection: through sexual contact; through parenteral exposure by intravenous drug abusers who share needles; through blood products, particularly in patients with hemophilia who received clotting factor concentrates; and, perhaps, through mothers who are Haitian or intravenous drug users to their infants. The existence of a cluster of AIDS cases linked by homosexual contact is consistent with an infectious-agent hypothesis.

The cluster may represent a group of homosexual men who were brought together by a common interest in sexual relations with many different partners or in specific sexual practices, such as manual-rectal intercourse. Frequent social contacts among some patients enabled them to identify other patients by name. Although these men were sexual partners of each other, nonsexual activities, such as drug use, may have contributed to the development of AIDS.

If the infectious-agent hypothesis is true, Patient 0 may be an example of a "carrier" of such an agent. He had had sexual contact with eight other AIDS patients and was the possible source of AIDS for at least three of them. Two of these three men had been his partners before he had overt signs of Kaposi's sarcoma. The existence of an asymptomatic carrier state of AIDS has been suggested by a report of AIDS-like illness in an infant who had received a platelet transfusion from a man who had no symptoms when he donated blood, but had AIDS eight months later. Furthermore, abnormalities in T-lymphocytes have been described among asymptomatic homosexual men in New York City and among persons with hemophilia. Whether these immune abnormalities are a reflection of "asymptomatic AIDS" or are unrelated to AIDS is not yet known.

The estimated mean latency period of 10 to 11 months for the six AIDS patients described in this study is similar to the estimated mean latency period for the development of Kaposi's sarcoma among renal transplant recipients. Kaposi's sarcoma developed in 15 renal allograft transplant recipients an average of 15 months following renal transplantation in one study, and 20 Kaposi's sarcoma patients showed signs of Kaposi's sarcoma an average of 16 months after transplantation in another.

The observation of a cluster formed on the basis of reported sexual exposures reinforces case-control study findings regarding the importance of sexual activities in the development of AIDS among homosexual men. Sexual partners of AIDS patients appear to be at increased risk for AIDS. This conclusion is reflected in interim Public Health Service recommendations for the prevention of AIDS: "Sexual contact should be avoided with person known or suspected to have AIDS. Members of high-risk groups should be aware that multiple sexual partners increase the probability of developing AIDS".

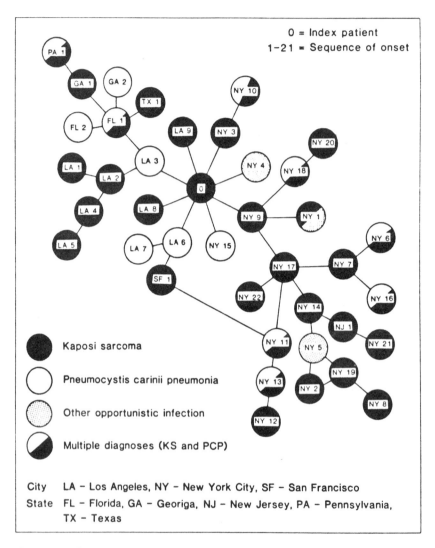

Figure 1. Sexual contacts among homosexual men with AIDS. Each **circle** represents an AIDS patient. **Lines** connecting the circles represent sexual exposures. Indicated city **or** state is place of residence of a patient at the time of diagnosis. "0" indicates Patient 0 (described in text).

IV. Stopping AIDS

The Editors

No one who is not infected with HIV today need become HIV positive tonight. Enough is known about transmission to devise ways of stopping the spread of AIDS.

Accidental infection even among health workers, is extraordinarily rare. We can be certain that casual contacts are not spreading AIDS, because of the 40,000 cases now reported in the USA, there are no old people, or 8 year old children or 30 year old virgins that are going down with AIDS without apparent cause.

AIDS is spread, and will continue to be spread unless society takes appropriate action, by blood, needles and sex. The blood transfusion service, at least in developed countries, is now adequately protected by the routine screening of every unit of blood.

Intravenous drug abusers must kick their habit or at least stop sharing dirty needles. IV drug users are also infecting their sex partners and therefore any children they may have are at risk. A greatly expanded effort is needed, especially in the USA that addresses the difficult task of treating drug addicts. In Holland, and several other countries, addicts are permitted to exchange old needles for sterile new ones at pharmacies.

There are probably other factors influencing transmission that are as yet poorly understood. There are proven cases where individuals have become infected with HIV after a single act of intercourse and others where an infected individual's sexual partner has remained free of the disease after a thousand or more unprotected intercourses.

All types of sexual activity can transmit the infection but some activities are more dangerous than others. Anal intercourse is more dangerous than vaginal intercourse and vaginal intercourse is more dangerous than oral/genital sex.

The risk of transmission can be reduced by using condoms and/or spermicides although like most things in medicine, these measures are not going to give one hundred percent protection against infection. Using condoms or spermicides when an individual may be at risk of HIV infection is rather like wearing a seat belt — if you are a bad driver a seat belt won't guarantee you won't kill yourself but it makes it less likely. Paradoxically, any use of so-called safe sex practices is enormously beneficial to society as it greatly slows the spread of disease, even though it may not give the individual complete protection.

If people are going to change their sexual behavior and adopt the use of barrier methods of contraception more widely, then they must receive clear information in a vocabulary they understand from informants they trust. In the long term, millions of lives depend upon the realism with which messages are transmitted. Sex education in school, beginning in the years before most individuals are sexually active, is essential.

Most people in society accept that such steps have to be taken, but a minority give a greatly inflated value to the marginal costs of distributing free needles for drug addicts or condoms to teenagers. In fact, all the data suggest that it is not the availability or the non-availability of needles or condoms which encourages the risky behavior, but a much broader set of factors that are more deeply rooted in our modern society. The lack of school discipline, the absence of chaperonage, the mobility of young people, particularly in the United States where the adolescents drive cars at the age of 16, together with important historical causes that have lowered the age of puberty, all contribute to the current problem of teenage sexuality. IV drug abuse is concentrated, although by no means exclusively limited to, inner city minority groups who live in harsh conditions with few employment opportunities.

A case might be made that in certain areas all pregnant women should be tested and advised of their status so they can make an informed choice about continuing the pregnancy so these women can make appropriate plans. The US military has begun compulsory testing of all service personnel and recruits. Prison populations may be protected if tests are performed. However, beyond these groups there is a strong consensus among public health workers that mandatory testing would be counterproductive. The more strongly an individual believes that AIDS is a self-inflicted disease, concentrated in deviant minorities, the more likely that individual is to call for mandatory testing. However, just as the US has no way of closing its borders to illegal immigrants, so it would have no way of ensuring universal testing, even if it were technically feasible. Moreover, those most likely to have the disease would also be those who would be most likely to avoid compulsory testing. There would be trade in forged certificates. Even if a more focused testing were performed, for example at the time of marriage, then at the present time it would only pick up one-tenth of one percent of all those with HIV infection and there would be 25 false-positives for every case that was detected.

At first sight testing might appear to protect health workers from accidental HIV transmission, but in realtiy, care has to be universally exercised: knowing some people were positive might encourage the careless to drop their guard against those they *thought* were negative — and might be newly infected, or have, in some way, escaped testing.

The public health community is virtually unanimous that testing is important but that it must be voluntary, confidential and linked with responsible patterns of counseling.

Now is the Time to Prevent AIDS

Editorial in *The American Journal of Public Health*
February, 1987

D
rug abuse and acquired immunodeficiency syndrome are two of the most critical public health problems receiving justified public attention in the United States. What actions should public health officials, educators, community organizers, clinicians, and others take to control and ultimately prevent these problems? Delineating effective, understandable, and appropriate actions and messages will be difficult, and delivering them may be even more so, but the severity of the problems justify even partially successful efforts.

The cumulative number of cases of AIDS is expected to increase from 27,000 in 1986 to 270,000 by the end of 1991. These cases will be largely unpreventable because, barring progress in therapy, they will occur primarily in individuals already infected with HIV. Public health actions must be taken to prevent HIV infections and AIDS during the next decade.

Public health professionals should not be deterred by the need for long-term efforts and long-range benefits. Changes and improvements in managing other major health problems include: the decline in cigarette smoking among adults, the increase in positive health behaviors related to several coronary artery disease risk factors, the changing perception of drunk driving as a public health problem, etc. Many changes took decades to develop. For example, the Surgeon General's first report on smoking was issued in 1964. Very basic behaviors, such as dietary habits, or smoking, may be easier to alter than those that place an individual at risk for infection with HIV: sexual behavior and drug use. Major public health problems related to these behaviors trouble our society deeply including: unintended pregnancy; sexually transmitted disease; and drug addiction. It may be tougher to convince people to use condoms than to quit smoking cigarettes.

For the prevention of sexually transmitted HIV infection, there appears to be a receptive audience and means to reach it relatively easily. This cannot be said about intravenous drug abusers not enrolled in treatment programs or incarcerated.

Their typical social isolation, criminal status, and lack of education compound to work against their access to positive health information. Nonetheless, controlling HIV infection in IV drug abusers serves not only their own interest but also that of the non-IV drug abusing heterosexual population.

IV drug abusers constitute by far the largest HIV-infected heterosexual population in the United States. HIV is clearly transmitted through heterosexual contact. So far, the epidemic in heterosexual IV drug abusers has been concentrated geographically in metropolitan New York and northern New Jersey. Predictably, the majority of children with AIDS have had drug abusing parents. The epidemiology points out the initial target populations, and the Surgeon General has recently issued a new report that outlines the message. IV drug abusers in the rest of the nation may not have HIV infection rates as high as those in the Northeast, but the potential for further spread is obvious. The need for accurate, quantitative information on drug abusers, their behaviors, and risk factors is acute and chronic. Public health authorities at all levels — international, federal, state, and local — should support efforts to obtain systematically gathered and scientifically analyzed information on drug abuse and drug abusers.

Action cannot await additional data. We must wrestle with this problem now if we are to have any hope of overcoming it. Suggestions of how to do this include:

1. Enlisting reformed drug abusers as peer counselors or community educators.

2. Expanding drug-abuse treatment clinics both in size (number of "treatment slots") and scope.

3. Reducing risk by instructing abusers on needle decontamination techniques or, as the Dutch have done and the Scots proposed, making clean equipment available to abusers who cannot be dissuaded from injection.

This last suggested means must be considered carefully and undertaken only as part of a "needle exchange" program, otherwise the net effect may be simply to increase the number of infected needles in the community.

Voluntary HIV-antibody testing and prevention-oriented counseling should be offered to all IV drug abusers and their sexual partners. Female IV drug abusers and female sex partners of males at risk for HIV infection should be offered family planning services in addition to the other prevention services. Education of all children should begin in the schools as soon as good lesson plans can be developed.

AIDS will be with us for years, unfortunately. How soon we take definitive action may well influence the course of this public health problem for many decades to come. Our actions should be balanced between those steps that will provide us with future guidance and those that by current consensus will benefit our communities. We cannot wait any longer.

* * * * * * * * * *

As of June 30, 1985, there were 15,254 cases of AIDS in the United States.

a. Diagnostics

New Questions About AIDS Test Accuracy

Deborah M. Barnes
Reprinted with permission from *Science, Vol. 238; 884-85*
November 13, 1987

According to recent testimony before a House subcommittee, blood tests for AIDS among low-risk individuals are even less accurate than critics have previously feared. In particular, an inexperienced laboratory's ability to do the Western blot assay — held by many to be the gold standard confirmatory test for having antibodies against the AIDS virus — is now under attack. At this point, however, it is difficult to evaluate the true extent of the problem because no one knows precisely how many blood tests for AIDS are being performed by highly qualified versus substandard laboratories.

Nevertheless, two striking findings emerge from the hearing. First, the Western blot test, at least in the wrong hands, is not as reliable as many have assumed. And second, laboratory proficiency in performing AIDS antibody tests, especially the technically difficult Western blot, is highly variable and sometimes completely unacceptable. At present, these problems are compounded by the lack of quality control and differing standards for interpreting test results. An added concern is that the problem of false test results may worsen as a growing number of inexperienced laboratories enter the for-profit AIDS testing market.

Whether or not these issues will have any impact on President Reagan's proposal for states to do routine testing of marriage license applicants, patients entering hospitals, and prisoners is still unclear. But politicians opposed to the notion of federally mandated testing can use the "accuracy-in-testing" issue as ammunition.

The accuracy of AIDS testing was explored at a hearing last month by the subcommittee on regulation and business opportunities of the House Committee on Small Business chaired by Representative Ron Wyden (D-OR). "I think we are going to need more testing," said Wyden in an interview with *Science*. "I am not anti testing. But to me the prerequisite is to increase the accuracy of testing." Wyden also stated that he would support legislation now being drafted by Representative Henry Waxman (D-CA) that calls for increased federal funds for voluntary testing and counseling, as well as protection of confidentiality and nondiscrimination of people who test positive.

Most blood tests for AIDS measure antibodies against human immunodeficiency virus (HIV), the virus that causes the fatal disease. At present no method exists for measuring the virus directly. The first in a series of blood tests is an ELISA, or enzyme-linked immunosorbent assay, which measures total antibodies against HIV. If a first and second ELISA are positive, then typically the blood is tested by Western blot, which is designed to confirm or deny the presence of antibodies against specific viral proteins.

Under ideal laboratory conditions both the ELISA and Western blot are capable of achieving greater than 99 percent sensitivity and specificity, which means that the tests correctly identify blood samples with and without antibodies more than 99 percent of the time. But studies indicate that in many laboratories, these tests are not performed under ideal conditions. Neither the exact number of laboratories performing inaccurate tests nor the number of inaccurate tests in known.

Lawrence Miike of the congressional Office of Technology Assessment (OTA) presented the most alarming analysis of the current state of AIDS testing. He estimates that among people at very low risk for AIDS, nine out of ten who test positive would not really be infected with the virus, a so-called false-positive result. But Miike himself has not actually measured the false-positive rate. Instead, he used published data on the prevalence of HIV infection in various populations and projected a series of test error rates based on laboratory proficiency data compiled by the College of American Pathologists and the American Association of Blood Banks.

The pathologists' College monitors the performance of most major laboratories in the United States, approximately 800 of which voluntarily participated in their recent evaluation of HIV testing. Miike's estimate of the false-positive rate is significantly higher than previous reports have indicated, perhaps because it is based on actual laboratory performance data rather than on estimates that assume ideal laboratory performance. Miike calculates that in a population at high risk for AIDS — with 10,000 of 100,000 (10 percent) persons truly infected with the virus — 984 of the 10,000 (9.8 percent) would be missed if laboratories performed according to the College of American Pathologists' analysis.

But the perception of how inaccurate the tests are depends, to some extent, on how the numbers are calculated and presented. For example, the study cited by Miike assumes that in a low-risk population of blood donors from the Midwest, about 10 of 100,000 are infected with HIV, a prevalence of 0.01 percent. Miike estimates that one of these 10 people will be missed after both ELISA and Western blot screening, and that an additional 80 will be falsely identified as HIV-positive. Thus, 80 of 89 people identified as positive are false positives, an error rate of 90 percent. But another way to express the same data is to say that 80 people out of 100,000 will be falsely identified as positive, an error rate of only 0.08 percent.

Miike's method of presenting error rates leads Herbert Polesky, director of the Memorial Blood Center in Minneapolis, who also testified at the hearing, to protest the OTA's use of the College of American Pathologists' data. "I think people are overreacting to the data," he said in an interview. "The error rate for false positives is probably about 5 or 6 percent and in the worst case it is probably twice that." He emphasizes that blood tests to detect HIV — particularly the ELISA screen — were originally designed to keep the blood supply safe. In that context, errors in identifying a blood sample as positive when it is not are acceptable, as long as all of the truly infected blood is correctly identified. But when the same system is applied to test large numbers of people at low risk for AIDS, the false-positive rate becomes unacceptable.

This problem has led many to question whether it is possible to do widespread screening for HIV infection accurately. Donald Burke of the Walter Reed Army Institute of Research in Washington, D.C., told House members that it is not only possible, the Army has been doing it for two years. "I share the view that testing people in low-risk populations is more likely to yield false-positive results," said Burke in an interview. "But I am a strong advocate of testing in low-risk populations. It can be made to work. We made it work."

Since October 1985, the Army has screened more than 1.4 million civilian applicants for military service and 800,000 personnel in training and on active duty. Overall, the prevalence rate for HIV infection is about 1.5 percent (1.5 people in 1000 tested), and the false-positive rate is extremely low. Burke testified that the Army analyzed a low-risk population similar to the one described by Miike and identified 15 of 135,000 people as positive for HIV antibodies. Further tests showed that one of them was not truly infected, a false-positive rate for the Army of 1 in 135,000 or 0.001 percent. (However, if Burke analyzed the same data by Miike's method, 1 of 15 or 6.7 percent would be expressed as false positives.) Burke cites the Army's rigorous control and regular checks over the laboratory that processes its samples as important factors in the accuracy of their tests.

Despite this record of accurate HIV screening, Burke also testified that many laboratories have performed too poorly to be considered for the military contract to analyze blood samples. Over the past two years a total of 19 different laboratories have applied for the contract to test Army applicants and personnel for HIV. Ten of the 19 (59 percent) on at least one occasion could not analyze test samples to a level of 95 percent accuracy and were therefore rejected.

Miike says that the problem with Western blot inaccuracy is twofold. First, the number of commercial laboratories doing the Western blot testing is increasing rapidly so that a greater percentage are inexperienced. In 1985, for example, only 18 laboratories did Western blot testing; today about 70 perform the tests. A second problem is identifying the criteria that indicate a test is positive. Until recently, some laboratories considered that having antibodies to one protein from the AIDS virus, either p24 or gp41, meant that a tests should be considered positive. Now, most laboratories require that a combination of antibodies to two or three different viral proteins must be present to constitute a positive test.

What it all amounts to, says Burke, is that no one is willing to accept responsibility for overseeing the quality of tests for HIV. "Right now there is no attention paid at a federal level that testing should be done as well as possible." The Food and Drug Administration (FDA) only reviews products (as opposed to laboratory procedures) that are identified in applications for licenses. The Centers for Disease Control does not monitor the accuracy of laboratory procedures, either. In short, no federal oversight is currently in practice.

As things now stand, FDA has approved only one Western blot test kit or product, which is made by Du Pont. The kit is so expensive — it costs about $45 to assay a blood specimen compared to the Army's carefully monitored $4 procedure — that very few commercial laboratories are using it.

Most of the witnesses at the recent hearing recommended that HIV testing accuracy should be improved and subjected to stiff quality-control measures before widespread testing — voluntary or routine — occurs.

b. Treatment
The Efficacy of Azidothymidine (AZT) in the Treatment of Patients with AIDS and AIDS-Related Complex A Double-Blind, Placebo-Controlled Trial

Margaret A. Fischl, Douglas D. Richman, Michael
Greico, Michael S. Gottlieb, Paul A. Volberding,
John M. Leedom, Jerome E. Groopman, Donna Mildvan,
Robert T. Schooley, George G. Jackson, David T. Durack,
Dannie King, Oscar L. Laskin and the AZT Collaborative
Working Group

Reprinted with permission from the *New England
Journal of Medicine, Vol. 317; 185-91,*
Copyright 1987 Massachusetts Medical Society
July 23, 1987

The acquired immunodeficiency syndrome (AIDS) is character-ized by severe immunodeficiency, life-threatening opportunis-tic infections, neoplasia, and a fatal outcome. The underlying immune defect in AIDS is caused by infection with a human retrovirus — human immunodeficiency virus (HIV). In addition, infection with this virus frequently causes a debilitating condition known as the AIDS-related complex. Strategies for the treatment of patients with AIDS or AIDS-related complex have focused on the development of drugs with activity against HIV *in vitro* and on agents that may restore immunity.

Azidothymidine (3'-azido-3'-deoxythymidine; zidovudine [Re-trovir], or AZT) is a thymidine analogue that inhibits HIV replication *in vitro.* AZT is phosphorylated by cellular enzymes and, as 5'-triphosphate, inhibits reverse transcriptase and terminates viral DNA-chain elongation. In Phase I studies, AZT was found to be well tolerated over a six-week period. In addition, some subjects had clinical and immunologic improvement characterized by an increase in the number of T helper cells, development of delayed hypertensivity reactions, and weight gain. On the basis of these findings, a multicenter, double-blind, placebo-controlled trial was initiated to evaluate the safety and efficacy of AZT in the treatment of a well-defined group of subjects with AIDS or AIDS-related complex. Before the study began, an independent board was established to review the study data for unacceptable toxicity or unequivocal benefit. The study was terminated prematurely because there was a significant difference in mortality between the AZT and placebo recipients. This report presents the clinical and laboratory data, which demonstrate the efficacy of AZT in this study population.

Patient Population — The study population consisted of two groups of subjects — patients with AIDS and patients with AIDS-related complex. Those with AIDS were eligible for the study if they had had a first episode of *Pneumocystis carinii* pneumonia histologically confirmed within the preceding 120 days. They were excluded if they had had multiple episodes of *P. carinii* pneumonia or any other opportunistic infection or any neoplasm. Patients with AIDS-related complex were eligible if they had either unexplained weight loss (defined as more than 6.8 kg or a 10 percent loss of total body weight within the 90 days before enrollment) or documented oral candidiasis and at least one of the following signs and symptoms: unexplained fever, extrainguinal lymphadenopathy, oral hairy leukoplakia, unexplained night sweats, herpes zoster, or unexplained diarrhea. The criteria for eligibility also included a hemoglobin level of 9.5 g per deciliter or more, a total granulocyte count of 1000 per cubic millimeter or more, a platelet count of 75,000 per cubic millimeter or more, a serum aspartate aminotransferase level of less than three times the upper limit of normal, a serum creatinine level of less than 2.0 mg per deciliter (180 umol per liter), an absolute number of cells of the CD4 surface phenotype of less than 500 per cubic millimeter, skin-test anergy, serum positive for antibody to HIV, and no recent history of therapy with antiretrovial agents, immunomodulators, or systemic antimicrobials. Subjects were asked not to take any medications without consulting the investigator. Short-term (<72 hours) use of aspirin or acetominophen was allowed for analgesia or fever. Specific licensed drugs were also permitted after the investigator consulted with the sponsor (Burroughs Wellcome Co.). Antimicrobial prophylaxis for the prevention of opportunistic infections was not allowed.

Study participants were recruited from 12 medical centers throughout the United States. The study was approved by institutional review boards at each participating center, and all subjects gave written informed consent.

Evaluation of Subjects — Clinical and laboratory evaluations included a medical history, a physical examination, neuropsychiatric assessment, and the following laboratory studies: measurement of hemoglobin, hematocrit, mean corpuscular volume, white-cell count, differential white-cell count, platelet count, reticulocyte count, erythrocyte sedimentation rate, serum electrolytes, serum glucose, blood urea nitrogen, serum creatinine, bilirubin, serum aspartate aminotransferase, alkaline phosphatase, vitamin B-12 , and folate, and serologic tests for hepatitis B, cytomegalovirus, and Epstein-Barr virus. Immunologic assessment included T-lymphocyte phenotyping by direct immunofluorescence with monoclonal antibodies of two-color flow cytometry on either whole-blood or Ficoll-Hypaque-separated mononuclear cells, quantitative immunoglobulin determination, and measurement of delayed cutaneous hypertensivity reactions (defined as >10 mm of induration) to four antigens (trichophyton, tetanus toxoid, candida, and purified protein derivative). Blood was also collected for pharmocokinetic studies, for detection of anti-HIV antibody by enzyme-linked immunosorbent assay, for measurement of serum p24 antigen levels, and for isolation of HIV from peripheral-blood lymphocytes. All subjects were evaluated twice before enrollment, weekly for the first eight weeks of the study, and biweekly thereafter. Neuropsychiatric assessments were repeated bimonthly, and immunologic and virologic studies were repeated monthly. Patients who were withdrawn from the study were followed periodically for any opportunistic infections or neoplasms and for survival.

Criteria for Response — The effects of study treatment on the clinical condition, immune function, and viral replication were monitored. Clinical end points used to assess the efficacy of AZT included survival, occurrence and frequency of opportunistic infections, occurrence of AIDS-associated neoplasms, Karnofsky performance status, body weight, and the number and severity of symptoms.

Treatment Regimen — The study was designed as a double-blind, randomized, placebo-controlled trial intended to last 24 weeks. Subjects were stratified into two groups according to the absolute number of peripheral-blood T cells with CD4 surface markers; one group consisted of subjects with 100 or fewer CD4 cells per cubic millimeter, and the other group had 101 to 499 cells per cubic millimeter. A computer-generated code for each center was used for randomly assigning subjects in each group to receive either AZT or placebo. A capsule consisting of 250 mg of AZT or placebo was administered orally every 4 hours throughout the 24-hour day. The placebo was indistinguishable in appearance from AZT and was similar in taste. Drug therapy was temporarily discontinued or the frequency of doses decreased to one capsule every eight hours or longer if severe adverse reactions were noted. The study medication was withdrawn if unacceptable toxic effects or a neoplasm requiring therapy developed. Subjects in whom an opportunistic infection developed were withdrawn from the study only if therapy with another experimental medication was required or if antimicrobial therapy might have resulted in serious additive toxic effects.

Statistical Analysis — Data were analyzed with the Statistical Analysis System (SAS). Stratified Wilcoxon's rank-sum tests were used to analyze comparability at base line, number of symptoms, Karnofsky performance status, weight, number of CD4 cells, and clinical data. The Mantel-Haenszel method for ordered ontingency tables with standardized midranks as scores implemented in procedure FREQ of SAS was used in analyses of dose reductions, severity of opportunistic infections, skin-test conversions, blood transfusions, and adverse reactions. Techniques for analyzing survival data were used in analyses of mortality, opportunistic infections, and Kaposi's sarcoma. The Cox regression analysis as implemented by SAS procedure COXREG was used. If there were too few treatment failures to permit the use of this method, an accelerated failure-time model was fitted with LIFETEST procedure of SAS. All P values were two-tailed.

Data were analyzed according to treatment group, diagnosis at entry into the study, and number of CD4 cells before treatment.

RESULTS — Two hundred eight-two subjects were enrolled in the study between February and June 1986. All but 13 participants were men. One hundred sixty had AIDS, and 122 had AIDS-related complex. One hundred forty-five subjects were assigned to AZT (85 had AIDS and 60 had AIDS-related complex), and 137 to placebo (75 had

AIDS and 62 had AIDS-related complex). The subjects in both treatment groups were comparable in age, body weight, Karnofsky performance score, number of symptoms, and mean number of CD4 cells
at entry (by Wilcoxon's rank-sum test). The only significantly different pretreatment variable was the number of days since the diagnosis
of *P. carinii* pneumonia in subjects with aids (77.5 days in the AZT
group vs. 86.6 days in the placebo group, P<0.04). This difference
was not considered relevant since neither mortality nor the development of an opportunistic infection during the study correlated with
the number of days since the diagnosis of pneumonia.

One hundred ninety-four subjects were still participating in the
study when it was terminated in September 1986. Twenty-seven
subjects had completed 24 weeks of the study, 152 had completed 16
weeks, and the remainder had completed at least 8 weeks. The mean
and median durations of participation were 120 and 127 days, respectively, in the AZT group, as compared with 116 and 120 days in the
placebo group. Sixty-one subjects (21 in the AZT group and 40 in the
placebo group) were withdrawn from the study before its termination. The main reasons for withdrawal were for occurrence of opportunistic infections (29 subjects), progressive Kaposi's sarcoma (1),
general debilitation (7), adverse reactions (5), the patient's request
(15), or noncompliance (4).

Survival — Nineteen subjects in the placebo group and 1 in the AZT
group died during the study (P<0.001 by the Cox regression model).
The immediate causes of death in placebo recipients were *P. carinii*
pneumonia (8 subjects), disseminated *Mycobacterium avium-com-
plex* infection (4), cryptococcosis (2), cerebral toxoplasmosis (2),
disseminated cytomegalovirus infection (1), B-cell lymphoma (1),
and severe debilitation with wasting (1). The immediate cause of
death in one subject receiving AZT was disseminated cryptococcosis.
Of the 20 subjects who died, 11 (10 placebo recipients and 1 AZT
recipient) had stopped taking the study medication 8 to 111 days
before death.

The probability of survival for 24 weeks among the subjects in the
AZT group was 0.98, as compared with 0.78 in the placebo group
(P<0.001). This increased likelihood of survival was comparable in
both the subjects with AIDS and those with AIDS-related complex
who received AZT. Two placebo-treated subjects with AIDS-related
complex died with opportunistic infections during the first three
weeks of the study. When these two subjects were excluded from
analysis, the probability of 24-week survival among subjects with
AIDS remained unchanged. The probability of 24-week survival

among subjects with AIDS-related complex was 1.00 in the AZT group, as compared with 0.83 in the placebo group (P<0.05).

A statistically significant decrease in mortality among recipients of AZT was found both for subjects with a CD4 cell count of 100 or fewer cells per cubic millimeter (P<0.001) and for those with a CD4 cell count above 100 (P=0.028). Similarly, the probability of 24-week survival was also significantly different in AZT and placebo recipients when subjects were grouped according to the pretreatment number of CD4 cells.

Opportunistic Infections and Kaposi's SArcoma — For the purpose of this study, opportunistic infections were considered to be those that met the Centers for Disease Control criteria for the diagnosis of AIDS. Twenty-four subjects in the AZT group and 45 in the placebo group contracted such infections during the study. One subject in the AZT group and five in the placebo group had more than one opportunistic infection. Opportunistic infections occurred throughout the study; however, no significant difference in the frequency of infection in the AZT and placebo groups was noted until after six weeks of therapy. (See Fig. 1 at end of this Chapter.) Furthermore, no opportunistic infection occurred in subjects with AIDS-related complex after six weeks of AZT administration, whereas 12 episodes occurred in subjects with AIDS-related complex after six weeks of placebo administration (Fig. 1).

The probability that an opportunistic infection would develop during the 24-week study was significantly lower in the AZT group than in the placebo group. Similarly, the probability of an opportunistic infection was also significantly different in AZT and placebo recipients when subjects were grouped according to diagnosis before entry (AIDS or AIDS-related complex).

The types of opportunistic infection noted during the study did not differ significantly between the AZT and placebo groups. The most common infection was *P. carinii* pneumonia, which accounted for more than 50 percent of all opportunistic infections.

Kaposi's sarcoma developed in 16 subjects during the course of the study. Ten cases occurred in the placebo group (seven patients with AIDS and three with AIDS-related complex), and six in the AZT group (three patients with AIDS and three with AIDS-related complex; P>0.20).

Clinical Status — The mean pretreatment Karnofsky performance scores in the AZT and placebo recipients were the same — 90. A significant difference between the groups in the change from baseline performance score was noted as early as 4 weeks of therapy (mean change from base-line score: AZT recipients, -0.3; placebo recipients, -2.2; P<0.05) and became more evident during the first 12 weeks (AZT recipients, ˇ1.3; placebo recipients, -5.2; P<0.001). This difference was related mainly to progressive deterioration of the condition of the placebo recipients. By week 16, however, there was no significant difference between the performance scores of the two groups (P>0.05). Similar differences between the AZT and placebo groups were noted when subjects were grouped according to pre-entry diagnosis (AIDS or AIDS-related complex).

No significant difference in performance score was noted between AZT and placebo recipients with more than 100 CD4 cells per cubic millimeter before treatment (P>0.2). However, statistically significant differences in performance score between AZT and placebo recipients with fewer than 100 cells per cubic millimeter before treatment were noted during most of the study (at week 4, P=0.01; week 8, P<0.001; week 12 P<0.0001; week 16, P=0.002; week 20, P<0.05; and week 24, P<0.2).

The mean body weights of AZT and placebo recipients at enrollment were comparable (AZT group, 68.9 kg; placebo group, 68.4 kg). Overall, subjects given AZT gained weight during the study, whereas subjects given the placebo lost weight. Significant differences between the groups were observed as early as week 4 (mean change in body weight: AZT recipients, ˇ0.5 kg; placebo recipients, -0.1 kg; P<0.05). Weight differences became more evident during the first 16 weeks of the study (mean change in body weight: AZT recipients, ˇ2.0 kg; placebo recipients -1.3 kg; (<0.001) and less evident thereafter. Similar differences between AZT and placebo recipients were noted when subjects were grouped according to pre-entry diagnosis of AIDS or AIDS-related complex. Subjects with more than 100 CD4 cells per cubic millimeter before treatment had small differences in weight whether they belonged to the AZT or placebo group (P>0.4); among the subjects with 100 or fewer CD4 cells per cubic millimeter, those receiving AZT had the greatest and most persistent weight gain.

Immunologic Data — The number of CD4 cells was significantly increased in subjects receiving AZT as compared with those receiving placebo (P<0.001 by Wilcoxon's rank-sum analyses). In general, subjects receiving AZT had increases in the number of CD4 cells, as compared with those receiving placebo, in whom a decline in the number of CD4 cells was most frequently observed. The earliest difference in the number of CD4 cells was noted at week 4, and differences persisted throughout most of the study.

The increases in the number of CD4 cells in patients receiving AZT were also statistically significant when subjects were grouped according to pre-entry diagnosis. However, after 12 weeks of therapy, a gradual decline in the number of CD4 cells was noted in those with AIDS who were receiving AZT and who remained in the study; after 20 weeks, a return to base-line values occurred in many of these subjects. This decline in CD4 cells appeared to coincide with the development of neutropenia. In contrast, in subjects with AIDS-related complex who were receiving AZT and who remained in the study, increases in the number of CD4 cells persisted throughout most of the study. Although a decline in the number of CD4 cells was noted after 20 weeks of AZT therapy among subjects with AIDS-related complex and a pretreatment CD4 cell count below 100, the mean count did not decrease to pretreatment levels, as in many subjects with AIDS. It should be noted, however, that the number of subjects completing 24 weeks of the study was small, as reflected in the decreasing level of statistical significance for CD4 cell counts in the latter weeks of the study. Furthermore, subjects with progressive disease who were removed from the study were more likely to have low CD4 cell counts. This was, particularly apparent in the placebo group. For example, the sudden increase in the mean CD4 cell count at week 24 among subjects with AIDS-related complex who were receiving placebo was directly related to the loss of placebo-groups subjects with progressive disease, who were more likely to have low counts, rather than to a true increase in the mean number of CD4 cells.

Thirty-seven of 129 subjects (29 percent) in the AZT group acquired reactivity to at least one skin-test antigen, as compared with 11 of 117 (9 percent) in the placebo group (P<0.001). Similar results were observed when subjects were grouped according to their pretreatment diagnosis or pretreatment CD4 cell count (Table 5).

Virologic Data — HIV was isolated at entry in 57 percent of the AZT group and 58 percent of the placebo group. No statistically significant differences in isolation rates were noted between the two groups during the study. However, 17 of 33 AZT recipients tested had negative cultures at week 20, as compared with 5 of 19 placebo recipients (= 0.056). There were too few subjects at week 24 of the study to allow statistically valid conclusions about an antiviral effect.

Thirty-six AZT recipients and 40 placebo recipients were found to have detectable serum p24 antigen. Of these, 28 in each group had both a serum specimen obtained at entry and specimens obtained later in which changes in antigen level could be evaluated. Statistically significant decreases from the serum level of p24 antigen at entry were found among AZT recipients at weeks 4,8 and 12 (overall, $P<0.05$). Similar trends were also noted at weeks 16 and 20, but the numbers of subjects were small for statistical analysis.

Discussion — In this study, AZT decreased mortality and the frequency of opportunistic infections in a well-defined group of subjects with AIDS or AIDS-related complex during a period of up to six months. The most striking difference between AZT and placebo recipients was a significantly lower incidence of death. The causes of death in subjects receiving placebo were progressive AIDS-related disorders, demonstrating that the administration of AZT can forestall the progression of HIV-related complications for at least the duration of observation in this study. This effect was most apparent among subjects with AIDS who had recently recovered from their first episode of *P. carinii* pneumonia and subjects with AIDS-related complex who had 100 or fewer CD4 cells per cubic millimeter before treatment. Because the study was terminated early, more definitive results on subjects with AIDS-related complex who had more than 100 CD4 cells per cubic millimeter before treatment were not available. Further studies will be needed to determine whether AZT will similarly benefit patients with other opportunistic infections fulfilling the definition of AIDS, or patients with less severe manifestations of HIV infection. It is likely that patients with other AIDS-defining opportunistic infections or those with recurrent episodes of *P. carinii* pneumonia will be debilitated and will more frequently require antimicrobial or other medical therapy. Therefore, tolerance to AZT and the efficacy of the drug may well be different in these patients. In addition, HIV infection is a chronic and probably lifelong infection, and treatment will therefore have to be extended for longer periods. Since the present observations were made over only 24 weeks, the long-term benefits and toxic effects of AZT in this patient population still need to be defined.

Opportunistic infection did occur less frequently among subjects receiving AZT and is the most likely reason for the decreased death rate in this group. No significant difference in the types of opportunistic infections was noted between AZT and placebo recipients. The most common infection was *P. carinii* pneumonia, which accounted for more than half the opportunistic infections. Since antimicrobial prophylaxis for the prevention of *P. carinii* pneumonia, which accounted for more than half the opportunistic infections. Since antimicrobial prophylaxis for the prevention of *P. carinii* pneumonia was not allowed, it is possible that coadministration of AZT and appropriate antimicrobial agents might have further decreased the incidence of opportunistic infections. Although several drugs, including acyclovir, trimethoprim-sulfamethoxazole, aspirin, and acetaminophen, were administered during the study to AZT recipients for the treatment of opportunistic infections, pain, and fever, only acetaminophen was associated with increased toxicity. Because information about drug interactions with AZT is limited, caution must be used when administering any concomitant medications.

Although recurrent opportunistic infections were noted in subjects receiving AZT, the rate of death related to opportunistic infections was much lower in this group than in the placebo group. The decreased case fatality rate for opportunistic infection suggests that subjects receiving AZT had a better outcome because the drug enhanced their immune systems. The alternative explanation — that AZT exerted a direct antimicrobial effect — is unlikely, given the lack of *in vitro* activity against the pathogens isolated. These results clearly support continued use of AZT despite the occurrence of opportunistic infections.

After six weeks of AZT therapy, no opportunistic infection occurred in the subjects with AIDS-related complex. This low incidence was notably different from the incidence among the placebo recipients with AIDS-related complex who acquired opportunistic infections during the study. On the basis of these findings, it is likely that continuing therapy beyond the six-month study period could have increased the difference between the placebo and AZT groups, particularly among subjects with more than 100 CD4 cells before treatment. The finding that AZT delayed progression to AIDS and resulted in sustained increases in levels of CD4 cells in many patients with AIDS-related complex, suggests that AZT may be particularly beneficial to patients with less severe HIV infection. The relative ratio of benefit to toxicity during early chemotherapeutic intervention in patients with less severe HIV infection is important, and further studies in such patients are needed.

Several indications of general clinical improvement, including a higher Karnofsky performance status and body weight, were noted early in the study among AZT recipients. The toxicity of AZT and the subsequent reduction of dose may have resulted in the failure of treatment to sustain these positive benefits in some patients. The smaller differences between the AZT and placebo groups after 20 weeks of therapy may also have been partly artifactual. The number of subjects receiving study medication for 20 weeks or more was small.

In addition, Karnofsky performance status and body weight were not recorded for subjects who were hospitalized. Because hospitalization was more frequent among subjects receiving placebo, the difference between the two treatment groups was reduced by the resulting loss of data on placebo recipients who were hospitalized.

Subjects receiving AZT had improvement in at least two measures of immune function, which may have contributed to the clinical benefits noted. Statistical differences in both skin-test reactivity and the number of CD4 cells were noted as early as 4 weeks and persisted through 20 weeks of therapy. The absolute number of CD4 cells decreased after 20 weeks in many subjects with a diagnosis of AIDS before treatment, suggesting that the initial beneficial immunologic effects of AZT may not be sustained. The decline in the CD4 cell count was often associated with neutropenia and may have reflected a cumulative toxicity of AZT or a required reduction of dosage. Sustained increases in CD4 cells were more likely to occur in subjects with AIDS-related complex, among whom neutropenia was less frequent. Because varying does schedules of AZT may offer a greater benefit, the relative efficacy and toxicity of varying doses and dose schedules are being evaluated.

The reduction in circulating levels of viral p24 antigen in the AZT group but not the placebo group over the course of the study strongly suggests that the antiviral activity of AZT *in vivo* parallels its activity *in vitro*. The quantitative relation between the amount of circulating virus and p24 antigen, however, has not been established.

The lack of a measurable effect on virus isolation from peripheral-blood lymphocytes may have been due to the activation of latent virus in cells by the culture techniques or by the failure of AZT to inhibit all virus replication. Nevertheless, the ability to culture virus from any patients after several months of therapy indicates that such patients are still infectious and should be counseled to continue to follow appropriate practices to prevent the transmission of HIV.

The study demonstrates that an antiretroviral agent can benefit patients with HIV infection. Although the use of AZT is associated with toxicity, overall the drug decreased mortality rates and opportunistic infections in two groups of patients with advanced HIV infection; the risk:benefit ratio was therefore in favor of the patient. Further studies will be needed to define the optimal dose of AZT and to understand the full range of benefit in the various stages of HIV infection.

Addendum — At the termination of the trial in September 1986, all study participants receiving AZT or placebo were offered the opportunity to receive AZT in an open-label study. As of April 30, 1987, the mortality rate among the original 145 AZT recipients was 6.2 percent after 36 weeks of AZT therapy and 10.3 percent after 52 weeks. Among the original placebo recipients, including those who later received AZT for less than three weeks and thus were unlikely to derive benefit from it, the morality rate at 36 weeks after entry into the study was 39.3 percent. AZT administration was therefore associated with a fourfold-to-sixfold reduction in the mortality rates in the study population at nine months.

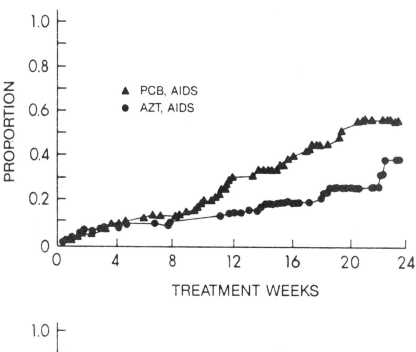

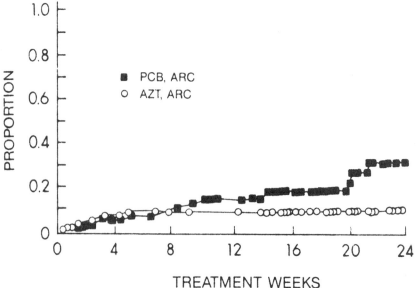

Figure 1. Proportion of Patients in Whom Opportunistic Infections Developed during the Study (Kaplan–Meier Product–Limit Method).

The upper panel shows infection among patients with AIDS who were receiving AZT or placebo (PCB), and the lower panel shows infection among those with AIDS-related complex (ARC).

AIDS Victims Grasp at Home Remedies and Rumors of Cures

Jane Gross
Reprinted with permission from *The New York Times*
May 15, 1987

Desperate AIDS patients are turning to home remedies, grasping at rumors of new treatments and worrying about how to raise money for the one drug that has proved effective against the deadly disease.

Like terminal cancer patients, these frightened men and women are casting about for cure or comfort, or at least for a measure of control.

And as time passes and the death toll mounts, they seem to grow angrier at the health-care establishment, more independent in their treatment decisions and more frantic in their search for something — anything — that might prolong life and reduce suffering.

"We're talking about thousands of exceedingly desperate people," said Dr. Michael Lange, an infectious diseases specialist at St. Lukes-Roosevelt Hospital Center. "They are poor souls who want to take something, to at least have the feeling they're trying."

When AIDS patients gather, the talk these days is of chemotherapy and antibiotics, of anti-viral drugs and immune system stimulants, of macrobiotic diets and meditation tapes.

To most laymen, AZT or AL-721 are mysterious acronyms, and aerosol Pentamidine and folic acid are part of the arcane language of medical books. But to the thousands of people suffering from acquired immune deficiency syndrome, they are commonplace, the diction of desperation.

"It used to be that people discussed their disease," said Lews Katoff, an AIDS patient and an official at the Gay Men's Health Crisis, a New York City AIDS services group. "Now, they discuss their treatment."

Typical is Tim Cooley, who said he "wasn't even a vitamin person" before his diagnosis. Now, Mr. Cooley carries a pill box in his pocket that emits a series of insistent beeps every four hours so he knows it is time to take AZT, folic acid and an antidepressant.

These are not the first pills and potions Mr. Cooley has tried, and he doubts they will be the last.

The only federally approved drug available to AIDS patients is azidothymidine, or AZT, which blocks the ability of the AIDS virus to multiply. Last month, the Burroughs Wellcome Company began selling the drug, under the name Retrovir, to 5,000 patients who had received it free in trials. They will pay about $10,000 a year, which poses little problem for the well-to-do, the well-insured or the indigent, but is likely to be a serious hardship for those who fall in between.

It is too early to tell how widespread that hardship will be, since many AZT patients have yet to exhaust their last month of free medication. Already, however, government officials, hospitals, physicians and pharmacists are devising innovative ways of paying for the precious blue-and-white capsules for those who do not have health insurance covering outpatient medication or who are not eligible for Medicaid.

In the New York area, pharmacists have so far been moderate in their markup policies. While Federal health officials say pharmacists often mark up the price of drugs by as much as 100 percent, they are charging around $230 for a vial of 100 AZT pills that cost $188 wholesale.

Many hospital pharmacies are charging $191, under the terms of a markup agreement with the wholesaler. A few Greenwich Village pharmacies are selling AZT at cost to anyone who states that he is needy, with no documented proof, and others are arranging weekly payment schedules.

"I don't feel I should take advantage of them," said Alvin Teichman of Arrow Pharmacy, on Ninth Avenue at 58th Street, near St. Luke's-Roosevelt and its heavy AIDS caseload.

Certain private hospitals, including St. Clare's Hospital and Health Center, on West 51st Street at Ninth Avenue, are raising money from benefactors to guarantee that no clinic patients are forced off the medication, which is matched in price only by a handful of drugs, such as interferon, cyclosporine and human growth hormone.

At the city's 11 municipal hospitals, no one seeking AZT is turned away, regardless of insurance status, as a result of an emergency $6.4 million budget allocation from City Hall.

"We bill, but there's no follow-up, no dunning letters," said Paul Moore, the director of the City Health and Hospitals Corporation's AIDS initiative. "You can't get blood from a stone."

On a national level, led by Representative Henry A. Waxman, a California Democrat, and Senator Lowell P. Weicker, a Connecticut Republican, there is a bill pending to set up an emergency fund of $30 million for distribution to needy AIDS patients. The measure, part of a larger appropriations bill, calls for individual states to set up formulas for dispensing the AZT aids.

Then, there are private strategies: A man in New York was sent AZT pills by a friend in California, who found he could not tolerate the drug's toxic side effects. A Manhattan internist bought Burroughs Wellcome stock, then set aside his dividends to help needy patients. Another doctor is similarly using money left to him in the wills of patients who died of AIDS.

For some AIDS patients, the problem solves itself when their resources are so depleted that they qualify for Medicaid, the public assistance program that in most states has agreed to cover the cost of AZT. "It's a humiliating procedure," said Dr. Lange of a process known as "spending down," in which a person exhausts his assets. "And it's morally wrong that people have to do that."

For many patients who take AZT, and many more who do not, other medications and preparations have gained popularity. Three of the most widely discussed at the moment are AL-721 or its analogues, derived from egg lecithin and believed by some to interfere with the AIDS virus: DNCB, a photographic chemical that its users think enhances the immune system when painted on the skin; and the aerosol form of Pentamidine, an antibiotic that prevents a sever form of pneumonia that is the leading cause of death among AIDS sufferers.

"The kinds of things we're doing would have seemed off the wall six months ago," said John Gamrecki, an official at the People with AIDS Coalition, a support and services group in New York. Mr. Gamrecki paints his ankles with DNCB and spreads egg lecithin on his morning toast, while complaining that it looks like "the hardened chicken fat you find on the casserole the next morning."

For the moment, inner-city drug abusers, who with homosexuals are at significant risk for AIDS, have neither the information nor the money to pursue such strategies. But among homosexuals, such information is a subject of obsessive interest for those who are sick or caring for others, and it sweeps through the community.

"ASK AROUND!" Michael Callen wrote in a new 145-page manual for newly diagnosed AIDS victims. "Network with other people with AIDS. The PWA grapevine is as reliable and speedy as any around."

A recent issue of Newsline, a newsletter published by the People With AIDS Coalition, was largely devoted to medical matters. It announced clinical trials of a new immune-system stimulant, reported on the distribution of an underground analogue of AL-721, compared AZT prices at various pharmacies and advertised the "guided visualization" tapes of Louise Hay, who conducts therapy weekends, and the yoga workshops of Swami Satchidananda.

Similarly, the bulletin board at the Gay Men's Health Crisis often carries pleas for drugs unavailable in this country, which are tacit testimonials. "Looking for ribavirin," said a typical index card. "I RAN OUT!!! If anyone knows where even a small supply might be available soon, please call Jeff."

With the knowledge gathered from the grapevine, people with AIDS alter the usual relationship between doctor and patient. "The educated person with AIDS knows more that the average physician," said Mr. Katoff. He added that his doctor "doesn't have a vote, he has an opinion" in treatment decisions.

In the manual, "Surviving and Thriving with AIDS," Mr. Callen personified the try-anything approach in a chronicle of his own experimental treatments:

"I've taken isoprinosine, been plasmapheresed (a form of blood cleansing where plasma and immune complexes are removed), taken naltrexone, been burned by DNCB, gotten transfusions of packed red cells, gotten gammaglobulin, taken Bactrum, dapsone and acyclovier (IV and oral) and whip up daily in my blender the poor man's AL-721 (lecithin, oil and juice). "See recipes on pages 57 and 58".

Among certain AIDS patients, such a regimen is considered a badge of courage. "People who don't do it are either intimidated or fatalistic," said Mr. Katoff, who takes AZT and aerosol Pentamidine. "I deal with problems actively and I view this thing as a challenge, a kind of adventure. Also, enough people have died to prove that doing nothing doesn't work."

Mr. Cooley says his "nibbling" at experimental treatments once seemed like a way to fend off death. "Now, I know I'm dying," he said. "It's not so much a question of fighting the disease, but of getting to that point in the most comfortable way."

But experimentation seems a luxury of the middle class at a time when the victims of AIDS increasingly are poor blacks and Hispanic people.

"Does an 18-year-old-black kid know egg lecithin from a hole in the ground?" said a homosexual man who was stuffing envelopes at the PWA Coalition one recent afternoon. "And if he knows, does he have $200 to pay for it?"

If a patient's condition improves, for whatever reason, the regimen of the moment seems a miracle cure. Mr. Katoff said he felt stronger within days of starting AZT treatment, able to jog five miles for the first time since he got sick, and less absent-minded.

"The thought of running out is terrifying," he said of the AZT. "It has a magical quality to it, whether you view it as black magic or white magic."

"At first, I tried to be unemotional about it," said Dr. Richard Hersey, a physician who stopped practicing medicine after learning he had AIDS and who also takes AZT. "But there's no question, if you're doing O.K. you start thinking it would be risky to be without it."

Some health-care experts worry that AIDS patients have become the latest prey for snakeoil salesmen who deplete their dwindling resources with empty promises.

But many of those facing what seems to be certain death take a different position. They argue that some drugs ease their suffering, that others add months to their lives and that the rest, however worthless, bolster their spirits. Over and over, like a refrain, these men quote from Dylan Thomas, promising themselves and anyone who will listen that they will not "go gentle into that good night."

"It would have been very hard a year ago to be in this situation and have a burning desire to live," Mr. Katoff said. "When there was nothing to try, there wasn't much choice but to go quietly. This way, at least, I have a feeling of control."

c. Prevention

Sex in the Age of AIDS Calls for Common Sense and "Condom Sense"

Marsha F. Goldsmith
Reprinted with permission from *JAMA*
May 1, 1987

Any Maypole erected today ought to be covered with a condom. That's the conclusion one might well reach after talking with physicians and others concerned with the expression of sexuality in 1987. Sheathing the ancient fertility symbol would negate its *raison d'etre*, but it would surely focus attention on the horrific truth that the male member now may convey the seeds of death as well as of life.

Getting people to recognize this fact and take the necessary steps to protect themselves and/or their partners from sexually transmitted diseases (STDs) — foremost among them acquired immunodeficiency syndrome — during coitus was the aim of a recent conference in Atlanta. The meeting was the first of its kind to be held in this country, according to its sponsors, the Centers for Disease Control (CDC), American Social Health Association, and Family Health International.

Participants in the conference, titled "Condoms in the Prevention of Sexually Transmitted Diseases," presented evidence of efficacy and arguments for use of a device that was first mentioned in Egyptian papyri, according to introductory speaker Michael Rosenberg, executive director of the American Social Health Association. Tracing its development means relying on much that is anecdotal, but the subject has been investigated seriously in Himes' *Medical History of Contraception*, and not so seriously in P. Sinclaire *Johnny Come Lately*.

Rosenberg says the first indisputable published reference to prophylactic use derives from the Italian anatomist Falloppio, who in the mid-16th century wrote about a linen sheath moistened with lotion for protection against venereal infection. Shortly afterward, 16th century French essayist Michel de Montaigne voiced a still-current complaint when he called such a sheath "armor against enjoyment, gossamer against infection."

The origin of the word condom is unknown, although one often-told story is that a (French or English) Dr. Condom gave his name to the penis cover he devised to curtail the proliferating bastard progeny of England's King Charles II. By the 18th century, such writers as Casanova and Boswell recorded their own use of condoms — usually made of the cecum of sheep or other animals — and although they were rather costly, they were used widely by the upper classes throughout Europe.

The vulcanization of rubber in the mid-19th century allowed condoms to be made of that material and brought their price within reach of many more people. Although occasional moralists inveighed against their use from the beginning and preached self-control as the only barrier to infection (they didn't even mention contraception), according to Rosenberg, the copulating populace embraced condoms so heartily that by the 1930s more than 300 million — by then mostly made of latex — were sold annually in the United States.

With the advent of other methods of contraception and of cures for venereal infection, interest in and use of condoms in this country declined drastically — until fear of AIDS influenced their recent much-publicized resurgence. Rosenberg said the actual production of condoms worldwide today is unknown, but manufacturing capacity is about 5 billion devices annually. In the early 1980s, about 5 million were manufactured annually in this country. Although the figure is undoubtedly higher now, no accurate data are available.

According to the most recent detailed survey, they are used most in Japan (among spouses of half of all married women of reproductive age) and least in Africa (less than 1 percent of spouses of such women). In the developed world overall, the rate of condom use was about 13 percent — which is also approximately the rate in this country. Frequency of use was not recorded.

Most condom manufacturing and importing countries have national standards for quality control. At Ansell, the largest US producer, for example, Bradley Pugh, vice president for research and development, oversees quality-control testing that includes stretching every condom produced over a metal form and passing high-voltage electricity through it. "If there are any holes," he explains, "it will burn right through." In addition, a random statistical sample of condoms in every batch made are filled with water, to see if they will leak. "Both electrons and water molecules are much smaller than HIV [which at 120 nm in diameter is a small-sized STD infectious agent, compared with the largest, *Neisseria gonorrhoeae* at 1000 nm, and with tiny hepatitis B surface antigen at 22 nm]," Pugh says, "and when they don't get through, we're sure the HIV can't get through." (Sperm, incidentally, are huge compared with STD agents; a single sperm is 3000 nm in diameter.)

Condom size and width standards vary slightly among different nations, Rosenberg says. Only two sizes are produced here, although conference speakers said there should probably be three or four to ensure good fit for penises of various configurations. The smaller size is promoted in this country as "offering a snugger fit for greater sensitivity." One company calls them "Huggers." In this regard, another conference speaker said that the promoters of condom use must take into account men's insecurities. "Perhaps," she suggested, "they could be marketed in sizes like olives: super, colossal, jumbo."

Styles, at any rate, vary greatly. They may be dry or lubricated, plain tip or reservoir end, straight or shaped, smooth or textured, and natural or brightly colored. Packaging appears to be important in attracting users and gaining market share, and the 50 or so brands sold by the five condom companies in the United States come wrapped in everything from discrete gold foil that makes them look like special after-dinner mints to glamorous erotic photos with coy copy to match.

All but about one percent of condoms made in the United States are of latex and sell for about $1.50 to $2.00 for a pack of three.

Increasingly, latex condoms are being offered for sale in this country in such places as university bookstores and dormitory and restroom vending machines, as well as by mail order. Many are distributed free by public or private clinics. Speakers in Atlanta said that while there have been laws against the public sale of condoms in parts of the United States, they were unaware of any legal restrictions against their sale here today. In Europe, they have long been readily available in such venues and at newspaper kiosks, tobacconists, and vending machines near pay telephones and bus stops.

In Great Britain, according to conference speaker Malcolm Potts, president of Family Health International, condoms are often purchased at barbershops. There, he says, after the customer has had his hair cut, the barber's murmured question, "Will there be anything else, sir?" is understood to mean "Do you wish to buy any condoms?" This civilized procedure allows shy persons, rather than making a perhaps difficult request, simply to murmur in return the number required and pocket a package of protection. The small number of natural-membrane condoms manufactured in the United States are made of lamb cecum imported from New Zealand. They are three or four times the price of latex condoms and, though often much preferred by the relatively few men who are familiar with them, may offer less protection against disease.

Attempting to appeal to the unprecedented variety and sophisticated demands of consumers now suddenly interested in their product, the four old-line US condom manufacturers have their research and development departments working to produce condoms that look, smell, taste, feel, and of course perform their prophylactic function better than these products ever have before.

Until the recent revival of interest, so slumbrous had the industry become that there was little (internal) technological innovation or (external) product assessment. The only reference in the literature that addresses the question of quality and cost of competing brands, and then only indirectly, is a preference survey published in *Consumer Reports* in October 1979. Conference speakers said it is inapplicable to the situation today, and agreed that an up-to-date evaluation of condoms from both the user's and the scientist's point of view is long overdue.

Some scientists have begun this process. Admonitions to employ condoms so as to enjoy "safer sex" are based on more than wistful wishing. They are based on several studies that have demonstrated the impermeability of condoms to STD agents. For example, Marcus Conant, professor of dermatology at the University of California at San Francisco, and colleagues have conducted studies that prove condoms to be effective barriers against the transmission of herpesvirus and human immunodeficiency virus.

Recently, Conant concluded a laboratory study of 12 varieties of latex and natural-membrane condoms as barriers against the transmission of herpesvirus 1 and 2, cytomegalovirus, and HIV. None of the viral agents passed through the latex, he said in an interview, while there was occasional leakage with he natural condoms. "This leads to the recommendation that people should use latex condoms for sexual intercourse with persons at high risk, such as homosexuals in San Francisco," he said. "Heterosexuals in the Midwest with few partners, on the other hand, might feel comfortable using the natural type."

Lest this option seem irresponsible, Conant emphasizes that risk factors are just that; people have to make a choice about their sexual behavior, and outside of a long-term monogamous couple — both of whom are know to be free of HIV — there is no such thing as completely safe sex anymore: "If one chooses to be sexually active with more than one partner, one tries to minimize the risk."

Concerning the "failure rate" of condoms used for contraception — 10 percent is an often-cited figure — Conant says flatly that a study has never been done. His clinical impression is that noncompliance with recommendations for proper use of condoms, rather than product failure, is responsible.

When the issue is pregnancy, people either forget to use a condom and then, when interviewed, "forget" that they forgot, or they indulge in extended foreplay before putting on a condom, or they remove it carelessly, or the condom breaks. When disease transmission is the issue, unprotected foreplay again may be at fault or the couple may engage in other intimacies, such as oral sex, without using a condom.

Although family planning experts say breakage is rare, there have been some reports in the literature concerning a high rate of condom tearing, particularly during anal intercourse. According to Mary Guinan, the CDCs acting assistant director for science, there are no established data on the breakage rate, nor on whether condoms made of thicker latex are less likely to tear than the superthin ones. A study that would address these issues is needed, she says.

According to Conant, who is also in private practice in an area that borders on Haight-Ashbury and the Castro district in San Francisco, "an even bigger issue is what happens when people fall in love." People who are extremely careful in their sexual behavior and use condoms when they are dating various members of a group will abandon all caution, and all barriers, he says, when they meet their "one true love, because how can you believe that this wonderful person can give you this terrible thing?" People have got to believe it, he says, and the strictures apply to heterosexuals as well as homosexuals.

Theresa Crenshaw of San Diego goes a step further. "For the sake of health, casual sex and multiple partners must be abandoned," she said in testimony presented to Congress this February at hearings on condom advertising. Admitting that "condoms in combination with spermicides are a valuable resource in our fight against AIDS," Crenshaw emphasizes the importance of behavior modification over resignation to the threat of AIDS and calls for avoidance of sexual activity with any partner outside of a "committed relationship." The message Crenshaw and her group stress is that "sexual behavior can change, but not unless we expect it and recommend it."

With technical work performed in the laboratory, Susanne Scesney made three determinations, as described in an interview: (1) latex condoms are impenetrable to HIV; (2) the spermicide nonoxynol 9, as proved earlier, kills HIV *in vitro*; and (3) when a condom containing nonoxynol 9 in the tip is torn, the spermicide kills the virus in two-thirds of all cases. Gantz said that why the virus survives in the other one-third of cases is unclear, but nonoxynol 9 is a sticky substance that must adhere to the virus to kill it, and in those cases it may not have reached all of the virus present.

The real question, of course, is whether condoms are protective against HIV and other STDs *in vivo*. The answer appears to be yes. The Swedish experience of aggressively promoting condom use and seeing an 80 percent decrease in the incidence of gonorrhea and the experience of the US armed forces in World War II, which learned, perhaps to its surprise, that servicemen given condoms came down with much less venereal disease than those given moral lectures (whose venereal-disease rate went up), are but two examples. There are many others.

In addition, the CDC, in its *Sexually Transmitted Diseases Summary 1986*, advises using condoms to prevent infection with *Chlamydia trachomatis, Ureaplasma ureallyticum, Trichomonas vaginalis, Candida albicans*, herpes simplex virus types 1 and 2 (when lesions are on the penis or the female genital area), human papilloma virus, *Treponema pallidum, Haemophilus ducreyi*, and human T-cell lymphotropic virus type III/lymphadenopathy-associated virus.

So the case is pretty well proved. All that remains to be done is to get people to use condoms — properly.

At the Atlanta meeting, ideas for how to do so abounded. Their very number made it obvious that there was no one simple strategy for so profoundly affecting human sexual behavior. Suggestions ranged from holding workshops, as is done in San Francisco's gay community , on "The Ins and Outs of Condom Use," to teaching communication skills because "to get the condom out of someone's pocket or purse and onto the penis, someone has to say something" (a somewhat dubious assertion, some thought), to encouraging focus groups that would emphasize such positive facts as "using a condom can help make intercourse last longer," to producing video instructions with actors using language to appeal to those blacks and Hispanics who contract AIDS in disproportionate numbers. One speaker suggested — not very much in jest — that the millennium would arrive when all cigarette vending machines were replaced with ones dispensing condoms.

Perhaps the overriding thought to emerge from the conference was that to get everyone who should do so to use condoms, the emphasis on HIV prevention should be removed from groups at risk and placed on risk behavior.

Conant, who has been battling the AIDS epidemic from the very beginning, spoke for all when he said, "Physicians must persuade every patient to practice safer sex. We'll lose lots more kids if we don't take what we've learned in San Francisco and apply it elsewhere."

The Wisdom of the Despised

Peter Jenkins
Reprinted with permission from *New Statesman*
November 14, 1986

Tony Newton, minister of health, is at the despatch box in the Commons. He shows the House (612 male MPs, 23 female, and they're all there, heaped to the rafters) how to conceal a condom in the mouth and roll it — this in mime, in the natural absence of a volunteer — over the penis of a man who is paying for oral sex but refusing to wear a sheath, so that the man never suspects it has been done.

The radio audience laments that the Commons isn't televised, but Lady Trumpington, Health undersecretary of state in the Lords, repeats the demonstration for some 1200 peers, 450 of whom have never before set foot in Westminster, and before the TV cameras. Health workers applaud the two ministers without a shadow of a smile. The rest of the nation divides into po-faced outrage and dying with laughter.

Better to die of laughter, on the whole, than of AIDS contracted through an open sore in the mouth. No, the scene hasn't been performed in our Parliament. But the trick of mouthing and palming a sheath onto an unwilling man, and removing it before he's in a state to be attentive, *was* shown by a woman prostitute at the European Parliament in Brussels during the second World Whores' Congress. She was dealing with the fact that prostitutes everywhere have to comply or pretend to, with the demands that they know are compounding their risk of contracting or transmitting the AIDS virus. "We have to speak out now about the high-risk groups among heterosexual men", says Michele Logan, a young British ex-prostitute whom we invited round to the *New Statesman* for an AIDS talk. And she didn't mean needle-users or bisexuals.

Michele works with the International Committee for Prostitutes' Rights (ICPR) which organized the two Whores' Congresses, and was at both of them. Condoms and the widespread reluctance of many individual "punters" (prostitutes' customers) and groups of "punters" to use them when paying for penetrative sex, were on the minds of this year's several hundred delegates, including guest venereologists, from 17 countries. Continental "eros centres" (e.g. Hamburg) "are run by men who pay taxes to government: prostitutes are *discouraged* from insisting that men wear condoms". In several Swiss cantons, medical checks on prostitutes are compulsory: "that deludes men into believing they don't *need* to wear sheaths".

And Britain? Michele pounces on "police who harass prostitute women the moment they find condoms on them. It's the same with hotel security. They'll check on a woman because they suspect she's a prostitute, because of her red shoes or whatever, you know, forcibly search her bag which is illegal, and if they find condoms, call the police. This has really got to change: let's get the facts about what goes on out from under the carpet".

"There are entire cultural groups of men, Muslims, Rastas," she goes on, "who from religious or whatever motives insist that if they're paying they don't and won't use a sheath whatever the act. Far Eastern men tend to carry condoms with them" — she speculates that modern population control programmes and former epidemics of venereal disease under military occupations are the reason — "so what is it with these Western boys? Western governments cheerfully shove contraception on the Third World. Why not on the men at home? In Jamaica they try to make sheath-wearing viril: *If you want to be a man, strong and safe, use Panther condoms.* You see the ads everywhere. You can, you have to, shift behaviour."

"Ask a prostitute her profession, and time and again what it really is is *addict*. A habit to finance, general poverty, a pimp — which is comparatively rare in Britain — time and again will force an individual prostitute or those in a business quarter of prostitution to take the cash and risk an "unprotected" man even when she knows much more about sexual health than the punter." Michele hands me the list of resolutions passed by the international gathering of "whores" in Brussels. They include:

— Addicted prostitutes (male as well as female) who use needles must have access to legal inexpensive needles in order to prevent the spread of disease, specifically hepatitis and AIDS (some 50 percent of intravenous drug-users in Edinburgh are estimated to by HIV positive and many are of necessity on the game);

— Codes for mandatory use of condoms by clients should be enacted (as by-laws at local authority level, presumably, were it to be done in Britain) to be enforced by worker organizations not by state authorities [that is, through prostitutes being able to turn to their own organizations or 'non-judgemental' health workers];

— Prostitutes and ex-prostitutes to be employed in training health workers about the realities of prostitution health issues.

In America, 7 percent of the 26,878 AIDS cases registered between 1981 and end-October 1986 have been women; 700 have died; 15 percent of the women with AIDS are understood to have contracted it from heterosexual contact, and 71 percent of those specifically from heterosexual contact with an intravenous drug user. Infection through prostitution is an unquantifiable but certain contributory factor. Beyond the diagnosed AIDS cases lies a vaster pool of women who must, if the findings of restricted surveys are to be trusted, now be HIV-positive. Again, a disproportionate number can be expected to be in prostitution and quite unable to leave it.

Michele tells me that in one or more localities in California the experiment has been tried of wiring the premises of identified HIV-positive prostitutes so that if they leave the building an alarm sounds in the police station. Or was it just a proposal? Federal health officials in Washington, addressing themselves to prostitute *and* client, though in oddly disparate form, have just urged that no man who has been with a prostitute in the last six months donate blood; and no man or woman who has been an active prostitute at any time since 1977 do so either.

The Philippines has just formally asked the USA to send "only AIDS-free troops" since "bargirls" near US bases were found to by HIV-positive (America is screening the military now). In Sydney, the Australian Prostitutes Collective is now state-funded so that it can and does distribute free condoms and safer-sex advice to the male "punters" in the Kings Cross red light district. The latter tactic, in which government or its agencies overtly recognises, fosters and funds mutual self-help among prostitutes so that they are as well armed as possible to turn away the money and insistence of the willfully "unprotected" man is unquestionably what a "great and good prostitute" would press on this week's Cabinet committee on AIDS — or on the public if given a seat on the successor body.

In Britain, nine women and seven men are so far known by the DHSS to have contracted AIDS after heterosexual contact. The Michels of the world need to be heard from, loudly.

AIDS and the Communities

June E. Osborn

Reprinted with permission from the *Congressional Record*
November 19, 1987

For the first time in human history, we have all the information we need to avoid an epidemic by personal decisions about behavior. There will never be a better vaccine than that! We should celebrate the fact that in just six short years, biomedical and epidemiological scientists have constructed a firm foundation of abundant data on which to build carefully focussed policies which are responsible to the precise contours of the epidemic. The good news is that our seemingly extravagant investments in basic research were in the nick of time, and we are in a position to respond to a major plague without panic and without resort to draconian extremes of social action.

But we have quite an agenda! We need to find ways to educate our people to those things that are risky and those that are not. We need to find ways to provide many levels of care to young adults stricken in the prime of life. We need to be addressing cruel questions about housing and employment and insurance and provision of health care for persons with AIDS, about burnout and postgraduate education for health care professionals, and about realistic and unreasoning fears of health care workers — the list seems almost endless.

Immersed as I am in these matters, I find it startling that much of the political dialogue about AIDS has little to do with the realities of the epidemic, its control and its containment. Instead the proposals put forward in the name of public health and public policy seem to ignore all that we have learned about the virus and its modes of transmission and, worse yet, to be predicated on stark unrealism. The general public indulges itself in complaints about the tastelessness of condom advertising and perseverates about the ephemeral risk of mosquitoes: and many public policy makers seem to be operating on the notion that we are coping with a short-term or finite problem; that the good old days will return in 1991 or soon thereafter.

Let us dispense with those dreams quickly; AIDS is here to stay! It is like the day after Pearl Harbor — the world has changed and will never be the same again. AIDS will be a fact of life for our children's children; we can exert great influence on how dominant a force it will be, but we cannot make it disappear. The awful projections of a quarter of a million Americans dead or dying of AIDS by 1991 are based on sufficiently valid data that, while they might be low, they will assuredly not be high. And nothing says that there won't be a further stepwise increase in 1992 and beyond. In the absence of public education and effective warnings — a national effort still not launched in the US, more than six years into the epidemic.

While the options of quarantine, of universal mandatory testing, or of "not delivering health care" are easily invoked, they are in reality unthinkable. If we have learned one thing in the twentieth century, it should have been that there are no "others" — that to declare one group of lesser value or beyond help is to degrade us all in intolerable ways.

For instance, let's look at quarantine more closely. In America we are talking about as many as two million individuals in whom infection and infectiousness are lifelong. They do not represent a threat to others except by the closest kind of consensual behavior; and yet in vague opinion polls, quarantine has sometimes had the support of 25 percent or more of the American people. The logistics would be daunting, to say the least; how would we do that, even if we could find an appropriate island or enclave? Would we feed them? Would we have them make license plates for a living? We would certainly have to guard them to keep them from slipping out; and I guess we would also have to guard the guards, since the temptation to slip in would always be there for family members, loved ones or individuals whose responsiveness to pathos or sexual allure might overcome their caution. This all sounds so perverse that I hate to discuss it but the winds of society are blowing strong in this irrational and dangerous direction, and silent contemplation of such atrocious options haunts the public policy debate in significant ways.

Indeed, I am suspicious that some thought of quarantine lies in the back of the minds of policy makers who seem to be positively possessed with the tenacious wish to screen. When pressed to justify their position, advocates of mandatory or very widespread antibody testing to detect asymptomatic infected individuals fall back on the rationale that it would be desirable to know with greater accuracy how many people are infected. Since they aren't doing much with the information we already have in hand, I find that argument peculiarly unconvincing; and anyway, we don't have to violate people's privacy and autonomy to do that; we can get a very good idea of virus prevalence through anonymous samplings of collected sera.

But a more fundamental argument arises concerning mandatory testing; given that the very restricted modes of transmission are consensual and private in nature, limitation of virus spread is based of necessity on voluntary changes in behavior. Since intravenous drug use is already illegal, the use of mandatory urine testing for drugs is an interesting "trial run." Thus far the chief results of such programs of which I am aware are — first — a black market in "negative" urine and — second — (in reaction to that) a level of intrusion in observing the donation of the urine to verify its authenticity that makes one shiver at the implication for AIDS control.

Mandatory premarital screening would detect fewer than one-tenth of one percent of those currently infected, and the cost of doing it right would exceed $100 million.

The very gravity of our epidemic situation it seems to me, demands that we be honest in our critical assessment of past policies. If we are honest with ourselves, then in point of fact I think penicillin rather than public health officialdom, deserves the credit for curtailing syphilis; and the explosive spread of antibiotic-resistant gonococci and the advent of chlamydia and a host of untreatable sexually transmitted diseases among both homosexuals and heterosexuals should warn us not to be so uncritical of past strategies. Even in the instance of smallpox — the only disease we have ever managed to eradicate — it is clear that administrative brilliance and focussed efforts based on a refined knowledge of the virus' properties and modes of spread accomplished in a decade what a vaccine had failed to achieve in nearly two centuries.

Let me be very clear; the horror of AIDS and its inexorable progress to an unpeaceful death is such that any political or ethical analysis would mandate whatever public health policies were best designed to abort the epidemic at the earliest opportunity. But even our immigrant screening plan is "off the wall" and dangerous in its thoughtlessness, for AIDS is, after all, the only category I know if in which we are net exporters, not importers, and that policy, which goes into effect Decmeber 1, is likely to provoke retaliation so massive that we will all do well to remember the stimulus and try to avoid similar zenophobic nonsense in the future. As to civil liberties and public health, it is a happy fact that the data lead to the conclusion that wise policies will optimize them both.

Just so you don't go away saying that I saw no use for the antibody screening test, let me describe what I believe to be its proper uses. First, mandatory screening of the donors of blood and blood products and of organs/tissues/cells is clearly important and warrants the investments in its deployment that have been made. Second, I am fully in favor of voluntary testing in the context of counseling, confidentiality and anonymity.

We should facilitate the use of the test, but there is much work to be done here, for many communities have located their alternative test sites in the heart of the inner city or in the sexually transmitted disease clinic, and the social disincentive to use their services can be quite strong for the worried well. Furthermore, the medical profession is not yet well educated about the epidemic. Bisexuality, closet homosexuality and the patronization of prostitutes — not to mention experimental use of illicit intravenous drugs — are not common topics of discussion in the present day patient physician relationship; and the CEO of a company may well hesitate to confide in his physician with whom he also plays golf on Wednesdays. Our policies should recognize this and facilitate realistic testing opportunities so that worried individuals can learn their status and behave responsible toward their loved ones, as most wish to do.

In short, we haven't tried the voluntary approach to control of the virus of AIDS nearly as energetically as I believe we must. Our data tell us that in both the US and Europe, when high risk individuals have been educated to recognize the specific behaviors that put them at risk, the results in terms of behavior modification have been truly astonishing. Compared to prior efforts at any sort of health education, much less sex education, the magnitude of change has been dramatic. And there is a special urgency about individuals who have yet to adopt lifestyles; about adolescents and children. We need their willing attention, not their surly compliance; the tone of our preventive programs will do much to determine which we get.

The central point about testing is that the antibody test is most useful as an adjunct to behavioral counseling, not the converse; and change in intimate sexual and drug-using behavior is far less likely to occur under mandate than it is by voluntary participation and cooperation. The human resources necessary for effective counseling are in short supply right now, what with blood screening and alternative test site needs; and wasting such resources on poorly targeted mass programs is hardly wise.

Let us look at some other things we should be doing, besides optimizing the use of the antibody test through well-conceived programs of voluntary participation. Well, obviously we should have been conducting public education campaigns long since; in fact, I find myself quite embarrassed when I am at the World Health Organization in Geneva to try to explain to my colleagues from other industrialized countries that we have yet to mount a coordinated program of public education in the United States. With two dozen or two hundred cases, the vast majority of countries who can afford to have deployed the full power of their media and government access to warn their people of the new threat; and we, with 43,000 cases, 1-2 million infected, and the experience from which they are all learning, have been officially mute!

Would you believe that October is US AIDS Awareness and Prevention Month? Have you heard so much as an official whisper? Isn't it embarrassing. The federal government seems to be too impoverished to buy prime TV time, so they tried radio; and the pamphlet that was to have gone to every household in the land has once again flunked the censors and had to be withdrawn. Oh how I wish we would at least do it right if we are going to be this late about it. People ask me sometimes how much I think would be "enough" in a public education campaign. I tell them that I don't want us public health people to seem greedy, so I would settle, for starters, for equal time with the US military recruiting advertisements. We could even borrow the Army's theme song — "Be all that you can be" — for while they are talking about what to do with a kid's future, we are talking about whether that kid has a future.

Our official silence is almost eerie — for there is an urgent duty to warn. We must be sure that the elegant science which has brought us so far so fast in understanding transmission patterns of HIV is not neutralized completely by a moralism which rejects discussion of any options except monogamy or chastity. I know of no society in which those are the sole patterns of sexual behavior, and ours is surely not going to be the first. Failure to warn about the new virus and its lethal consequences is an extraordinary punishment for unapproved sexual activity. We do need some media time, for there is really quite a lot to talk about. While we would like everyone to conform to the safest of sexual mores and to abstain from drugs, I honestly don't think we need to restrict our messages during precious media minutes simply to tell them that. Anyway, Secretary Bennett has now helped us out with his own pamphlet which is rather exclusively devoted to extolling the virtues of the moral life.

But the average age of onset of sexual activity in some surveys is sixteen; we have the worst epidemic of teenage pregnancy in the industrialized world; and given those realities, alternatives do need to be discussed. Condoms, for instance, are quite effective (although not foolproof) in preventing the spread of the virus of AIDS during intercourse when used appropriately; and it is hard for me to believe, when condoms are among the perilously few defenses we have to turn to in limiting the spread of a killer, that someone could perceive silence as an ethically defensible stance. Not only do we not have national educational programs about this, but our public laws — enforcing an unreal morality — mitigate against prudent behavior; for instance I am told that there are still many cities where a woman found carrying a condom could be arrested for prostitution!

What about drug users? and needles — how about free needle exchanges? As commonly happens with a good catch-phrase, the notion of "free needles" sets morals aflame and distorts the discussion. It is contended that easy access to needles and syringes would encourage drug use. I don't know whether it would or not — some European countries have needle exchanges which have worked well and have not had that effect. Clearly the issue is not a simple one, but the fact is that drug use is the open avenue to the epidemic's future and we should not spend time quarreling but find out! It was with that in mind that the Institutes of Medicine/National Academy of Sciences study group recommended that this issue be put to experimental test.

The needle argument is a distraction of course, from the shocking omission in our so-called "war on drugs". What sort of a moral crusade is it when no accommodation is made for prisoners of war. There are not now enough treatment slots in the United States to accommodate those addicts who already "want out." Can you imagine putting a heroin addict on a six-month waiting list when she seeks treatment?

It has been said that we haven't yet made an impact about AIDS on drug users; but how would you ever know when there is no opportunity for them to react? I believe we should not consider our policies even vaguely rational with respect to the AIDS epidemic (not to mention the drug epidemic) until the treatment centers have openings going begging and until sexual partners of addicts are found, organized and mobilized into self-help groups.

I have spend quite a bit of time on drugs, for it is difficult to overemphasize the role drug users will play in the future of the epidemic. By 1991 the percent of women involved will have increased from 76 percent to 90 percent, with drug use or sexual partnership with a drug user as the major vehicle. More than 90 percent of pediatric AIDS will be the direct or indirect result of drugs. Even in the context of female prostitution, the likelihood of a prostitute being infected and therefore potentially infectious tracks dominantly with IV drug use.

The challenge to health care is so large a topic that I cannot grapple with it meaningfully in a brief overview. The provision of beds may present a bit of a problem as our numbers of AIDS cases increase tenfold; but the hospitals had overbuilt in recent decades and we may be able to reopen some old wards if we can figure out the financing. But ominously, there are many places where AIDS patients are unwelcome; the reason given is fear, and yet there is the strongest kind of evidence that they present far less threat to their caretakers than do persons infected with half a dozen more familiar pathogens. Indeed, if health care workers were well protected against hepatitis B, their protection against HIV would be one hundred times greater than required, for the virus of AIDS is a puny thing indeed when it comes to transmission.

Even if acute care hospitals can get their act together, there is another kind of problem with provision of health care. AIDS patients don't really need to be hospitalized for the rest of their lives once the diagnosis is made. They can continue to function, to create and to contribute to society if they are supported in ways molded to their needs, which will change gradually over time. There need to be options which can account for this; outpatient care for those who can function; home care for those whose only medical need for the moment is intermittent intravenous therapy; long-term care for those whose debility is substantial but whose acute care needs are very limited; and finally, hospice care for those who have nearly reached the end of the dreadful road and should be helped to die with dignity. And all along this continuum of care there must be compassion, for to withhold it and allow the institutionalization of blaming the victim is to wound our society seriously if not mortally.

This is really a familiar list of needs, for our elderly register almost exactly the same set of requirements to complete their lives optimally — and yet we lack the institutions to meet these needs, and even where they exist, AIDS patients are being turned away out of misplaced fear. That is only a sample of a daunting health care agenda, and we had better hop to it, for even the short-term coping strategies are being swamped as the numbers of AIDS cases increase inexorably. We should fear the consequences of inaction, for it may be hard to reconstruct our jerry-built health care system once it is overwhelmed.

Our generation has spent much time worrying about thermonuclear bombs, for good reason. But while we were doing so, less than thirty years ago, a veritable microbiological bomb was quietly detonated in our midst. Now it is up to us to see whether we can mobilize what we have learned — and ironically, in an era in which science and technology have been turned to with almost blind confidence, it will be our challenge to face this new pandemic microbe without immediate recourse to drugs or vaccines.

Teaching Children about AIDS

Surgeon General C. Everett Koop
Reprinted with permission from *Issues in Science
and Technology*
Fall 1987

The AIDS epidemic officially began only six years ago, when the U.S. Public Health Service published the first five reports of persons struck down with *Pneumocystis carinii* pneumonia. These cases, involving "otherwise healthy homosexual males" living in Los Angeles, were considered "clinically unusual." Just *how* unusual is now a matter of history.

Today, the total number of AIDS cases on record in the United States is over 40,000. And the curve is rising dramatically. One or more cases have occurred in every state; in each of 17 major cities, the count has already topped 300. By 1991, according to estimates from the Centers for Disease Control, the number of AIDS cases may exceed 270,000.

This is a terrible disease, for which we do not yet have a cure. Nor do we have a vaccine, and one probably won't be generally available before the end of this century. Meanwhile, the mortality rate for AIDS is virtually 100 percent; over half the recorded victims of the disease are already dead, and the rest probably soon will be. The only thing we have that may work — and I repeat: "*may* work" — is education, education, and more education.

The AIDS virus — also known as the "human immunodeficiency virus," or HIV — is transmitted from one person to another in blood or semen. In other body fluids, such as tears, saliva, sweat, and urine, the virus particle count is too low or is absent altogether. Hence, we have no substantiated cases of AIDS virus being transmitted in water glasses, on toilet seats, by sneezes or coughs, and so on.

Certain sexual practices engaged in mainly by homosexual and bisexual men often produce semen *and* blood that are passed between partners. These men are the persons most at risk of catching AIDS, not because of their particular sexual orientation, but because of their sexual behavior *within* that orientation.

But practices can be changed. In fact, after several years of intensive AIDS education directed to homosexual and bisexual men, it appears that they have become more cautious and, as a result, the transmission of other diseases such as syphilis, gonorrhea, and hepatitis has, in fact, decreased. Because they each have a shorter incubation period than AIDS, we can track these diseases more easily for short-term data. We can only assume that the transmission of AIDS within this group has probably decreased as well.

The need to change practices is exactly the same issue for intravenous drug abusers, who constitute the second largest group of AIDS victims. The ones who use their own clean needles for each "fix" are killing themselves by abusing potent, addictive, illegal drugs. But they probably won't kill themselves through an AIDS-related disease.

Drug abusers tend *not* to be this fastidiously hygienic, however. About 90 percent of all heroin addicts borrow used and dirty needles, as well as other contaminated drug paraphernalia. These addicts are making absolutely sure that they die as early and as uncomfortably as possible. And when they engage in sex, they're shortening the lives of other people as well.

It's clear that if every homosexual and bisexual man used a condom during sex from this day forward, and if every IV drug abuser used only a clean needle for each fix, the epidemic of AIDS would slow down in these populations, gradually reach a steady state, and finally begin to recede as those who are already infected die off and no new victims take their places.

But that's only a theory. The reality is far more grim. Some homosexual and bisexual men have changed their sexual practices, but not all of them have. And we have no idea how many drug addicts may have heard our "clean-needle" message of AIDS prevention. Nor do we know how many have actually processed that information, and, as a result, changed their behavior. So, the theory remains just that: a theory. The AIDS epidemic, in reality, is not going to level off and recede for many years to come. And the percentage of completely innocent victims of the disease could become increasingly significant. The overall number of AIDS cases will probably increase ninefold over the next five years, but the number of cases involving heterosexuals will increase about 20-fold.

At present, about 4 percent of all reported AIDS victims are heterosexuals — men and women who are neither homosexual nor bisexual nor IV drug abusers. Apparently, their only high-risk activity was to have had sexual relations with someone who was infected with the AIDS virus.

A common example could be that of a heterosexual man who has sex with an HIV-infected prostitute, then goes home and has sex with his unsuspecting wife or with other women, all of whom could receive the virus from him. Nothing very kinky about it, nothing very exotic, but all very tragic.

The tragedy is then compounded when one of these women becomes pregnant and passes the virus on to her newborn infant either in utero or in the birth canal during delivery.

It's true that the number of children born with AIDS is still quite small. They constitute just over one percent of the total number of all AIDS victims. A couple of years ago, however, *there weren't any*. Now, there are 470. In fact, some hospitals — in New York, New Jersey, and Washington, D.C., for example — have had to set aside isolation wards to take care of the rising number of infants infected with the AIDS virus (and who are frequently abandoned or orphaned).

Over half the babies born with AIDS are black. Another 25 percent of all babies born with AIDS are Hispanic. And just to increase our sense of horror at what is happening in the black and Hispanic communities, we suspect that these cases are vastly underreported.

What we're seeing with AIDS, therefore, is more tragic evidence of the demography of high-risk pregnancies and birth. In our society, such pregnancies are most likely to occur among black women under the age of 19 who are poor, not ready for work (usually without a high school diploma), and without ready access to sound health care.

This fact is in addition to what is emerging with more and more clarity regarding the incidence of AIDS among black adults. In the population generally, one of every eight Americans is black. But among Americans with AIDS, one of every four is black. Also, about a third of all black AIDS victims are IV drug abusers, which is also disproportionate.

This is catastrophic news for the black community, which already is under great economic and social stress. And it's also more evidence of the apparent inability of U.S. society in general to make much headway in helping young people control their own destines.

In the absence of a vaccine or any miracle drug to stop AIDS, the best thing society can do to contain this epidemic is to present scientifically accurate and personally sensitive information about AIDS to our children. The objective is to make them a lot more responsible in their relationships than their elders have been. And before AIDS education even begins, a child should be given information relative to his or her own sexuality.

I've recommended that this be done in the context of a comprehensive school health curriculum, so that children may make the same kinds of intelligent, life-saving choices regarding their own sexuality as we hope they will in regard to their own dental health, their ability to handle anger and stress, their rejection of cigarettes and other drugs, and so on.

Instead of calling it "sex education," I'd like it called something like "studies in human development." Children should be learning all about themselves — about their unbelievable complexity, and especially about their own great value. If they are properly taught their own worth, we can expect them to treat themselves, and others, with great respect.

Human development instruction should keep pace with — and not anticipate — a child's own development and curiosity. It should begin in infancy, taught by parents through overt instruction and good role modeling, and by enlightened teachers armed with facts and useful materials.

Education in this country has traditionally been the responsibility of states and communities. That tradition should continue, but the federal role — getting factual, scientifically accurate information into the hands of local teachers — is also important. This year the Public Health Service is investing a million dollars in just such an activity. For example:

— Last December our CDC, the lead agency in our educational efforts, brought together an ad hoc group of advisors drawn from organizations such as the American Academy of Pediatrics, the National Congress of PTAs, the National Education Association, the School Board of the City of New York, and so on. This group produced a set of guidelines — which are responsive to, and consistent with, the needs of the community — for teaching about AIDS in the nation's schools.

— Under a grant from CDC, the Indiana Department of Health and Indiana University have jointly produced a manual on AIDS for students and teachers, copies of which are available from CDC in Atlanta.

— Cooperative agreements are being established with state education departments and local school districts to support their efforts in mounting programs to teach about AIDS. That program should be in place early this school year.

In these and related activities, there are some basic concepts in human development that ought to be conveyed. For example, I think children ought not to be afraid of sex. Still, I think it makes sense to suggest to them, as they approach pubescence, that abstinence at their time of life is by far the preferable option. Abstinence is in fact the only option that really prevents sexually transmitted disease.

But children grow up, and, as adults, not too many of them choose to be sexually abstinent all their lives. So what's next? I've advised that the next-best protection is a faithful, monogamous relationship; one in which they have only one continuing sexual partner who is equally faithful. Paraphrasing Lee Iacocca, I say: If you have a monogamous relationship, *keep it*; if you don't have one, *get it*.

But, again, not everyone is fortunate enough to achieve such a relationship. Many men and women who take marriage vows may practice monogamy, but not all of them do. So the next concept is: When in doubt, protect yourself. If you don't know what you're doing and with whom you're doing it, then don't do it. But if you go ahead anyway, then you must be absolutely certain that your partner is free of the AIDS virus. Otherwise, if you're a man, use a condom from start to finish; if you're a woman, make sure your partner uses a condom from start to finish. A condom is not perfect. But it's the best thing available for people who neither abstain nor are monogamous.

That's my basic message on sex and AIDS education for children. In my report of October 1986, I devoted fewer than 200 words to the subject. But for some people, those were 200 words too many! Because they believe that sex education in school will lead to promiscuity, they prefer that such instruction be given at home. I agree, but the fact is that most parents do not provide sex education to their children, so schools and churches must do it instead.

I'm sure that some of the controversy about sex education and AIDS education reflects genuine concerns by parents and school officials regarding course content. But the discussion also reflects the continued ambivalence and confusion in our society about male-female relationships in general.

There is more to human relationships than just "good sex," and young people ought to be told that. We should encourage them to seek out relationships that are sensitive and affirmative — equitable relationships in which both adults are mutually loving, caring, respectful, and considerate.

We all want such relationships. But many people settle for much less. They tend to overemphasize sex because it's easier and can be accomplished with very little thought. This is the distorted message, delivered by so much of our popular media as well, that sex is most often a casual and even gratuitous act in which no one gets hurt, no one gets pregnant, and no one takes responsibility.

I suggest that we teach AIDS education at an appropriate moment within the context of a total sex education curriculum. But more fundamental is the *social* context that embraces sex education itself. And this is where we have to reach beyond the biology staff and secure the help of psychology and sociology staff as well.

The larger social context is the one in which men and women relate to each other generally in our society. And here, the evidence is not very inspiring.

Earlier this year, for example, I was briefed on a study — done for our National Institute of Mental Health by Dr. Mary Koss of Kent State University — that involved a representative sample of about 6,000 men and women who attend 32 colleges across the country.

Although these subjects were reasonably well-educated, middle-class individuals from workaday American families, 25 percent of the college men said they had committed some form of sexual aggression against a female companion one or more times. About 8 percent of the sample had tried to rape or *had* raped their companions. And half of them said that, given the chance, they'd do it again.

Twenty-five percent of this representative sample comes to 740 men. But 25 percent of the total male enrollment in U.S. higher education today is a *million and a half* men — a million and a half young men for whom male-female relationships are not caring, not respectful, certainly not loving, and hardly equitable.

Thus our job in the long run is to get through to these young men — and young women — and many millions more who are adolescent and pre adolescent, and try to instill in them more positive and humane values. And our job right now is to advise them as follows: That they should be abstinent; if not abstinent, then monogamous; and if not monogamous, that at least supercautious.

We must tell young people the truth about AIDS and about the way it's spread. We must talk sense to them, and their parents, and their teachers. This is no rose garden. But we've got to make the effort. We have to educate and inform them, even though we do so in the midst of all the other complex aspects of sexual relations in America. Their lives are at stake, and so is the physical and spiritual life of this country.

* * * * * * * * * *

In January 1986, the World Health Organization reported the disease in 113 countries, reporting over 51,000 cases of AIDS.

V. The Epidemic Comes Home

The Editors

AIDS does indeed have the world surrounded. A look through the headlines of the world press for any one day would be convincing evidence that some sort of terrible and mysterious scourge was raging through each and every society. Those societies which have already been profoundly impacted are struggling with the rising toll of dead and dying while those yet to be touched are closing borders, testing in their airports and circling the wagons around the heartland.

The articles in this section deal mostly with the intensely human side of the tragedy of AIDS. Most history books contain the political proclamations and tales of the great battles and the generals who won them. It is only recently that even some of our text books are carrying small paragraphs about the "little people" — the people who suffered sometimes immeasurable pain and torment under the hooves the the white horses and B-1 bombers which blazed their ways into the documentary family alblum of great nations and some not so great nations. In Africa many tin-hat dictators have strutted along the dusty roads of the countryside while just beyond the flag-wavers thousands and millions of their "subjects" lived in the most miserable and un-forgiving conditions of deprivation and disease.

It is perhaps this pattern of our remembered past which is now coming home to haunt us — thousands and millions of poor and nearly destitute "subjects" living in the "inherited dust storm" of the battles of the mighty who rode out and tilted at imaginary windmills while the graneries in their homeland rotted and the grain in the fields was consumed by marauding soldiers and field rats.

The personal stories told by the writers in this section are of those who were left behind — those who were (and still are) closed out of access to good and decent housing, medical care and even social treatment. The women of New York whose bleak lives are testament to the ill-treatment of their men, their society and sometimes "the system" is only the tip of the iceberg of the millions of "stories" which are being lived out in the grimy, mean streets of the inner cities, the urban shantytowns and dusty rural roads of the world.

The army colonels, the populist demagogues, the bureaucratic maze and the under-financed health care systems of some of the rich and liberal countries have left in their wake an underclass of citizen who — for one reason or another — often doesn't give a damn about the body politic, the public health or even their own life and death.

How will we reach them? How will we be able to save their lives if they do not care and if they have been driven into a despair of drugs in order to forget their pain and indulge in the frenzy of "the moment" of sexual pleasure and mind-fogging behavior when the moment is maybe all they have — or at least all that they can see from their disadvantaged position at the bottom of the heap?

We must, as a compassionate society, help them for their own good above all other motivations. But it is also easy to understand the stampede which may descend upon them in the attempt to cure them of their diseases before they leak out into "our" world.

The AIDS epidemic is coming home. It is in the house down the road, around the corner and perhaps even now, next door. We are reaping the sins of our fathers in a sense of the word which defies cliche.

In this endeavor it may be important to go back and read Surgeon General Koops message one more time: "education, education and more education", may be the only weapon we have right now which will serve our community to the greatest advantage in the months and years to come. We are in the path of a steamroller which is without a driver and is powered by forces which we do not yet understand and is on a tragectory which even our most sophisticated computer modeling techniques cannot quantify.

a. The Human Dimension

Into That Good Night
Reprinted from *America*

P aul felt lousy.

No particular aches or pains. Just an overall, washed-out feeling. Twenty-four was too young to feel so tired, he thought. Better see somebody. Better get it checked out.

A few days later, doctors at St. Vincent's Medical Center gave him the diagnosis. Paul had AIDS. And probably less than eight months.

In the weeks that followed, the full fallout of the disease began to descend on his world. His employer let him go. His landlord threatened to evict him. Many of his friends simply walked away.

All the while, Paul grew weaker, and the knowledge that he was dying began to sink in with horrifying weight.

One day in his room at St. Vincent's, Paul opened his eyes to see a stranger at his bedside.

"Paul, I'm Sister Patrice Murphy," she said. "I'm with the Supportive Care Program here. I thought maybe we should talk."

In the months that followed, they would talk a great deal.

As with so many of the terminally ill patients the SCP cares for — usually patients dying of either cancer or AIDS — Sister Patrice and her colleagues visited Paul and his family regularly, both in the hospital and at home.

They talked about death and quality of life and about the stages of the disease Paul could expect to face. They helped him write letters, and attended to the dozens of details he could no longer handle alone.

Mostly, though, they listened. "Often, the best thing we can do is just to be there for them," says Sister Patrice. "To let the person talk or rage or cry or say nothing. To let them come to terms with death in their own way without making them do it alone."

When death comes, the patient's family and friends are invited into a bereavement group, where they can share their feelings with other survivors and help each other cope with the pain of losing a loved one.

Two days before he died, Paul handed Sister Patrice a note. Too weak to speak, he had scrawled a simple message. "Thank you. It's going to be OK. Don't worry anymore."

Toward a Spirituality for Victims of AIDS

by James Stulz
Reprinted with permission from *America*
June 28, 1986

Any epidemic poses challenges for the society within which it erupts. There are more sick persons to be cared for and more grieving relatives and friends to be comforted. In the past, church organizations were the principal providers of health care, and they met these challenges in a way that today's secular agencies cannot. The church added a spiritual and prayerful dimension to its response to epidemics. In the 16th century, for instance, the Forty Hours devotion often included prayers for protection from the plagues, and saints like Camillus of Lellis (1550-1614) and John of God (1495-1550) founded congregations of nurses to serve the plague-stricken.

AIDS and ARC together constitute a 20th century parallel to the medieval plague. Patients are said to have AIDS when they develop one or more of the diseases that the Atlanta Centers for Disease Control lists as life-threatening for those infected by the AIDS virus. Persons with ARC are those whose immune systems are damaged but who have not developed one of the illnesses on the Atlanta Center's list.

There are currently far more people with ARC than with AIDS. Although many of them may never develop AIDS, they are in a position of maximum risk for that disease. ARC may manifest itself in such minor ways as a low fever or swollen lymph nodes, although it has also been known to have such severe effects as paralysis. Nevertheless, ARC is not judged to be life-threatening in the manner of AIDS.

Unless otherwise note, however, "AIDS" will be understood in this article to refer both to AIDS and ARC.

The AIDS epidemic is a contemporary challenge at many levels to the church as well as to civil society. But insofar as it affects homosexuals, this modern plague is a new and special challenge for a church that has long failed to minister to the needs of homosexuals. Nowadays, the spread of AIDS is evoking some positive responses from the church. In New York and San Francisco, for instance, former convents have been converted to hospices for those dying of AIDS. But besides medical care, the victims of AIDS also need help in developing a religious outlook, a "spirituality" as it may be called, that will enable them not only to endure their illness but even derive grace from the experience.

For some time, I have been working as a member of a volunteer home-care group that serves AIDS patients. Many of these have been or are members of the same Catholic parish as myself. From my conversations with them, the following reflections have been distilled. They are fragments that might be tentatively synthesized as a step toward a spirituality for victims of AIDS.

Since there is still no cure for AIDS, those who contract it have a devastating foreknowledge of pain, suffering and death. They can place this within a Gospel perspective by recalling the agony Jesus suffered in the Garden of Olives when He foresaw His own suffering and death. Most deaths from AIDS occur among men in the age range from the 20s to the 40s. That means they share another experience with Jesus. He died, humanly speaking, before His time. Like Him, they too are deprived of living to old age.

Christians believe that the cross of Jesus was redemptive and that all other human suffering is capable of bringing about redemption. Of course, similar concepts are found outside Christianity. Classical Greek tragedy, for instance, distinguished the "pathos" of mere brute pain from "tragedy" that requires a consciousness of suffering and a deliberate choice to live it through.

For many of us, admiration of the Greek notion of tragedy and assent to the Christian teaching of the redemptive value of suffering remain at a purely cerebral level. There is a truth here that we admit on faith, though reluctantly, but then put safely aside. A man with AIDS, however, can experience this truth in his very flesh even as Jesus did. Indeed, many AIDS victims report that their experience of the disease has somehow been positive. They report a new and intuitive grasp of the real necessity of suffering, the necessity of the cross — a truth they have experienced not only on the level of faith, but in their flesh. This is not to imply that they are mentally unhealthy people who delight in pain, but rather that they have come to understand the place of suffering in God's scheme of things. Some people with AIDS have been able to give far more than a notional assent to Paul's words: "In my own flesh I fill up what is lacking in the sufferings of Christ for the sake of His body, the Church."

In the daily life of a person with AIDS, as with all sick people, there is the possibility of experiencing Jesus' redemptive suffering and love in the spirit and in the flesh itself — in the whole person. With this kind of offering of the whole self, the job of the Lord's presence becomes full. Homosexuals who have AIDS, formerly apparent outcasts from the church, can have — through their physical suffering and foreknowledge of future pain and death — the full experience of the joy of sharing intimately in the redemptive work of Christ.

For those seeking to put the experience of AIDS within a religious framework, a first step is to go in this way to the heart of the meaning of the cross, of the Christian doctrine of redemption, of the knowledge of Jesus as Saviour and Redeemer. This approach is justified not only by Christian faith, but also by the lived experiences of some AIDS patients. Pastors would do well, then, to explore and nourish this resource when they minister to persons with AIDS.

Besides that joy they feel occasionally when they can experience their sharing in Christ's redemptive work, people with AIDS have also reported, like others with life-threatening illnesses, that they experience greater joy than ever before in God's creation. They speak of being moved to spontaneous tears by the beauty of a sunset or by music. They say this is not a desperate clinging to the world, but rather an enhanced appreciation of God's work in that world. This may be accounted another spiritual insight fostered by the experience of a fatal disease.

AIDS patients have also spoken of a heightened appreciation of God's gift of life itself. Some have searched for symbols to celebrate that gift or for ways to enrich whatever life they have here and now. One man bought and wears a bracelet that is for him symbolic of the celebration of life. Another is going back to college, and a third is putting together on videotape a collection of vintage movies. Once again, they speak of being motivated not by a desire to grasp what life remains but by a sort of "Eucharistic" joy, an appreciation of God's gift of life.

For people with AIDS, suicide forcefully suggests itself as an alternative, and many have taken their lives when the disease became highly debilitating. The temptation to suicide might be met by emphasizing the conviction embodied in get Greek theory of tragedy — that human dignity comes from living out one's destiny, not in avoiding it. Christians, however, have a very different source of spiritual support in this extremity. They can try to make their own the redemptive prayer of Jesus in the Garden: "Father, if it is your will, take this cup from me; yet not my will but yours be done".

AIDS patients have said that they once understood the phrase, "Thy will be done," to mean something like "Grin and bear it," but that they have now come to feel in the fullness of their being — in flesh and spirit — that they desire God's will to be done in them. Christian spirituality has always taught people to make an offering of their lives to God each day. A Carmelite variation on this classic theme calls for offering oneself as a "victim soul" and thereby making a special sort of total gift. People with AIDS, like all those who are fatally ill, have a compelling opportunity to offer even more than that to the Lord as they face what will probably be a difficult dying. More urgently than the rest of us, they can offer the Lord both their life and their death.

These are grand ideas: the total offering of oneself to God, redemption through suffering, sharing in the work of Christ and His church, cultivating joy in the gift of life, and choosing life, however difficult it may be, rather than suicide. But persons with AIDS must often endure debilitating weakness, constant fever and diarrhea for many months before they experience the pain of a life-threatening illness. Grand ideas seem to evaporate when one is worn out by a constant struggle with feelings of weakness and sickness. We all know how mean our thoughts can be when we have no more than a common cold.

AIDS patients may find it easy to summon the courage to say "Thy will be done" during the periods when they feel relatively well. When they feel sick, however, and must face mysterious medical procedures, they are likely to become frightened and depressed. In trying to bring spiritual help to these people, we must remember that the human person is necessarily complex and therefore experiences life at various levels. No matter how healthy our spiritual state may be, we still have to deal with our emotions and the psychological suffering that can accompany them. But that psychological pain is also part of the cross that one had offered to share in those hours that were dominated by Christian insight.

Those afflicted with AIDS need somehow to remember that their will remains intact even when they are torn by depression and fear. On the cross, Jesus cried out: "My God, my God, why have you forsaken me?" But we know that He only felt forsaken. So too, people dying of AIDS may need to remember that even though they feel forsaken, God has not abandoned them.

People with ARC need particular spiritual emphasis of their own because their situation is not as threatening as that of the AIDS patient. Although they are often somewhat debilitated, severe sickness is not imminent. They live with anxiety and uncertainty, however, because they are urgently aware that they belong to a high-risk group. They often say: "I would almost rather get AIDS. That way, I would at least know and could plan my life. The uncertainty is terrible."

These people might reflect that they will have the opportunity to carry the cross when, and if, AIDS develops. For them here and now, however, anxiety and fear are the stuff of life, and it is in the present moment that one shares in the life of Christ.

In fact, the threat posed by ARC has actually brought homosexuals together in prayer. In private encounters as well as in public ceremonies like the numerous healing services that are regularly held in San Francisco, homosexuals are joining in the laying on of hands and in praying for one another's healing. Where once they met socially and for sex, now certain homosexuals who think they have the gift of healing, meet for prayer and services of healing and their friends who have AIDS or ARC. It is striking to see a spiritual community being formed within the homosexual population where it probably had never existed before. It is also heartening to see that this prayer community has links with the Catholic Church, which has a centuries-old tradition of prayer for healing.

Within the church there has been prejudice against homosexual people. But the AIDS epidemic has created a role for homosexuals in the church and in Christian life. Those who have contracted AIDS or ARC have an opportunity to share in a special way in the redemptive work of Jesus and of His church. It is urgent that they be helped to understand this opportunity and to seize it.

The Bleak and Lonely Lives
of Women Who Carry AIDS

by Jane Gross
Reprinted with permission from *The New York Times*
August 27, 1987

The number of women in New york City who are infected with AIDS virus but free of the symptoms of the disease has now reached 50,000. Eighty percent are black or Hispanic.

And they have become the primary carriers of the disease from the world of drug abuse to the larger community, making their education an increasingly urgent task.

Their lives — chaotic and impoverished — are confounding public health officials as they seek to contain a widening epidemic than now hits hardest in neighborhoods where drugs are rampant.

According to the doctors, nurses and social workers who counsel the women aware of their infection, many of them, particularly the drug addicts, react with passivity and denial. They are not using condoms that can arrest the spread of AIDS. And they are becoming pregnant despite the knowledge that they could infect a fetus, and bearing children, many of whom will die.

But another category of these infected women, the sex partners of men who have injected drugs, are behaving far more responsibly — protecting their mates and avoiding or terminating unwanted pregnancies. To these women, the counselors are preaching the feminist message that women can take control of their lives, even in the face of poverty, illness and death.

Health officials say the vast majority of infected women, both those in the inner city of all races and the few others who have acquired the virus from bisexual men or from blood transfusions, are unaware they carry and can spread AIDS. The disease has already killed more than

700 women in New York and more than twice that number nation-wide. With the passage of time, scientists are becoming persuaded that all of those infected will eventually develop the symptoms and die.

Poor women often do not know that AIDS is transmitted by hetero-sexual sex, so health officials are seeking to promote counseling and voluntary testing, particularly at family-planning clinics where such programs are largely unavailable.

"These women live in environments where they can't escape men who are drug abusers," said Dr. Sheldon Landesman, who is directing a study on AIDS and women at the State University of New York Health Science Center in Brooklyn. "And once large numbers of non-drug addicted women get infected, the ballgame's over."

Like so many of the infected women, Laura found out she harbored the AIDS virus after the last of her three children was born with the deadly disease.

"My first reaction was to put a pillow over the baby's face and to blow my brains out," she said in an interview in her room in a welfare hotel.

According to Laura's account, corroborated in large part by her social worker at a Bronx hospital, she was infected by a drug-abusing boyfriend. She is not herself an addict.

Laura's last name has been omitted. She is afraid of being located by her boyfriend, who she says beat her repeatedly.

Laura's boyfriend, the father of the sick child, was in jail at the time she and the baby were diagnosed. "If I had him in front of me, I'd have killed him with my bare hand," she said. "I'd feel better if I'd gotten the disease from drugs instead of from some low-life."

A 26-year-old high school dropout, Laura was told the devastating news about a year ago and it turned upside down a life that was already precarious.

Since then, she has been hospitalized twice in psychiatric wards.

She has placed all three of her children in foster care with relatives, because she was unable to cope with mothering them.

She returned to her boyfriend when he was released from jail because she was "afraid of being alone the rest of my life," then had unprotected intercourse and got pregnant.

He was still using drugs, stealing her welfare checks and beating her. So Laura fled, sleeping for several days on roofs and in stairwells before seeking help from her social worker.

Laura then had an abortion, and later a tubal ligation.

For a while, Laura abstained from sex, then she met a man and broached the subject of AIDS and condoms. Horrified, he disappeared.

Now, she said, she is dating another man who does not know she carries the virus, but who agreed to use condoms because he knows she spent years with a junkie and is therefore at risk. Laura fears the relationship will eventually be crippled by her dishonesty, but says she won't chance losing him because she can barely imagine life without a man.

"I finally met my Prince Charming and what can I give him?" she said.

Laura's social worker runs a support group for women whose lives have been scarred by AIDS. Here, with chairs drawn into a tight circle, working-class women and those on public assistance trade autobiographical stories, as college-educated, middle-class women did a dozen years ago, during the heyday of consciousness-raising groups.

"It helped me to realize I'm somebody," Laura said.

For now, Laura is free of the wasting symptoms of AIDS, but understands that in all likelihood she will get sick and die.

"I read the odds and the percentages," she said. "I know what will eventually happen. I'm scared, don't get me wrong, but as long as my kids are safe I can lie down and be at peace. I just hope I don't suffer much, but I try not to think about it a lot. The way I ruined my life, I know one thing — I'm not going up there to God."

More immediate for Laura is the sting of being shunned by some relatives. "I have an uncle who won't sit in the same room," she said. "I guess he's afraid he'll breathe my air. There are family things I'm not allowed at when he's there."

Laura's room in the welfare hotel is decorated with pictures of her children, clustered around her in happier times. Hanging from the mirror is a pair of baby shoes.

Laura writes letter to the children, intended for delivery after her death, that explain why she gave them up and how much she loved them. "The hurt I'm bringing to everybody else is what really bothers me," she said.

In some ways, Laura's situation represents a best-case scenario, since she has placed her children in stable homes, is using condoms and is not bearing children.

Far more common are the unruly lives that doctors and nurses grapple with in studies of women and AIDS now under way at Montefiore Medical Center in the Bronx and the Health Science Center in Brooklyn.

Studies such as these have helped establish the infection rate among women in New York City. Similar national data are not available, although experts estimate that at least 100,000 women nationwide probably carry the virus. While women represent 7 percent of the AIDS cases across the nation, they represent 11 percent in New York, where the drug abuse is endemic.

At the Brooklyn center, Dr. Howard Minkoff, director of obstetrics, is now treating 15 infected women who have each had one baby with AIDS and are in the midst of pregnancies.

At the Bronx hospital, according to Verna Robertson, a nurse practitioner involved in one AIDS study, none of the infected women use condoms all the time and more than half who become pregnant have their babies, despite being informed that there is a 50-50 chance the newborn will have the terminal disease.

"Translating awareness into behavior is most difficult," said Dr. Peter A. Selwyn of Montefiore. "Nobody has any magic solutions."

Among the infected women involved in these studies is Judy — her real name has been changed to protect her privacy — who is in a methadone program, expecting a baby and living in an abandoned building with a man who abusers her. "This AIDS is nothin'," Judy told her counselor. "I gotta worry where I'm gonna sleep tonight and whether he's gonna beat me."

Counselors who work in the inner city say these women and others believe themselves to be powerless to change their lives. "There's the sense that fates and destinies are in control," said Susan Homan, coordinator of the Brooklyn study.

Dooley Worth, who does similar counseling on the Lower East Side, says: "All the problems they live with on a day-to-day basis wind up making them so passive. For them, passivity is a means of coping."

For a woman infected with AIDS, or Acquired Immune Deficiency Syndrome, most counselors urge three behavior changes: using condoms, avoiding pregnancy and staying free of drugs. The last, they find, is the easiest.

"They feel they have more control over that than the sexual part," Ms. Robertson said. "You see, that's just dealing with their own behavior, not someone else's or the pressures of a relationship." Health experts report that all women have great difficulty persuading men to wear condoms but that such conversations are especially troublesome for Hispanic women, who account for more than a third of the local female AIDS cases.

According to Miquel Arenas, the director of an AIDS testing center run by the New York City Health Department, Hispanic men often refuse to use a condom and sometimes are abusive if asked. Mr. Arenas traced this attitude to "the sense of masculinity" that is so important to Latin men and the pervasive influence of the Catholic church in the barrio.

In the black community, there has been a longstanding discussion about whether encouraging the use of condoms is a form of population control.

"It can sound genocidal, or at least insensitive," said Suki Porfts, the director of the Minority Task Force on AIDS.

At Montefire, Dr. Selwyn said he agonizes over the implication of this sort of reproductive counseling. "When you're talking about AIDS and women, you're talking about blacks and Hispanics," he said. "There are people out there who would find it suitable if these women stopped having babies altogether. It is too easy to feed into those racist agendas."

The real danger, Dr. Selwyn said, is that counselors will ignore the hobbling circumstances of these women's lives. "Any intervention program must appreciate their situations," he said. "If you come in with a heavy-handed message, that is unacceptable for ethical and social reasons, and also won't have the desired effects."

Dr. Selwyn and his counterparts in Brooklyn described an attitude that would predispose a woman to continue a pregnancy even in the face of AIDS. In poor black and Hispanic communities, these experts say, women often depend entirely on their men and their babies for both pleasure and self-esteem.

"Reproductive and sexual relations are a very important part of their lives," said Dr. Minkoff. "It's not like they can say, 'I'm depressed so I'll go to Bloomingdale's.' "

"If they have a child, they're respected and valued."

The women sometimes explain that they want another child to leave something behind in the face of death, that they view a 50-50 chance of having a healthy baby as acceptable odds. But, counselors say, these explanations usually do not surface until a pregnancy has proceeded past the point when abortion is possible.

"They wind up having babies more by default than intent," Ms. Robertson said.

Rhonda, a 24-year-old Harlem women, was tested for the virus under prodding by physicians who were caring for her husband, a one-time drug user who already had an advanced form of AIDS.

She is one of the small number of women — several hundred out of the 50,000 who are infected — who have turned to the City Health Department for extended counseling.

"We're only seeing the most motivated ones," said Ms. Worth, whose counseling groups, at the Stuyvesant Polyclinic, are run in conjunction with the city.

The counseling begins either on a telephone hot line or at one of two city sites where 1,437 women have been tested for the virus, with 36 of them showing evidence of infection. Overall, 50,485 people have been tested city-wide, including those tested by their private physicians. Data are not available about the sexual breakdown of those tested or the percentage who are infected.

Experts have now extrapolated that 50,000 women are infected, most of them untested and unaware. They represent 3 percent of the city's women of reproductive age. The infection rate is thought to be 50 percent among women who use drugs and 20 percent among those whose mates are addicts.

Counselors at the test sites talk at length with their patients both before their blood is drawn and when they return several weeks later for the results. But, experts acknowledge that it usually takes weeks or months for the shock of a diagnosis to sink in, so the most useful counseling must come later.

Mr. Arenas, the director of a city test site, gives his patients information on follow-up care to pursue after their minds have cleared. But, since patients are identified only by a three-digit number, to maintain privacy, there is no way to keep in touch with them.

Most of them just get lost," Mr. Arenas said.

For the few who seek follow-up counseling, like Rhonda, there are common stages of denial, anger and a sort of uneasy acceptance. Often they talk of suicide, their counselors said, but they rarely kill themselves. Instead, slowly and painfully, they figure out whom to confide in, how to conduct their relationships with men, how to provide for the future of their children.

"As one of them said to me, 'Nothing about my life will ever be the same'," Ms. Worth said. "Getting by, day by day, that's the hard part."

Once the women understand that death is not necessarily imminent, they struggle with the agony of not knowing what will happen next. "I look in the mirror every day and ask myself 'Do I look sick?' " said Rhonda. "Every time I get a cold, I think I'm going to die."

Ms. Worth said the women in her group worry that every symptom is "the beginning of the downward trajectory." But, this reaction seems to be limited to the middle class. Among the poorest women, who are often indifferent or ignorant about health care, there is no demonstrated concern about their physical well-being, experts say.

Another telling difference between women of various socioeconomic backgrounds is their comfort in a group-therapy setting. Ms. Ports of the Minority Task Force noted that poor women, unlike gay men or women of the middle class, "are not able to talk it out, talk it out endlessly."

In counseling groups, a limited kind of control is offered as an antidote to the uncertainty and powerlessness that come with an AIDS diagnosis. Women are urged to eat well, get a lot of rest, exercise and stay off drugs, if they are former addicts. "People need to be able to feel they can have some impact," Ms. Worth said.

There was a time when counselors assured people that a positive test did not mean they would get AIDS. These days, they do not say that and instead skirt the issue.

As the epidemic progresses, it has become clear that virtually everyone who is infected will become gravely ill: "There is a persistent toll of morbidity and mortality that does not let up with time," said Dr. Stephen C. Joseph, the City Health Commissioner.

"I don't tell people they're not going to get sick," Mr. Arenas said. "But I also don't say everyone eventually gets AIDS. That would not serve any theraputic purpose."

Despite limited success in educating the women at highest risk, Dr. Joseph and others are determined to persevere, since their infection is the primary bridge that transports AIDS from the gay and drug-abusing worlds into the larger community.

Public health officials have been criticized in some quarters, including among feminists, for directing their preventive education at women, but Dr. Joseph defends this strategy as realistic and practical.

"Let me expose my own bias here," he said. "I think women generally have a more sharply defined sense of the future than men. And I think they tend to be more responsible about health issues. This is where we stand a chance of having some success."

* * * * * * * * *

Doctor With AIDS Permitted to Practice at Cook County
Reprinted with permission from *The New York Times*
July 14, 1986

CHICAGO, July 7 — County officials voted Monday to allow an AIDS-stricken physician to continue seeing patients at Cook County Hospital, but with sharp restrictions on which examination techniques he would be allowed to use.

It was disclosed in February that the physician, whose identity has not been made public, suffered from acquired immune deficiency syndrome.

On a 14 to 2 vote, the hospital board adopted a resolution that allowed the physician to continue work at Cook County but barred him from performing "invasive procedures" such as hypodermic injections and throat, rectal and vaginal examinations.

Objections to the decision were voiced by the Illinois chapter of the American Civil Liberties Union, which said the restrictions were unduly severe.

"He can't even check a patient for a sore throat," said an A.C.L.U. spokeswoman, Penny Strong, who said the group would urge the physician to take the matter to court as a discrimination case.

b. The Ethical Dimension

Only a Moral Revolution can Contain this Scourge

Immanuel Jakobowits, the Chief Rabbi, London
Reprinted with permission from *The Times*
December 27, 1986

I have delayed publicly expressing a view on the awesome menace of AIDS now hanging like a monstrous medieval plague over mankind, despite pressures from within my community and beyond to make some authentic Jewish pronouncement. This is due not merely to the fact that most authoritative Jewish statements on the moral issues were made thousands of years ago.

The earliest sources of Jewish law and morality are quite unambiguous. The Bible brands homosexual relationships as a capital offence (Lev. 20:13), and execrates any sexual licentiousness as an abomination, whether in the form of premarital "harlotry" (Deut. 23:18) or of extra-marital adultery (Lev. 20:10). Equally stern are the warnings of national doom consequent on any defiance of these principles: the land itself will "vomit out" peoples violating these injunctions (Lev. 18:28-29).

My hesitation in adding a Jewish voice to the many religious and moral statements already widely publicized, and worthy of endorsement, has been accentuated by the uncompromising nature of these biblical strictures. The difficulties go beyond the dilemma of choosing between soothing platitudes and unpalatable truths.

I am still racked by doubts on how to react to such a horrendous threat, how to address an age not exactly attuned to the puritan language of the Bible, how to transcend the perplexities which baffle medical and government experts, and how to present deeply held convictions without causing offence, panic, or disdain for the very teachings I espouse.

There are questions to which I simply know of no categorical answers. Some are practical: is it right to advocate "safe sex"? Or, should all citizens be subjected to screening tests to identify carriers and if so, how is this information to be used? Some questions are theological: can a disease like this, patently discriminating against certain sections of society, be attributed to divine wrath, or altogether be adjudged in moral terms?

And some are purely human: how can one reassure without spreading complacency, warn without condescension or self-righteousness, and highlight the horrific without inducing immunity to shock by horror? Altogether, are habits and behaviour susceptible to change by moral exhortation, by publicity campaigns, or even by medical information?

Inscrutable as the answers may as yet be, and rudimentary as may be our understanding of the long-term effects of AIDS and its spread, not to mention the prospects of halting its ravages, certain facts seem incontrovertible as a basis for some conclusions in the light of Jewish insights and moral principles.

Both at the individual and the public level, we are certainly never entitled to declare a particular form of suffering as a punishment for a particular manifestation of wrongdoing. We cannot more divine why some people endure terrible ills without any apparent cause than we can comprehend why others prosper though they clearly do not deserve their good fortune.

Even less are we ever justified in being selective, subjecting some scourges to this moral analysis while exempting others (AIDS, yes; but earthquakes or floods or droughts, no). There is no such simplistic relationship between evil and misfortune, if only because there are too many exceptions. According to Jewish exegesis, the prophet Isaiah had his lips scorched because he sinned in saying, "I dwell in the midst of people of unclean lips" (Is. 6:5-6).

There is all the difference — even if the distinction is a fine one — between ascribing massive suffering to personal or social depravity as a divine visitation, and warning that such depravity may lead to terrible consequences. If I warn a child not to play with fire, and it ignores the warning and gets burned, the hurt is not a punishment but simply a consequence. If people recklessly indulge in infidelity and end up in the agony of a broken marriage, they suffer no vengeance; they simply pay the inevitable price for moral negligence or turpitude.

Public information campaigns should therefore be explicit and unequivocal: AIDS is the price we pay for the "benefits" of the permissive society which, helped by the pill, liberal legislation and more "enlightened" attitudes, has demolished the last defences of sexual restraint and self-discipline, leading to a collapse of nature's self-defence against degeneracy.

An even greater price in human misery than deaths from AIDS is being paid for violating the imperatives of sexual morality: the devastation of the family, with millions of casualties, especially among young people driven to vice and crime by the absence of a loving home.

The provision of condoms, condoning and facilitating sexual irresponsibility, is therefore hardly the answer, even if they temporarily reduce the transmission of AIDS. They would only increase the ravages of personal degradation and social disintegration. In any case, what has to be carefully weighed is individual safety against the erosion of public standards. The principle is illuminated in a striking precedent — Jewish law and thought must invariably search for guidance in earlier sources.

A leading 15th Century Spanish-Jewish scholar objected to the establishment of facilities for communally controlled prostitution to keep licentiousness from running wild — even if this objection meant failing to prevent married partners from committing the capital offence of adultery (as implied in the Ten Commandments, Judaism makes no difference between killing a person and killing a marriage). He argued that however culpable individual indiscipline is, its mitigation cannot be sanctioned at the expense of the slightest public compromise with the Divine Law.

True, in Jewish law, the saving of life overrides all religious precepts. But even this pro-life stance has three cardinal exceptions: forbidden liaisons, murder and idolatry are proscribed even at the cost of life. This, too, would seem to rule out recourse to any measures, such as condoms for unmarrieds, which would encourage indecent conduct, though the rule might be invoked to treat more leniently the distribution of clean needles for drug-abusers.

No less important than clean needles are clean speech, clean thoughts and clean conduct. What will be crucial is the cultivation of new attitudes calculated to restore reverence for the generation of life and the enjoyment of sexual pleasures exclusively within marriage. Nothing short of a moral revolution will in time contain the scourge.

The role of governments in achieving these objectives is admittedly limited. Morality cannot be legislated, nor can politicians and civil servants become preachers. But the administrators of our national affairs cannot remain morally neutral either when the eventual cost may be counted in millions of lives.

Governments can help to refine human behaviour — for instance, by opposing any legislation liable to weaken the bonds between husband and wife or parents and children. Equally, governments can, by the careful use of language in official speech and documents, eliminate from the common vocabulary the kind of euphemisms or misnomers that make perversions acceptable. I think of words like "gay" for homosexual, "heterosexual" for normal, "safe sex" for inadmissible indulgence, and "stable relationships" for unmarried couples.

The Jewish experience demonstrates that in the final analysis only spiritual power is invincible as a shield against lust. This is perhaps reflected in observant Jews, however addicted to smoking, finding the Sabbath prohibition against lighting a cigarette far more effective than the most alarming health warnings in securing complete abstention from smoking for one day in seven.

They have also discovered that a conscience so trained prevails even in the most intimate relations between husband and wife: the religious ban on any physical contact for some 12 days in every normal month, regularly rejuvenating the marriage through an iron self-discipline, achieves more than the most skilled marriage counsellor could in regulating the rhythm of love and longing. Natural urges can be bridled in submission to a higher law.

What is needed then, is a massive campaign mobilizing government resources and citizens of all faiths and of one to strive for moral excellence, to avoid the arousal of passions in literature and entertainment, to extol the virtues of fidelity, and to promote the utmost compassion for those struck by a hideous killer as a result of ailings which may not be theirs but the society's into which they were born, and which to ennoble is the charge of us all.

Every action to promote these ideals has now become a lifesaving operation — including saving marriages as the sole legitimate origin of all human life.

Note: Sir Immanuel Jakobowiz is the author of *Jewish Medical Ethics*.

When Doctors Refuse to Treat AIDS

Editorial in the *New York Times*. August 3, 1987
Reprinted with permission.

Fear of AIDS has produced its most painful symptom yet: doctors and dentists who refuse to treat patients they believe to be infected with the AIDS virus.

"I've got to be selfish," says the chief heart surgeon at a Milwaukee hospital. "I've got to think about my family. That responsibility is greater than to the patient."

Any physician who holds that belief needs a new profession. The tradition of medicine rests four-square on the opposite proposition that a physician's first duty is to his patients. And the duty can be carried out without irrational fear, since the evidence shows little chance of contracting AIDS in caring for those infected.

Those who openly refuse to treat people with the AIDS virus stand in sad contrast to the physicians and nurses who unhesitatingly cared for the first AIDS sufferers. These health care workers, in the years before the cause of AIDS was discovered, had abundant reason to fear contracting the strange disease and infecting their families in turn.

Because of their courage, it is now well established that health care workers run very small risk of contracting the AIDS virus from their patients, and that the risk is essentially nil if they follow the precautions advised by the Centers for Disease Control. Even doctors or nurses who accidentally absorb AIDS-tainted blood are unlikely to be infected. Of 886 health care workers exposed through cuts or needle sticks, only three have tested positive for the virus. All three had breaks in the skin through which the virus may have passed, and one was exposed to the patients's blood for 20 minutes.

How paradoxical, then, that armed with this wealth of reassuring evidence, a number of doctors are now behaving as if they are at grave personal risk. There is every reason for health care workers to be careful, and last week the Centers for Disease Control convened a meeting to review new guidelines on how they can best protect themselves. But concern is different from an irrational degree of fear.

So far only a handful of doctors have openly refused to treat patients. The American Nurses Association states that nurses "are not backing away from caring for AIDS patients. They have from the beginning and they will to the end."

But among dentists in Chicago, so few are willing to accept AIDS patients that the Chicago Dental Society is considering setting up a special clinic. And a quarter of 258 doctors in training at New York hospitals said recently they thought it was ethical to refuse to treat people infected with the AIDS virus. When even medically trained people ignore medical evidence and succumb to panic, they set a miserable example for others in society who must deal with the disease and its carriers.

Six percent of those who have contracted AIDS through sexual contact or sharing contaminated needles are in fact health care workers. Patients could just as well refuse to be treated by any hospital staff who had not been tested for the AIDS virus.

Instead of public and physician each irrationally demanding the other be tested or rejected, both would do better to reaffirm the terms of the old ideal, that doctors are honored for selflessly caring for the sick.

"Don't Tell Me on Friday"

Thomas Richards
Reprinted with permission from *British Medical Journal*
April 5, 1986

I am a gay man who discovered last summer that I had antibodies to human T cell lymphotropic virus III. For me there are two central strands to the question of whether or not people should be tested for such antibodies; firstly, will knowing that you are positive help your own health; and secondly, will it make you more or less likely to infect others?

Like many people, when I first discovered that I was antibody positive I felt shock and disorientation. I woke up in the mornings shaking, had problems sleeping, and lost my appetite. I wrote a will, drank heavily, and seriously considered suicide. I thought, like others, that I was bound to develop acquired immune deficiency syndrome. [The newspaper] *Capital Gay* recently reported that a Newcastle conference on AIDS had been told of six people who had killed themselves on discovering that they were positive.

But, through good counseling from both the doctor at the special clinic and a clinical psychologist, after three to four weeks I got used to being positive. I was put in touch with a gay self-help group in London called Body Positive. The support, both practical and emotional, that both the psychologist and Body Positive gave were all important for me. Where I should have been without their help I dare not consider.

Such help should, I believe, be available to everybody immediately that they find out that they have antibodies. This belief explains my title because people should not be given this news if an appointment with a psychologist cannot be arranged until after a weekend — the first 72 hours are the worst. Given the restricted counseling facilities that are as yet available, I think it inevitable that doctors are going to have to make full use of voluntary organizations such as Body Positive.

Knowing that you are positive gives you a chance to alter your lifestyle. It becomes more likely that you will adopt a healthier diet and cut down on alcohol, tobacco, or cannabis. As an actor I decided that stress was my main problem, and I took up yoga for the first time in my life with great success.

The most important question is — will knowing that you are positive alter your sexual behavior? Gays in this country have up until now followed a free and easy existence. All we risked living in the "fast lane" was, it seemed, the occasional social disease. Clearly we must adopt a more responsible attitude, and it does seem that gay men who are discovered to be positive and who are properly counseled do behave responsibly and change their sexual practices. They follow the "safe sex" guidelines suggested by organisations such as the Terrence Higgins Trust.

While in a perfect world all gay men should for the last two years have adopted safer sexual practices, including the use of condoms, this is not a perfect world and they have not. The reality is that at one o'clock in the morning after four or five pints in a gay pub or club, gay men go home with each other without checking that one of them had condoms.

I do not advocate the compulsory testing of gay men. But so long as we understand the test and its limitations and so long as good counseling is available, I think we should be encouraged to take the test — both for our own good and that of the community, gay and straight. The decision must, however, reamin a personal one. My experience — and that of St. Mary's Hospital — is that those who change their behavior most are those who are tested, found positive, and properly counseled.

Thomas Richards is a pseudonym.

VI. We Get Letters

The Editors

The "Letters to the Editor" page is a hallowed institution in societies which enjoy a free press. It is a forum in which everyone can express his or her views and display his or her intelligence — or lack thereof!

The Letters to the Editor sections of scientific and especially medical journals often comprise many pages and are an important and well-read part of the publication. And, in most journals the greeting used by the correspondents is not "Dear Editor", but a collegial "Dear Sir", as though the writer were talking directly to colleagues at the workbenches and blackboards of the laboratories of the world. And, indeed he is.

A lot of the work of medical science is conducted in the "Letters to the Editor" pages. The quiet and sometimes tedious sorting out of anomalies in the nature of things are often worked out in this "dialogue between and among peers." There is no better way for a researcher in New Zealand to converse with a colleague in Boston than through the pages of his professional journal. It is easy to spot a trial balloon when a letter begins ..."we recently saw a patient in our clinic who...." One can observe, through a regular reading of the letters pages, the development of a picture, the parts of which are supplied by individual, isolated scientists responding from every corner of the world.

One such communication in 1981 presented the enigma of five young, seemingly healthy men in Los Angeles who had what their physicians considered a rare form of pneumonia which was "unusual" among this group of patients. And, it was noted, all five men were homosexual. The stream of letters which followed this seemingly simple observation became a rushing torrent which — within a few months — set off a scientific explosion which resulted in the identification, isolation, and potential control of the first epidemic of a viral disease in the history of modern medicine.

It is true, to a certain extent, that scientific efforts impact on the public consciousness only as "breakthroughs" or as "breakdowns". This is probably due to the modern press more than to the nature of modern scientific research. most scientists do work in windowless labs set off in mountain and lakeside spedor. Some work in secrecy, but most do not.

It is not that the scientists don't want people to know what they are doing, it's just that thy learned long ago that most people just don't care what is going on in those faraway laboratories until something goes wrong.

As can be seen from a close scrutiny of the progress of the work on unerstanding the AIDS virus, many things went right. As a matter of fact, when the final medical history of the AIDS epidemic is written, the scientists of the entire world will be held up as exemplary international citizens working for the general good of the world's peoples. Most of the mistakes (which seem to fascinate the press and the popular imagination) have taken place on a political, policy and legal level. The shame of delay, obfuscation and downright subterfuge can be laid at the doors of the legislative buildings, not the medical research laboratories.

Another phenomenon (which we will explore in Volume II), is the powerful reactionary forces which progress and modernization unleash in a society. When the public is faced with a mystery (and a potential threat) as deep as the AIDS virus and its diseases, panic, confusion, blame, and the lower instints of man rampage through the society — and as a reflection of that society — through the "Letters to the Editor" of the popular press.

The history of epidemics shows that the first reaction — not only of the victims, but of the general population — is denial. It can't happen to me, and it isn't happening here — and if it is happening, it is because "somebody else" brought it here.

The picture from the medical press is, however, a calm and long-term view of a problem which will not just go away, but must be discovered, analyzed, documented and treated. The popular press cries for the destruction of the individual who has the disease, the scientist calls for the destruction of the disease and the virus which causes it.

Someday the "Letters to the Editor" in the medical journals will be discussing a new and different threat to the health of the human body, but you can bet that the popular press will still be discussing AIDS and how it was caused by a nation which accepted evolution, marxism, scientific materialism and a liberal interpretation of the Ten Commandments of Moses!

* * * * * * * * * * * *

Condoms and AIDS Prevention

To *The Lancet* March 7, 1987

SIR, — Professor Kelly and Dr. St. Lawrence (Feb. 7, 1987) urge those who partake in penetrative sexual activities to refrain because, they argue, condoms (sheaths) have a substantial failure rate and are unreliable. Their view can only fuel the negative response that condoms have received.

While at the Middlesex Hospital, London, in 1983-84, I with others faced the need to advise homosexual patients who were at risk of HIV infection. I shall never regret my decision to advise those who felt they could not avoid anal intercourse about the advantages of sheaths. One had to do something. There was no evidence that a sheath would help prevent transmission of the virus but sheaths had had a significant effect on other infections and the abandonment of barrier methods of contraception had played a part in the increases in, for example, Chlamydia trachomatis, papillomavirus, and herpes simplex virus infection. It was reasonable to assume, therefore, that whilst a sheath might not always work, it would impede the spread of AIDS.

Sheaths are available fully tested to British Standard BS3704 and thick enough to withstand anal intercourse providing they are put on carefully and a water-based lubricant is used. Some sheaths are spermicidally lubricated. Without a sheath the risk of infection has been estimated as about 1 percent for each act of anal intercourse with an HIV antibody positive partner. Even if sheaths fail occasionally their regular use should lower the rate of cross-infection with the virus.

Many homosexuals practice anal intercourse rarely or never, and many are monogamous. Of those who do not have a stable relationship and who also practice anal intercourse, some feel that to give up this practice would be to give up sex altogether. Advice therefore has to be practical, and it should include accurate and positive information about the use of condoms and about the risks of penetrative sex, especially receptive anal sex.

Lloyd Clinic,   S.J. Tovey
Guy's Hospital
London

* * * * * * * * * * * *

To *The Lancet*
March 7, 1987

SIR, — Although condoms are not 100 percent reliable, much better figures than those cited by Professor Kelly and Dr. St. Lawrence have been reported. In three large series the use-effectiveness of the condom ranged from 0.8 to 4.8 per 100 women at one year. To enhance contraceptive effectiveness condoms should be used with a spermicide, and such preparations probably protect against sexually transmitted viral infections. According to Hicks et al., "HIV is inactivated in vitro in one minute by 0.05 percent nonoxynol-9, a compound present at concentrations of 5 — 12.5 percent in several spermicides widely used in Europe." The argument that only radical changes in sexual mores will substantially reduce the spread of HIV is correct — but meantime the use of barrier methods must be emphasized.

Department Of Obstetrics   Michel Thiery
University Hospital
Gent, Belgium

* * * * * * * * * * * *

To *British Medical Journal*
October 26, 1985

SIR, — AIDS is recognised to be a sexually transmitted viral disease and many of those afflicted in Europe and North America are homo sexual men. Homosexual male communities have been addressed by pamphlets and advertising campaigns recommending diverse "safer sex" practices. Nearly all these efforts advocate, without qualification, use of the rubber condom, but little information is available about the efficacy of the condom as a viral barrier. We have found only two published studies on the testing of condoms with any virus. Barlow compared the incidence of diverse sexually transmitted disease, including herpes and warts, among a group of clinic attenders and a subpopulation of condom users. His data included too few patients to judge the viral efficacy of the condom. In a limited in vitro study, Conant et al, investigated leakage of Herpes simplex through two brands of condoms. Their methodology was reasonable, but the number of replicate tests of each brand was not given, and only two brands were studied, making the findings of little value to potential users. By contrast, large numbers of replicated (161) were regarded as essential for the physical testing of condoms by a respected American product testing institution, the Consumers Union. It reported laboratory testing of American brands of rubber and skin condoms and found significant leakage in some brands, as well as substantial differences among brands. The Consumers Union also reported variable degrees of deterioration in a third of the 21 rubber brands tested. Because of various failure rates in some brands, it is repeatedly recommended using a condom with a vaginal contraceptive jelly, cream, or foam and advised against using petroleum based lubricants because they weaken latex.

Condoms inflated with air or water are generally stable; leakage is slow. In view of the small molecular weights of water and of the gases in air, it seems logical that vastly larger viruses would disperse through the walls with difficulty. Therefore, we conclude that condoms are probably of substantial value as a prophylactic against transmission of diseases. In view, however, of the Consumer Union's findings and of many studies of condom failure rates, and since AIDS is a mortal disease, knowledge of the degree of virus leakage is essential. That information does not exist, although it could be obtained readily by laboratories working with the AIDS virus. We believe that there is an urgent need for such research on condom efficacy, including adequate replicate testing and adequate brand sampling. Meanwhile, even though we believe that condoms afford a substantial degree of protection and their use should be encouraged, that encouragement should be tempered with cautionary warnings discouraging increased sexual activity. Users should be told of the risks. "Safer sex" guidelines that we have seen rarely, if ever, provide instruction in the proper use of the condom. The Consumers Union reported that the commonly cited 10 percent "use failure rate" for condoms is significantly reduced when improper use is eliminated from data. Consequently, educational instruction in correct usage is important.

Bruce Voeller
The Mariposa Foundation
Los Angeles California

Malcolm Potts
Family Health International
Research Triangle Park, N.C.

* * * * * * * * * * * * * *

Condoms Prevent Transmission of AIDS-Associated Retrovirus

To *JAMA*
April 4, 1986

To the Editor. — The majority of cases of acquired immunodeficiency syndrome (AIDS) have occurred after exposure to seminal fluid, blood, or blood products. It has been recommended that individuals avoid contact with seminal fluid through the use of prophylactic sheaths, although the proof that the virus could not pass through these commercial products has not been established. In previous studies we demonstrated that herpes-virus could not pass through condoms. We have now performed similar studies to determine whether retroviruses would be retained by these materials.

Report of a Study. — For the experiments, both a mouse retrovirus and the AIDS-associated retrovirus (ARV-2) were employed. A solution of tissue-culture medium containing either 10(7.3) infectious mouse xenotropic type C retrovirus particles per milliliter or 10(6) infectious ARV-2 particles per milliliter was used. The plunger from a 12-mL syringe was placed inside the condom, to which was added 4 mL of the virus-containing medium. The condom was then placed inside the syringe barrel and the entire unit was submerged in a beaker containing 2.5 mL of tissue-culture medium supplemented with 10 percent fetal calf serum and antibiotics.

The procedure involved 15 cycles of aspiration and expulsion of the tissue-culture medium surrounding the barrel of the syringe. In this manner, tissue-culture fluid was drawn through the syringe in very close proximity to the condom, which was subjected to the pressure created by the aspiration of the plunger within the condom. The condom was subsequently removed from the syringe barrel and its distal surface containing the viral fluid was placed directly in the tissue-culture medium for 30 minutes on ice.

The tissue-culture fluid on the outside of the condom was then assayed for the mouse xenotropic virus on mink S + L-cells and on mink lung cells, as described previously. By this latter technique, the inoculated mink lung cells were passed weekly for three weeks and then assayed for infectious virus through focus formation in mink S + L-cells. Infectious ARV-2 was measured by induction of particle-associated reverse transcriptase activity and ARV-2 antigens in cultured mitogen stimulated normal human peripheral mononuclear cells.

Comment. — The Titers of the viruses before these experiments were substantial and were well above levels found in seminal fluid. Following the experiments, no infectious virus was found present in the tissue culture fluid placed in close contact with the prophylactics. These experiments, particularly those with the mouse retrovirus, which was present in exceptionally high titer, conclusively indicate that retroviruses cannot pass through the condom membranes. The data mirror the observations made with herpesvirus. These results should encourage persons known to be at risk for passing or contacting the AIDS virus to use condoms as a safety procedure.

University of California	Marcus Conant
at San Francisco	Denise Hardy
	Judith Sernatenger
	D. Spicer
	J.A. Levy

* * * * * * * * * * * *

AIDS and the Heterosexual Epidemic

To *The Lancet*
April 18, 1986

Sir, — Sir John Rawlins was concerned about apparent disparities in information on AIDS emerging from the medial profession (11 Apr, p. 970). Although it is unrealistic to expect the profession to speak with one voice on this matter any more than it does on any other, perhaps I can resolve some of the misunderstandings. Dr. Moss's point was that among heterosexuals the group most likely to become infected with the human immunodeficiency virus (HIV), and hence to pass it on heterosexually, are drug misusers; this relates to the probability of a sexual partner being positive.

The quotes from Professor Adler and myself relate to the risk of HIV transmission between a seropositve man and a seronegative woman during conventional vaginal intercourse. Both statements are broadly correct when applied to regular partners, but the interpretation that has been put on them leads to misunderstanding. Sexually active people, including drug misusers, appear to transmit infection to their regular heterosexual contacts in about 50 percent of instances (range 35 — 85 percent); this is similar to data for regular homosexual contacts. These figures therefore seem to be relevant to the vast majority of settings for potential heterosexual transmission.

In haemophiliacs the situation seems to be different, with only 5-10 percent of sexual partners becoming infected, and it probably cannot be used as a surrogate for heterosexual transmission generally. Firstly, some seropositive haemophiliacs may not be infected with HIV but only "immunised" with the virus that has lost viability but not antigenicity during processing of factor VIII; this might also account for the apparently lower rate of progression to the acquired immune deficiency syndrome in this group. Secondly, haemophiliacs tend to have fewer sexual partners, so they have a lower incidence of other sexually transmitted infections. This could reduce the number of target lymphocytes and macrophages in semen and hence reduce the amount of infectious virus in haemophiliacs; preliminary unpublished evidence supports this. Finally, few reports include sufficient data about the sexual activity between such couples, which may be pertinent.

It is a common fallacy to think that by counting the number of AIDS cases one has an estimate of the scale of the epidemic. Yet by the time the first cases of AIDS were reported in the USA in 1981 there was already a 24 percent seroprevalence of HIV infection among San Francisco homosexuals. There are now over a thousand heterosexually acquired cases of AIDS in the USA and probably 50-100 times that number of HIV positive. In Africa the scale is vast. We are certainly seeing cases of heterosexually acquired HIV infection and AIDS in the UK but fortunately the number is relatively small.

We thus still have time to establish new patterns of sexual behaviour that will limit the extent of the problem. Prevention means acting before you have a problem, which is why the government's education programme and its broad focus were correct and indeed farsighted. We, and other countries where the epidemic is relatively small, have a brief opportunity that we cannot afford to miss. In fact, there is a remarkable consensus on many points about AIDS and HIV among my colleagues, but the medical and lay media do not always reflect it.

St. Mary's Hospital   Anthony J. Pinching
Medical School
London

* * * * * * * * * * * * *

Lack of HIV Infection and Condom Use In Licensed Prostitutes

To *The Lancet* December 13, 1986

SIR, — Licensed prostitutes in West Germany have a human immunodeficiency virus (HIV) antibody prevalence rate of 1 percent and unlicensed prostitutes have a prevalence of 20 percent. This difference has not been explained although intravenous drug usage is more common in unlicensed prostitutes. Any data on variable rates may provide useful information to limit the spread of HIV infection.

448 licensed female prostitutes in Nuernburg, West Germany, were studied in March and April, 1986. The city has a population of about 500,000, with 25,000 US Army personnel. One percent of US soldiers presenting to the sexually transmitted disease clinic are Western blot positive and about 1.6 per 1,000 US soldiers are Western blot positive.

89 percent of the licensed prostitutes were tested for HIV antibody by enzyme-linked immunosorbent assay and positives were confirmed by immunofluorescence test. 50 percent of the prostitutes completed an anonymous questionnaire, providing demographic data and details on sexual practices.

No prostitute tested was anti-HIV positive by immunofluorescence. All prostitutes were German or other Western European. Their mean age was 30 years (range 18-62) and they had been prostitutes for 77 months on average (range 1-480). The mean number of clients was 13 per week (range 1-50). 21 percent regularly had US military clients and 2 percent of the prostitutes regularly had African clients. One was an intravenous drug user, 10 percent had tattoos, and 1.8 percent had had intimate contact with a person in an AIDS high risk group.

Thirteen percent practise open-mouth kissing with clients. Seventy-four percent occasionally to always masturbate clients, eighty percent with condoms; sixty-three percent occasionally to always perform oral sex, ninety percent with condoms; ninety-two percent occasionally to always have vaginal sex with clients, 97.5 percent do this with condoms; and 5 percent occasionally to always have rectal sex, 55.5 percent with condoms.

This heterosexually very active group of women has remained free from HIV infection. The demographic mix of their clients, the absence of intravenous drug abuse, and the frequency with which condoms are used for all sexual practices may be protecting these prostitutes from infection.

US Army Hospital   Gergory L. Smith
Nuernberg, W. Germany

Yale Univ. Medical School   Kevin F. Smith
New Haven, Conn.

* * * * * * * * * * * * *

Condom Use And HIV Infection Among Prostitutes In Zaire

To *The New England Journal of Medicine* February 5, 1987

To the Editor: Sexual contact, whether heterosexual or homosexual, is the most important mode of transmission of the human immunodeficiency virus throughout the world. Epidemiologic data, combined with the finding of HIV in seminal fluid, cervical secretions, and blood, provide a theoretical basis for the recommendation by the U.S. Public Health Service that use of condoms by homosexuals or heterosexuals may offer protection against HIV transmission.

A recent report presented experimental evidence that despite mechanical stresses, condoms provide an effective barrier against HIV. We report epidemiologic evidence that condoms may reduce the risk of HIV acquisition through sexual intercourse.

In late 1985, 377 female prostitutes were enrolled in a study of sexual practices and HIV seroprevalence in Kinshasa, Zaire (Project SIDA). Serum samples were considered positive if they were repeatedly reactive on the enzyme-linked immunosorbent assay and were confirmed as positive on immunoblot examination. Participants were interviewed by trained Zairian staff, and responses were recorded on standardized forms. Of 376 prostitutes who responded to questions about condom use, 88 (23 percent) reported that at least one of their sexual partners during the previous year had used a condom. Of these women, 85 quantified their partners' use of condoms. Seropositivity according to category of condom use was as follows: partners not using condoms, 26 percent (74 of 288); fewer than 25 percent of partners using condoms, 35 percent (19 of 55); 26 to 49 percent of partners, 32 percent (7 of 22); 50 to 74 percent of partners, none of 2, and 75 percent or more of partners, none of 6.

There was a significant difference in seropositivity among the eight women reporting condom use by half or more of their partners (none of 8, as compared with women reporting less frequent use (26 of 77, 34 percent) (P = 0.046). The two groups of women had similar numbers of annual and lifetime sexual partners, no differences were noted in the distribution of other potential risk factors for HIV, including types of sexual contact, age, previous injections, or blood transfusions.

Conclusive evidence to support the value of condoms in preventing transmission from infected partner to uninfected partner (man to woman, woman to man, or man to man) will remain difficult to collect, and retrospective studies such as ours, which rely on the participants' recall of specific sexual and contraceptive behaviors must be interpreted with caution. Nevertheless, the combination of experimental evidence and our preliminary epidemiologic data supporting the protective potential of condoms, along with evidence that they offer protection against other sexually transmitted viral diseases, suggests that the proper use of condoms may help prevent sexual transmission of HIV.

Jonathan Mann, M.D.
Centers for Disease Control,

Peter Piot, M.D.
Inst. of Tropical Med.

Henry Francis, M.D.
Nat'l Institute of Allergy
and Infectious Diseases

Robert Byers, PhD
Centers for Disease Control
Atlanta, GA, US

Pangu Kasa Azila, M.D., MPH
Ngandu Kabeya, M.D.
Dept. of Public Health
Kinshasa, Zaire

Thomas Quinn, M.D.
Nat'l Inst. of Alergy
and Infect. Dis.

Ngaly Bosenge, M.D.
Nzila Nzilambe, M.D.
Mpunga Kalala, M.D.
Dept. of Publ. Health
Kinshasa, Zaire

Robert L. Colebunders, M.D.
Inst. of Tropical Medicine
Antwerp, Belgium

James W. Curran, M.D.
Centers for Disease Control

* * * * * * * * * * * * *

Heterosexual Promiscuity Among African Patients With AIDS

To *The New England Journal of Medicine* July 18, 1985

To the Editor: The overview of the epidemic of the acquired immu-nodeficiency syndrome (AIDS) presented by Landesman et al. (Feb. 21 issue) stressed the important point that the disease may be spread-ing among heterosexual populations and its possible link to female prostitution. In this respect, data from Central African countries, where AIDS occurs almost exclusively among heterosexual people, are very indicative. We recently collected base-line information on the sexual life style of 58 African men with AIDS or the AIDS-related complex; the diagnoses were made in 33 in Kigali, Rwanda, and in 25 in Brussels, as previously reported. These data indicate that, as com-pared with healthy controls match for sex, age, geographic and ethnic origin, and annual income, the patients had a significantly higher median number of different heterosexual partners per year and also had more frequent contact with prostitutes. We defined regular con-tact with prostitutes as sexual intercourse with prostitutes at least once a month in the previous two years.

In addition, of 42 African women in whom AIDS or the AIDS-related complex had been diagnosed in Brussels and Kigali, 10 (24 percent) were professional prostitutes. In none of these women, nor in any of 33 Rwandan prostitutes studied prospectively did we find a history of addiction to parenteral or nonparenteral drugs. This is in sharp con-trast to the assertion of Landesman et al., that "A link between prosti-tutes who use nonparenteral drugs and HTLV-III serpositivity is also suggested from studies in Africa and Haiti."

In Central Africa, infection with HTLV-III or lymphadenopathy-associated virus is linked to heterosexual promiscuity and female prostitution. However, it is likely that other cofactors, yet to be determined, are necessary to permit the expression of the full-blown syndrome.

St. Pierre Univ. Hospital   N. Clumeck
Brussels   P. Van de Perre

Free Univ. of Brussels   M. Carael
Instit. of Sociology
Brussels, Belgium

Centre Hospitalier de Kigali   R. Rouvroy
Kigali, Rwanda   D. Nzaramba

* * * * * * * * * * * * *

AIDS and Sexual Behavior In Gay Men

To *American Journal of Public Health* December 1985

Although McKusic, et al., document a desirable trend with respect to high-risk sexual behavior among homosexual men in San Francisco, the overall results of their study are discouraging. Despite the authors' statement that men not in monogamous relationships made "substantial reductions in high-risk sexual activity," the proportion of respondents who had receptive anal intercourse (without a condom) with non-regular partners in the preceding year declined by less than 10 percent. The reductions in other high-risk practices were similar. In the context of the severity of AIDS, these changes are almost ludicrous. The study was conducted in 1982 and 1983, and it might be argued that further changes have been made subsequently; however, the authors' recent update showed similar results through 1984, and similar data have been reported from Chicago. Marked decreases in the incidence of gonorrhea in gay men in several cities have been cited as evidence of salutary changes, but gonorrhea is a self-limited infection whose incidence and prevalence may be greatly influenced by modes of behavioral changes, especially if fear of AIDS leads to more frequent medical examinations during which gonorrhea screening is performed. The prevalence of AIDS virus infection, by contrast, is cumulative, and much more substantive behavioral alterations are needed if the epidemic is to be curtailed. For example in Seattle, where up to one-third of gay men are infected with the AIDS virus, a marked reduction in high-risk sexual contacts from 10 to 2 partners annually still confers a 55 percent risk of exposure; in San Francisco, where two-thirds of gay men may be infected, there would be an 89 percent chance of exposure. We lack sufficient understanding of the determinants of sexual behavior to know why so many persons continue high-risk practices with multiple partners. One element, however, may be the absence of risk-reduction guidelines that are based on an objective interpretation of the available epidemiological data and that do not minimize the issues. Clearly gay men should be advised to abstain from all but monogamous sexual activity in permanent committed relationships. "Safe sex" guidelines for new or casual partnerships should be presented only as a distinct second choice; the prudent person does not take even a 1 percent chance of exposure to a deadly communicable disease. These are the guidelines of the Seattle-King County Department of Public Health, and they mirror the views — in private conversations, but not always in public forums — of most epidemiologists, biomedical AIDS investigators, and many gay leaders. By analogy, the fact that most persons who drink and drive do not heed our advice to stop does not deter us from giving it, and we do not tell drinkers they may drive if they use seat belts and stay under 30 miles per hours.

Seattle-King County Dept. of   H. Hunter Handsfield, MD
Public Health
Harborview Medical Center
Seattle, WA

* * * * * * * * * * * *

Transplacental Transmission of HTLV-III Virus

To *New England Journal of Medicine* May 16, 1985

To the Editor: Epidemiologic studies of the acquired immunodeficiency syndrome indicate a horizontal transmission primarily through blood, semen, and possibly saliva. Vertical transmission of the disease to children by transplacental infection has also been suggested. We report further evidence strongly suggesting the occurrence of vertical transplacental transmission of human T-cell lymphotropic virus Type III (HTLV-III).

We studied a premature child born by cesarean section after 28 weeks gestation to a mother with terminal AIDS. The mother died two hours after delivery. No opportunistic infection developed in the child, who had normal values for total T lymphocytes and lymphocyte subsets and no anti-HTLV-III antibody, as tested by the enzyme-linked immunosorbent assay in serum. He had not received blood or blood products. He died at 20 days of age with severe hydrocephaly and sequelae of intracerebral hemorrhages. Tissue samples were obtained at autopsy; light microscopical examination of the thymus, lymph nodes, spleen, and Peyer's patches was normal.

IgG against HTLV-I, HTLV-II or HTLV-III was chromatographically purified from plasma obtained from patients with AIDS or normal

Haitians, assayed for specificity by Western blot technique, conjugated with rhodamine, and used for identification of specific antigens in frozen sections of the child's thymus by means of direct, double-staining immunofluorescence.

IgG against HTLV-III yielded a positive reaction by Western blot with HTLV-III infected H9 cells. Rhodamine-conjugated IgG against HTLV-I or HTLV-II did not react with sections of thymus obtained from the patient. Rhodamine-conjugated IgG against HTLV-III did not react with sections of control thymuses but reacted strongly with the thymus of the infant, displaying a cytoplasmic fluorescence of cells mostly located around Hassall's bodies and lymphatic and blood vessels. This pattern of fluorescence remained unchanged after previous incubation of thymus sections with IgG against HTLV-I or HTLV-II. HTLV-III containing cells reacted with fluorescein-conjugated monoclonal antibodies against helper/inducer T cells (OKT4+, Ortho-mune), as demonstrated by direct double-staining immunofluorescence. In some sections of the deep cortex, however, HTLV-III expressing cells did not react with OKT4 monoclonal antibodies. These cells have not yet been identified.

Since the child was born by cesarean section and had no contact with his mother after gestation, these findings strongly suggest transplacental transmission of HTLV-III. In addition, expression of HTLV-III antigens in OKT4+ cells is further evidence for the lymphotropism of the virus.

Hopital Sainte-Justine   Normand Lapoint, MD
Montreal, Quebec   Jean Michaud, MD
                             Draska Pekovic, MD
                             J.P. Chausseau, PhD
                             Jean-Marie Dupuy, MD

* * * * * * * * * * * * *

Possible Transmission of a Human Lymphotropic Retrovirus (LAV) from Mother to Infant with AIDS

To *The Lancet* July 28, 1984

SIR, — Reports of acquired immunodeficiency syndrome or related syndrome in infants born to parents at risk for AIDS suggest vertical transmission of an agent, the main candidates being the human T-lymphotropic virus(es) known as LAV (lymphadenopathy associated virus) and HTLV-III. Evidence for the involvement of LAV in AIDS includes isolation of this retrovirus from stimulated T lymphocytes in patients with AIDS, a high prevalence of antibodies against the virus proteins in patients with AIDS or with a related syndrome, and a selective tropism of LAV for the T4 lymphocyte subset, with depression of cell growth and even a cytopathic effect. We now report a possible transmission of LAV from mother to infant in three unrelated families whose members have manifestations of AIDS or of related syndromes.

The immunological methods and the methods for isolating and characterising LAV, and studying antibodies by a radioimmunoprecipitation assay (RIPA) which detects IgG antibodies against LAV p25 protein and an enzyme-linked immunosorbent assay with purified viral antigens have been described elsewhere. No family had an AIDS risk factor other than ethnic origin and no infant had a history of blood transfusions.

In family 1, a 4-month old Haitian boy presented with lymphadenopathy. Hepatosplenomegaly, failure to thrive, and *Pneumocystis carinii* pneumonia were subsequently noted. Disseminated *Mycobacterium bovis* infection was diagnosed 4 months after inoculation with BCG, and neurological impairment with cortical brain atrophy was observed. Symptoms of AIDS progressively developed in his mother post partum. Only the non-identical twin sister remained healthy with normal immunological investigations. LAV was isolated from stimulated T-lymphocytes and detected by reverse transcriptase activity in cell-free supernatant in the infant with AIDS, in his mother, but not in his healthy twin sister. LAV antibodies were found in the whole family, except for the healthy twin.

In family 2, also Haitian, both parents exhibited symptoms of AIDS without any opportunistic infection. Their only child presented with diarrhoea a few days after birth and he had enlarged lymph nodes. LAV was not sought but LAV antibodies were detected in the serum of the patient and of his parents.

In family 3, a 1-month old Zairian infant had recurrent diarrhoea, severe sepsis, hepatosplenomegaly, and lymphadenopathy, followed by candid oesophagitis and interstitial pneumonia. Cytomegalovirus was isolated from blood at the age of 15 months. The father was healthy and immunological tests were normal. The mother had the first symptoms of AIDS less than 2 months after delivery and died 10 months later from multifocal infections. Immunological investigations during the first 4 months of life did not demonstrate immunodeficiency. Between 5 and 7 months, T3+ lymphocytes fell to 3 percent (of 700 lymphocytes/ul) and T4+ lymphocytes disappeared from her blood; the absolute number of B lymphocytes increased.

Despite hypergammaglobulinaemia, production of antibody to vaccinial and to viral antigens was defective. LAV-associated reverse transcriptase was detected in the supernatant of stimulated T lymphocytes from the mother but not from the father or from the child. Only the mother had LAV antibodies.

In the thirty-four published cases of AIDS or related syndromes in infants (including our three), the fact that first symptoms were present by one month of age in 25 percent of patients raises the possibility of in utero vertical spread. In family 2, transmission of LAV probably occurred in utero since the infant had the first symptoms of AIDS very soon after birth. In family 3, the lack of retrovirus detection and the absence of immunodeficiency in the father together with an early separation of the infant from the mother (before the infant was 1 month old) suggest a similar prenatal transmission. LAV was not isolated in this infant, probably because T4 lymphocytes, the target cells of this retrovirus, had disappeared. Impaired humoral immunity may also explain why antibody to LAV was not produced. The progressive decrease of antibodies to LAV in an AIDS patient with haemophilia B supports this interpretation. In family 1, a postnatal transmission could not be excluded because symptoms started later and because the father also had symptoms related to infection.

The IgG antibody to LAV found in infants 1 and 2 could not be of maternal origin because the titre remained stable up to 9 months after birth. Furthermore, the healthy twin had no LAV antibodies at 7 months of age. We do not know why the twin has escaped symptoms of LAV infection. Longitudinal studies in infants born to mothers at risk for AIDS and harbouring LAV are needed to confirm an in utero viral transmission. Another point is that the severity of symptoms of AIDS observed after pregnancy suggests that immunological changes during pregnancy may modify the host-retrovirus relation.

Hopital des Enfants Malades   Etienne Vilmer
Paris, France   Alain Fischer
                                     Claude Griscelli

Institute Pasteur   Francoise Barre-Sinoussi
Paris, France   Veronique Vie
                                     Jean Claude Chermann
                                     Luc Montagnier

Hopital Claude Bernard   Christine Rouzious
Paris, France   Francoise Brun-Vezinet

Hopital La Pitie Salpetiere   Willy Rosenbaum
Paris, France

* * * * * * * * * * * *

AIDS and Breast Milk

To *JAMA* January 24, 1986

To the Editor. — In the Aug. 16, 1985 issue of JAMA is a book review favoring the value of human milk banking. Recently Ziegler et al., reported a case where a newborn apparently contracted the acquired immunodeficiency syndrome virus through breast milk from his mother. The child was delivered by cesarean section and the mother contracted the AIDS virus after blood transfusion given in conjunction with her cesarean section. In the reported case, the blood transfusion was given after delivery, and the baby was breast-fed for six weeks. Thirteen months later, AIDS developed in the donor of one of the units of blood used for transfusion, resulting in testing of the mother and the child.

Both the mother and the child were then found to be HTLV-III positive. The mother had AIDS-related complex. The baby had a transient episode of failure to thrive and then developed lymphadenopathy and eczema but was otherwise well. The woman's husband and the other siblings were seronegative for the AIDS virus.

The AIDS virus has been demonstrated in semen, saliva, and tears. There is no reason to expect that the virus would not be present in breast milk of an infected woman. Ziegler recommends that until more studies are done on the possible transmissibility of the AIDS virus in breast milk, that lactating women who are in high-risk groups for infection with AIDS should be advised of the possibility of the transmission of this virus to their children.

We suggest that pending the results of these further studies, the same screening policies and procedures that are currently being used to ensure the safety of human blood be applied to human milk bank donors.

Martin Luther King Jr.   Jonathan Wasserberger MD
General Hospital   Gary J. Ordog, MD
Los Angeles, CA   John J. Stroh, MD
                               Subramaram Balasubramanaram, MD

* * * * * * * * * * * *

Isolation of AIDS Virus From Cell-Free Breast Milk of Three Healthy Virus Carriers

To *The Lancet* October 19, 1985

SIR, — AIDS in infants probably results, in some cases, from contact with maternal blood during delivery. However, transplacental transmission has been reported. Postnatal transmission was strongly suggested when AIDS developed in a breastfed baby whose mother had been virus-free at birth but became infected after a blood transfusion. While looking for HTLV-III/LAV carriers in families of patients with AIDS or AIDS-related complex we decided to attempt virus isolation from breast milk.

To detect virus, carriage lymphocytes were stimulated with phytohaemagglutinin (PHA) and cultivated for 4 weeks with recombinant interleukin-2 (Transgene). Extracts were taken twice-weekly for solid-phase radioimmunoassay with rabbit hyperimmune serum against HTLV-III, monoclonal antibodies directed at HTLV-III p24 and p15 and at p15 rabbit or antimouse Ig labelled with iodine-125. In the culture supernatants, virus-particle bound reverse transcriptase was assayed.

To detect virus in breast milk, a 1 ml sample was centrifuged for 20 minutes at 2300g. The layer between the lipid supernatant and the cell pellet was filtered through a 0.22 um Millex filter and was inoculated, half onto a 10 ml suspension containing 10 X 10(6) H9 cells and half onto lymphocytes preactivated with 5 ug/ml PHA and cultivated with IL-2. Cell suspensions were treated with 2 ug/ml polybrene and some lymphocyte cultures were also treated with 500 units/ml of antibody to a-interferon.

In family 1, the 5-month old infant was admitted to hospital with splenomegaly, intermittent fever, failure to thrive, and diarrhoea without pathogen isolation. She had not been given any blood product and was breastfed. The father was Belgian born, and the mother had been born in Zaire. In family 2, the index case was a 32-year-old Belgian man who had lived in Zaire for the previous 10 years and was admitted to hospital in Kinshasa in August, 1983, with diarrhoea, weight loss of 15 kg in 3-4 weeks, and adenopathy. He had received transfusions but no blood product. His health improved, he regained 5 kg, and he was symptomless when he came to hospital in Liege, where generalized lymphadenopathy was found. His wife was Belgian. She was delivered of a normal child who was breastfed for a month. The family went back to Zaire and has not been followed up. Family 3 was from Rwanda. The infant had a maculopapular rash at 2 months of age and began to show failure to thrive and fever. When 5 months old, she was transferred from Kigali to Brussels with interstitial pneumonia.

All five milk samples provoked appearance of HTLV-III antigens in 7-15 days when inoculated onto H9 cells. A strong cytopathic effect necessitated addition of non-infected H9 cells to keep the cultures growing. Filtered supernatants from the milk-inoculated H9 cells infected Hut 78 cells, and the appearance of RT activity, and Hut 78 cells proved no less sensitive to the virus cytopathic effect than H9 cells had been.

The milk samples were also inoculated to primary lymphocyte cultures grown with IL-2 after stimulation with PHA. Results were negative with milk from the two first mothers studied. When investigating the third case, we added IFN-a-antibody and twice isolated virus, indicating that IFN-a may prevent the growth of HTLV-III/LAV before establishment in a continuous cell line.

When the possibility was raised previously that breast milk could transmit AIDS, it was suggested that lymphocytes in milk might harbour the virus and so transmit infection even in the presence of serum and milk antibodies. Attempts to grow lymphocytes from milk meet with problems of bacterial infection. Our studies on cell-free filtered milk suggest that extracellular virus was present, probably in large amounts. Presence of free virus does not necessarily mean that breast milk is contagious, because to initiate infection the virus must first bind to receptors on cells such as T4 lymphocytes. Two mothers had antibodies to HTLV-III in their serum and antibodies or virus-antibody complexes in milk should now be investigated. Even so our findings may be clinically and epidemiologically important.

Institut Pasteur de Brabant   L. Thiry
Brussels, Belgium

Free Univ. of Brussels   S. Sprecher-Goldberger

Hopital St. Pierre   T. Jonckheer
Brussels, Belgium   J. Levy

Hopital de Baviere   P. Van de Perre
                                     P. Henrivaux

Univ. of Leige   J. Cgoniaux-LeClerc
Institut Pasteure de Brabant

Hopital St. Pierre   N. Clumeck.

* * * * * * * * * * * *

Breastfeeding and HIV Infection

To *The Lancet* August 15, 1987

SIR, — Concern has been expressed about the possible role of breastfeeding in the transmission of HIV infection. We have reviewed data on the first 83 infants enrolled in the European collaborative study of infants born to HIV-positive mothers. Eleven (13 percent) have been breast fed for 1 week to 7 months. Six infants have lost antibody, are clinically well, and have been negative on virus and antigen tests. Three infants are antibody positive and remain well, but they are still too young for us to be sure whether they are infected or retaining maternal antibody.

Two of the 11 breast fed infants are infected and have AIDS or AIDS-related complex. One has had lymphadenopathy, hepatosplenomegaly, and neurological signs since the age of 2 weeks, had a positive viral culture at 4 months, and had chronic parotitis at 9 months. The second child had generalized lymphadenopathy and oral candidiasis at 8 weeks and died of disseminated cytomegalovirus infection at 7 months. It is likely that both infants were infected in utero.

There is a single published report of HIV isolation from the non-cellular fraction of breast milk but unsuccessful attempts at isolation may have gone unreported. The only case-report attempting to link breastfeeding with transmission of HIV infection concerned a child breast fed for 6 weeks, whose mother presumably seroconverted after receiving a blood transfusion after a cesarean section. It was not until 13 months later that the blood donor was found to have AIDS. When the first immunological tests were done on the mother and her infant at 17 months, both were HIV positive, while the father and older children were antibody negative. Although other forms of close contact with mother could not be excluded, there were no other risk factors for HIV, and breastfeeding seemed to be the most likely route of infection.

At least 6 of our 11 breast fed babies have apparently escaped HIV infection despite feeding for up to 7 months. Although these numbers are too small to make any definitive statement, they do add to the impression that the relative contribution of breast feeding to HIV transmission is probably small compared with that of intrauterine transmission. Breast feeding shortly after acquisition of HIV, as in the case of post partum transfusions, may be a special case carrying a higher risk of viral transmission. To extrapolate from this special group to HIV-positive mothers who were seropositive before delivery is not justified in the light of current knowledge.

Since it is not possible to distinguish between intrauterine, intrapartum, and postnatal infection using current laboratory techniques, the level of risk involved in breast feeding can only be assessed by following up from birth cohorts of breast fed and bottle fed infants of HIV-positive mothers.

Institute of Child Health
London, UK

Y.D. Senturia
A.D. Ades

University of Padua
Padua, Italy

C.S. Peckham
C. Giaquinto

* * * * * * * * * * * * *

Female-To-Female Transmission of HIV

To *The Lancet* August 15, 1987

SIR, — Dr. Monzon and Dr. Capellan's report of apparent female-to-female transmission of HIV (July 4) has potentially serious implications for safe-sex guidance and demands close scrutiny. Women who are exclusively homosexual rarely have serious sexually transmissible infections other than genital herpes, which is acquired principally by receptive cunnilingus. However, syphilis, gonorrhoea, chlamydia, trichomonas, hepatitis B, and human papillomavirus may occasionally be transmitted orogenitally, digitally, or via shared sex toys and close traumatic genital contact.

The report suggests that HIV was transmitted orogenitally, but most safe-sex guidelines list cunnilingus as a medium to low risk activity, where low risk means "almost certainly no risk whatsoever". Although HIV can be isolated in low titer from saliva there is no good evidence to show that it could be of sufficient concentration or viability to be transmissible; active or receptive anilingus has not been associated with anti-HIV seropositivity in homosexual men, and there were no seroconversions among thirty doctors and nurses who had repeated lacerations and skin-puncture bites from a brain-damaged, HIV antigen-positive haemophiliac. While vaginal and cervical secretions can contain small quantities of HIV — and this is a proposed mode of female-to-male infection — orogential contact not involving semen is most unlikely to be responsible for HIV transmission between women or between men and women. However, when offering practical advice to those who are concerned about remaining theoretical risks of bidirectional infection from enthusiastic exchange of saliva and vaginal secretions, the use of a thin adhesive deformable barrier membrane might be recommended for safe cunnilingus and anilingus: at a practical demonstration of such a product, experienced users reported a moderate loss of sensitivity with good protection from body fluids.

In contrast to a previous, well-documented case, Monzon and Capellan do not seem to have asked about shared use of sex toys, biting, or other traumatic sexual practices causing vulval or vaginal bleeding. These are high-risk activities. Detailed inquiry is essential whenever HIV transmission is thought to have occurred in unusual circumstances.

Royal Northern Hospital   Peter Greenhouse
London, UK

* * * * * * * * * * * *

Drug Addiction and Fear of AIDS

To *The Lancet* January 17, 1987

SIR, — *Lancet* letters reporting a reduction in gonorrhoea and syphilis among homosexual men suggest that this might have been due to fear of AIDS. AIDS is a sexually transmitted disease for homosexuals, bisexuals, and heterosexuals, but it is essentially a parenterally transmitted disease and in Italy 44 percent of AIDS cases are in drug abusers; Italy also has a high proportion of paediatric AIDS cases (7 percent) and all have been born to women with antibodies to human immunodeficiency virus. We have seen a trend, similar to those reported for sexually transmitted disease, but in heroin addicts. Our infectious diseases department has recorded a striking fall in admissions for acute viral hepatitis in addicts in the last 18 months, especially in the second half of 1986. Over the same period increasing numbers of heroin addicts have been seeking methadone detoxification.

HEROIN ADDICTS WITH ACUTE VIRAL HEPATITIS ON SEEKING METHADONE TREATMENT IN 1985 AND 1986

	1985		1986	
	Jan–June	July–Aug	Jan–June	July–Dec
AVH	38	24	12	2
Methadone	25	37	50	75
HIV-Ab positive	19/63	17/61	18/62	31/77
	(30%)	*(28%)*	*(29%)*	*(40%)*

AVH = acute viral hepatitis. Methadone = under methadone maintenance therapy.

These results suggest a change in behaviour. Acute viral hepatitis is acquired during the first months of heroin abuse show a sharp reduction in incidence among addicts is likely to have been caused by the fear of AIDS, either discouraging young people from experimenting with drugs and/or inducing heroin addicts to use more sterile injection practices and to avoid the exchange of syringes. The rise in numbers of requests for detoxification demonstrates an increase in addicts trying to escape their addiction. We conclude that information campaigns and a fear of AIDS achieved a reduction in numbers in one group at risk for AIDS.

Ospedale Regionale, R. Pristera
Bolzano, Italy M. Casini
 F. Perino
 A. Degiorgis

* * * * * * * * * * * * *

AIDS and Health-Care Workers

To *The Lancet* January 24, 1987

SIR, — Dr. Searle's investigation (Jan. 3) of health professionals' attitudes towards AIDS reveals a disturbing degree of ignorance and misconception among surgeons and a mixed group of other consultants. One group of clinicians who have to make important decisions relating to human immunodeficiency virus infection yet have hardly any experience was not mentioned. Last year, in this department of obstetrics and gynaecology with thirteen junior staff, two of the four registrars, the senior registrar, and all six consultants had never seen or managed a patient with AIDS, while most other juniors had gained such experience in general or genitourinary medical posts. Indeed, medical students are more likely to have had contact with such patients than their obstetrics teachers.

Pregnancy accelerates progression from asymptomatic HIV infection to AIDS and AIDS-related complex faster than any other factor; maternofetal HIV transmission occurs in up to 65 percent of cases; and, in women who become pregnant when they have AIDS or ARC, maternal and fetal mortality approaches 100 percent. Antenatal, pre-conception, and family planning clinics are among the few clinical settings in which knowledge of a high-risk individual's HIV status is of value in directing management, although limited published experience and lack of treatment options currently restrict action to avoidance or termination of pregnancy in those who are seropositive.

In recognition of these risks, the Royal College of Obstetricians and Gynaecologists commissioned an expert review of AIDS in relation to obstetric care; despite this, at a meeting of the Royal Society of Medicine in May, 1986, most obstetricians appeared to support blanket antenatal HIV antibody screening without pre-test counselling, a policy that may be medicolegally unsound. Furthermore, of ten researchers presenting papers of obstetric relevance at the International Conference on AIDS in Paris, in June, 1986, all but one commented that their gynaecological colleagues' overriding concern was the risk of acquiring HIV infection from their patients, which is virtually non-existent.

All districts should formulate and implement a policy on antenatal management in the presence of HIV infection. However, those who have chosen the best policy — pre-test counselling for high-risk women — may be hampered by lack of specialised counsellors or the money to pay for them, a situation which must be remedied urgently. Whilst genitourinary physicians are happy to advise and assist in the management of HIV-affected mothers, they are too overstretched to cope with a flood of unnecessary counselling requests caused by inappropriate antenatal screening. Gynaecologists must recognise and train for their responsibilities in counselling and management of HIV infection, for all branches of medicine must share the increasing burden of HIV infection.

Royal Northern Hospital   Peter Greenhouse
London UK   Philip Palmer

* * * * * * * * * * * *

Seroepidemiology of Human Immunodeficiency Virus in Africa From 1970 to 1974

To *The New England Journal of Medicine* August 13, 1987

To the Editor: The acquired immunodeficiency syndrome was recognized for the first time in Africans soon after its appearance in the United States. The origin of AIDS remains enigmatic and controversial. Several investigators have questioned, mainly on the basis of false positivity, the validity of certain seroepidemiologic evidence suggesting that the disease originated in Africa. Nonspecific reactions due to cross-reactivity with other distantly related retroviruses and cellular antigens (DR4 and other HLA types), the "stickiness" of serum and high titers of antimalarial antibodies, and immune complexes have been shown to be fairly common sources of false positive results in the serum of Africans. Other studies do not support the hypothesis that AIDS originated in Africa or was present before the late 1970's.

From 1970 to 1974, a trial of a pneumococcal vaccine was conducted in black mine workers in South Africa. Alequots of serum collected during this trial were stored at -20C until November 1986, when they were tested for antibodies to HIV. Participants in the vaccine trial came from Mozambique (1191 subjects), Malawi (1080), South Africa (171), Botswana (32), Angola (29) and Swaziland (16). Initially, all serum samples were screened with the Abbott enzyme immunoassay for HTLV-III, but because this test yielded many false positive results, screening was done with the Wellcozyme antiHTLV-III test and all positive samples were subjected to further testing by indirect immunofluorescence (the H9/HTLV-III cell line was kindly supplied by Dr. R. Gallo), Elavia enzyme immunoassay, and Western blotting (duPont strips).

Of the 2,574 specimens tested, 11 were found to be positive with the Wellcozyme test; of these, 6 were confirmed as positive with indirect fluorescence. Most specimens had low titers. None of the 11 positive samples on the Wellcozyme test were found to be positive with the Elavia enzyme immunoassay or Western blotting. Two samples (one from a worker from Malawi and the other from Lesotho) that were positive on the Abbott enzyme immunoassay and indirect fluorescence but negative on the Wellcozyme and Elavia tests gave only moderate staining with Western blotting to P17, 24, 35, 41, 55,

65, and 120. These two samples were tested further with the Abbott antigen-capture test and were found to be negative.

This study has confirmed that in testing serum from Africans that has been stored frozen, false positive results and lack of uniformity in the results of various methods can be expected. The results of the present study fail to provide conclusive evidence of HIV infection in southern Africa in the early 1970's and are in keeping with those of Wendler et al., Levy et al, and Lyons et al. In a comparable group of mine workers surveyed in 1986, the prevalence of HIV infection was found to be 3.71 percent in Malawians and 0.07 percent in Mozambicans.

Institute for Med. Research   R. Sher
Johannesburg, S.A.   S. Antunes

Rand Mines   R. Reid
South Africa   H. Falcke

* * * * * * * * * * * * *

HTLV-III/LAV-Seronegative, Virus-Negative Sexual Partners and Household Contacts

To *JAMA* April 4, 1986

To the Editor. — Public concern about the transmissibility of human T-cell lymphotropic virus type III/lymphadenopathy-associated virus (HTLV-III/LAV) has been heightened by several reports suggesting the existence of an antibody-negative, virus-positive state in some asymptomatic sex partners of persons who are antibody positive. We recently evaluated 88 household members and/or sex partners of persons with hemophilia and found that only two nonhemophiliacs were HTLV-III/LAV antibody positive. We report herein the results of culturing peripheral blood lymphocytes of 20 of the nonhemophiliac contacts whose index hemophiliac was antibody positive.

Report of a Study. — These contacts included ten of 14 sex partners of 12 persons with either the acquired immunodeficiency syndrome or the AIDS-related complex, two of 16 sex partners of asymptomatic hemophiliacs, and eight household members who were not sex partners (four fathers, three mothers, and one brother of six asymptomatic hemophiliacs aged 5 to 13 years). Sex partners reported having vagnal or oral intercourse from fewer than once to eight or more times per month (median, four to eight times per month); other household members had nonsexual contact with the index hemophiliac. Participants were 15 to 71 years old (median 34.5 years).

Serum samples were collected under sterile conditions and cells were frozen and stored at -60C until tested. Serum samples were assayed for the presence of antibody to HTLV-III/LAV structural proteins by Western blot analysis using the methods of Tsang et al. Lymphocyte samples were cocultured with phytohemagglutinn-stimulated lymphocytes, to which 5 percent interleukin-2 had been added. Lymphocyte cultures were monitored for viral replication with immunofluorescence and particulate reverse transcriptase assays by persons who were unaware of the characteristics of the donors. When evidence of infection was noted by these methods, the cells were also examined by electron microscopy for viral particles.

Only one household member was virus positive. She was the wife of a hemophiliac patient with AIDS and, at the time of evaluation, she was both antibody positive and an AIDS patient. The remaining sex partners and household members had had no detectable HTLV-III/LAV antibody or virus.

Comment. — These results, in contrast to those of two frequently quoted reports, suggest that sex partners, as well as household contacts who are not sex partners of hemophiliacs, are seldom antibody negative and virus positive. However, virus may be present in the lymphocyte of some asymptomatic persons at titers too low to produce infectivity in culture. Furthermore, the number of persons tested in both studies is quite small and thus the significance of these disparate findings will be determined by further studies.

Centers for Disease Control   Terri McFadden
Atlanta, GA   Janine M. Jason, MD
                                  Paul Feorino, MD

* * * * * * * * * * * *

Minimal Risk of Transmission of AIDS-Associated Retrovirus Infection by Oral-Genital Contact

To *JAMA* April 4, 1986

To the Editor. — The San Francisco Men's Health Study is a prospective study of a population-based random sample of single men 25 to 54 years of age residing in the 19 census tracts of San Francisco with the highest incidence of acquired immunodeficiency syndrome. One thousand thirty-five eligible men were recruited. Participants visit the study clinic at six-month intervals, where they undergo a detailed medical and life-style interview and physical examination and provide specimens for laboratory study. Serological testing for AIDS-associated retrovirus (ARV) is performed on the cohort using the indirect fluorescent antibody technique.

Between June 1984 and January 1985 at the time of the first clinic visit, 214 exclusively heterosexual men were found to be uniformly seronegative for antibodies to ARV and will not be considered further in this communication. At that time, the overall seropositivity rate for the remaining 821 homosexual and/or bisexual men was 48.4 percent. Fifty-six of the homosexual and/or bisexual men studied gave a history of continuing to engage only in oral-genital contact but no rectal intercourse (either insertive or receptive) in the two years prior to entry into the study. An additional 15 men gave a history of having no sexual partners during the same two-year period. The ARV serological tests on these two groups of individuals compared with those who continued to engage in rectal intercourse revealed a very low rate of infection.

Since our cohort was recruited between June 1984 and January 1985, this two-year period goes back to late 1982, by which time 118 cases of AIDS had been diagnosed in San Francisco, the sexual transmissibility had been established, and educational efforts to alter risk behavior had been initiated. Compared with men who had no sexual partners in the prior two-year period, the men who continued to engage in oral-genital contact only did not have an increased rate of infection by ARV (P>.0001). Moreover, we found in a more detailed sexual practices interview at subsequent clinic visits that all of the 14 seropositive men had engaged in receptive anal intercourse prior to June 1982. In contrast, only 24 of the 50 seronegative men in these two groups had engaged in previous receptive anal intercourse (P<.001). These results may not completely exclude the possibility of transmission of ARV infection by oral-genital contact because they are based on a small number of observations. They do, however, show no excess risk of infection by this route and support the theory that anal-genital exposure is the major mode of infection. An extended report describing the distribution of sexual practices and ARV serology is in preparation.

Univ. of California at Berkeley   David Lyman, MD
                                  Warren Winkelstein, MD

Univ. of California at San
Francisco

Michael Ascher, MD
Jay A. Levy, MD

* * * * * * * * * * * * *

AIDS and Promiscuity

To *The Lancet* October 25, 1986

SIR, — The behaviour of the most promiscuous one or two percent may be more influential than the average number of partners in determining the rate of spread of venereal disease. This neglected aspect of infectious disease epidemiology may be important for measures to limit the AIDS epidemic. A risk of human immunodeficiency virus infection of 1 percent per sexual contact with an infected person is arbitrarily assumed in the following simple model, from which only qualitative inferences can be drawn.

Consider a population in which 98 percent have three sexual contacts every 100 days (low promiscuity) and 2 percent have three sexual contacts every 2 days (high promiscuity). If each sexual contact is equally likely to be with a member of the "low" or "high" population, the prevalence of HIV infection will increase in a way shown in the figure, rising from an assumed initial prevalence of 0.01 percent to 38 percent within 10 years. The increase is not exponential, since virtually all "high promiscuity" individuals are infected within 5 years and then constitute a constant source of infection for the rest of the population. (This roughly linear pattern has been observed in both San Francisco and New York.) If, on the other hand, the contact rate is wholly that of the less promiscuous 98 percent, the proportion infected even after 20 years would be less than 0.1 percent. The rapid spread of AIDS among homosexual men may thus have been due to the influence of a small minority who are very promiscuous. More radical changes in behaviour are, however, needed to control an established epidemic: if the more promiscuous 2 percent of homosexuals switch to the less promiscuous contact rate five years after the start of the epidemic, when the prevalence is 12 percent, the subsequent rate of increase is reduced by the prevalence would still be 30 percent after a further 10 years.

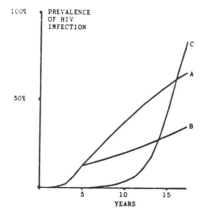

Prevalence of HIV infection, assuming risk of transmission of 1% per contact and initial prevalence of 0·01%.

(A) 2% have 1-5 contacts per day, remainder 1 per month.
(B) As for (A) the promiscuous 2% adopting the lower contact rate after 5 years.
(C) Annual change of regular sexual partner.

These calculations are not relevant to homosexual men who live with a regular partner. Unfortunately, a homosexual who has a series of monogamous relationships lasting a year may eventually be at greater risk than a "low promiscuity" individual who has one new contact a month. If the risk of infection is 1 percent per contact, the probability that the partner of an infected individual will become infected within a year is almost 80 percent, for intercourse three times a week. The prevalence in a population of couples who take a new partner annually, again assuming an initial prevalence of 0.01 percent, increases very rapidly. Venereal disease cannot spread in a strictly monogamous society, but if partners are changed occasionally the rate of spread of infections such as HIV, where the risk of transmission per contact is low, may depend largely on the frequency of intercourse. Paradoxically, therefore, the rate of spread can vary inversely with the number of different sexual partners.

This alarming prediction may be approximately correct for the regular partners of infected homosexual men, but the prevalence of HIV seropositivity in the wives or partners of infected haemophiliacs is only 10 percent or so. This suggests that a risk of infection per contact of 1 percent is much too high for heterosexual intercourse, at least for haemophiliacs. The risk is probably lower for vaginal than for anal intercourse, but it may be that only a minority of infected men are highly infectious (if so, contact tracing might provide an effective means of control). In the absence of studies on heterosexual transmission in the general population, it is impossible to predict whether

AIDS will soon spread rapidly into the heterosexual population, as it has in parts of Africa.

These speculative simulations indicate that a promiscuous minority probably played a major role in the emergence of the AIDS epidemic in homosexuals, and suggest that a similar epidemic could develop among single heterosexuals who have a series of monogamous relationships. The only firm conclusion, however, is that without better epidemiological data on transmission, contact, and seropositivity rates we cannot predict the eventual scale of epidemic or plan effective action to limit it.

Institute of Cancer Research   Julian Peto
Surrey, UK

* * * * * * * * * * * * *

Association Between HTLV-III/LAV Infection and Tuberculosis in Zaire

To *JAMA* July 18, 1986

To the Editor. — Immunosuppression caused by drugs, infections, cancer, or other conditions is known to increase the risk of tuberculosis. Studies of patients with the acquired immunodeficiency syndrome and of the incidence of tuberculosis in young men in selected US cities suggest that an increased risk of overt disease among persons previously infected with the tubercle bacillus may be associated with human T-cell lymphotropic virus type III.

Project SIDA is a collaborative AIDS research project in Zaire, involving the Zairian Department of Public Health, the Public Health Service, and the Institute of Tropical Medicine, Antwerp, Belgium. In March 1985, project researchers determined the prevalence of antibody to HTLV-III/LAV in 231 (84 percent) of the 274 inpatients of the tuberculosis sanatorium in Kinshasa, Zaire.

Of the 231 study participants, 159 (69 percent) had confirmed pulmonary tuberculosis. Of these 159, 96 (60 percent) were men and 63 (40 percent) were women; the median age was 29 years.

Of the 159 confirmed pulmonary patients, 53 (33 percent) were repeatedly HTLV-III/LAV seropositive by enzyme-linked immunosorbent assay; all of the 43 serum samples tested thus far have been confirmed by Western blot testing. In contrast, the prevalence of confirmed HTLV-III/LAV antibody in healthy hospital personnel 20 to 49 years of age in Kinshasa is 4 percent to 8 percent.

Among patients with tuberculosis, there was no association between HTLV-III/LAV infection and age, sex, a history of tuberculosis, extent of roentgenographic lesions, having received bacillus Calmette-Guerin vaccine, or date of diagnosis. Twenty-nine percent of patients who were HTLV-III/LAV seropositive and had tuberculosis also had an anergic reaction to 5 tuberculin units of intradermal tuberculin, compared with 19 percent of seronegative patients.

The presence of HTLV-III/LAV antibody in patients with tuberculosis was significantly correlated with a history during the past two years of severe weight loss (<10 percent of body weight) with or without prolonged fever (less than one month's duration) or chronic diarrhea (more than two months' duration). In patients with tuberculosis, lymphadenopathy on physical examination was equally common in those who were HTLV-III/LAV seropositive and those who were seronegative (35 and 32 percent).

Practitioners and public health workers, especially in developing countries where tuberculosis is a common disease, should be aware of the association between HTLV-III/LAV infection and tuberculosis. Infections with HTLV-III/LAV may substantially complicate both management of individual patients with tuberculosis and public health strategies for tuberculosis control in developing countries.

Project SIDA
Kinshasa, Zaire

Johathan Mann, MD Dixie E. Snider, Jr. MD
Henry Francis, MD Thomas C. Quinn, MD
Robert L. Colebunders, MD Peter Piot, MD
James W. Curran, MD Nzila Nzilambi, MD
Ngaly Bosenge, MD Matiatudila Malonga, MD
Dikilu Kalunga, MD Masaki Mu Nzingg, MD
Nkoko Bagala, MD

* * * * * * * * * * * * *

Prevention of AIDS: Lessons from Osler

To *The New England Journal of Medicine* June 12, 1986

To the Editor: In the absence of effective treatment for AIDS, efforts to contain the disease are focused on the control of transmission. Recommendations include a reduction in promiscuous behavior among homosexuals, and heterosexuals alike. Heterosexual contact with prostitutes is especially discouraged.

In 1892, Sir William Osler, in his classic textbook *The Principles and Practice of Medicine*, discussed prophylaxis for another sexually transmitted disease — namely, syphilis. The measures that he recommended for the prevention of syphilis are similar to those now being publicly advocated for AIDS, although described with much more elegance.

"Irregular intercourse has existed from the beginning of recorded history, and unless man's nature wholly changes — and of this we can have no hope — will continue. Resisting all attempts at solution, the social evil remains the great blot upon our civilization, and inextricably blended with it is the question of the prevention of syphilis. Two measures are available — the one personal, the other administrative.

Personal purity is the prophylaxis which we, as physicians, are especially bound to advocate. Continence may be a hard condition (to some harder than to others), but it can be borne, and it is our duty to urge this lesson upon young and old who seek our advice in matters sexual. Certainly it is better, as St. Paul says, to marry than to burn, but if the former is not feasible there are other altars than those of Venus upon which a young man may light fires. He may practise at least two of the five means by which, as the physician Rondibilis counselled Panurge, carnal concupiscence may be cooled and quelled — hard work of body and hard work of mind. Idleness is the mother of lechery; and a young man will find that absorption in any pursuit will do much to cool passions which, though natural and proper, cannot in the exigencies of our civilization always obtain natural and proper gratification.

The second measure is a rigid and systematic regulation of prostitution. The state accepts the responsibility of guarding citizens against small-pox or cholera, but in dealing with syphilis the problem has been too complex and has hitherto baffled solution. On the one hand, inspection, segregation, and regulation are difficult, if not impossible, to carry out; on the other hand, public sentiment, in Anglo-Saxon communities at least, is as yet bitterly opposed to this plan. While this feeling, though unreasonable, as I think, is entitled to consideration, the choice lies between two evils — licensing, even imperfectly carried out, or widespread disease and misery. If the offender bore the cross alone, I would say, forbear; but the physician behind the scenes knows that in countless instances syphilis has wrought havoc among innocent mothers and helpless infants, often entailing life-long suffering. It is for them he advocates protective measures.

Mayo Clinic   Marvin A. Vaughan, MD
Rochester, MN   James T.C. Li, MD

* * * * * * * * * * * * *

AIDS Information — Safe Sex

To *The Lancet* November 1, 1986

SIR, — "Safer sex" guidelines, such as those issued in the UK by the Terrence Higgins Trust and the Health Education Council, are crucial to the effort to limit the spread of human immunodeficiency virus. They recommend reducing the number of sexual partners and avoiding contact with potentially infected blood or secretions, with emphasis on avoiding penetrative intercourse unless using a condom. The campaign has been directed mainly towards sexually active homosexual men. Have these guidelines affected the sexual behaviour of this target group?

In the United States three surveys have demonstrated significant changes in gay male sexual behaviour during the AIDS epidemic. In a Canadian study gay men were found to have decreased their numbers of partners and changed sexual practices, but it is not clear whether the men had access to guidelines on safer sex In an attempt to assess the impact of guidelines we have done a survey of 326 gay men in the pubs and clubs of central London. Four interviewers, gay men themselves, approached a wide cross-section of men and asked questions about their sexual practices.

Three hundred-ten men (95 percent) had had information on safer sex; 250 (77 percent) said that AIDS had changed their sex life; 162 (50 percent) said they knew someone with AIDS, and 96 (29 percent) used condoms:

(1) How have you reacted to safer sex information?

Welcomed and followed it	75%
Seen it but had no effect	18%
Resented it	2%
Not seen it	5%

(2) Which of the following do you do?

Anal intercourse	53%
Orogential sex	79%
Oroanal sex	38%
Kissing	93%

Mutual masturbation	92%
Sadomasochistic sex	24%

(3) No. of sex partners in previous month

0	19%
1	41%
2-5	35%
6-10	4%
11-20	2%

(4) No. of sex partners compared with previous year

More	10%
Same	41%
Fewer	48%

Of the 174 men who have anal intercourse, 45 percent now use condoms, this figure is 59 percent in those men who had had intercourse with more than one person in the previous month. Knowing someone with AIDS significantly correlates with having fewer sexual partners than in the previous year (55 vs 40 percent; $p<0.01$). Of the 16 men (5 percent) who said they had not seen safer sex information, 3 said they used condoms, and this probably means that the message was passed along on the grapevine.

This sample of sexually active gay men reported changes in sexual behaviour, in part related to knowing someone with AIDS. The vast majority of gay men had seen safer sex guidelines, and many are attempting to follow them, by, for example, starting to use condoms. Our findings have appeared in simplified form in Capital Gay and are likely to have been read by up to 40,000 gay men and women. This may itself have had an educational effect, and we plan to repeat the survey in six months' time.

2, Chapel Cottages   S.W. Burton
East Garston   S.B. Burn
Berkshire, UK   D. Harvey
                            M. Mason
                            G. McKerrow

Testimony before the
Social Services Committee
on Problems Associated
with AIDS
House of Commons, London, 1986-1987 session

MEMORANDUM BY THE CONSERVATIVE FAMILY CAMPAIGN

We recommend a 10-point plan be enacted by Her Majesty's Government to curb the spread of AIDS.

1. AIDS should become a notifiable disease.

2. Testing for the disease should be offered nationally to every citizen on a voluntary basis in the first instance; and also be undertaken for all visitors to this country from known AIDS infected areas.

3. Victims of the AIDS virus should be placed in isolation hospitals. The Christian Hospice Movement should be actively encouraged and assisted so they may become the major caring vehicle running the isolation establishments which need to be funded and run in such a way that the last months of the victims lives are as dignified as possible.

4. The 1967 Sexual Offences Act should be repealed thus re-criminalising homosexuality. We believe this will contain homosexual acts, and by making homosexuality illegal once again, schools will have to teach all young people what the law is. This would have a considerable effect on stopping young boys and girls choosing a homosexual or lesbian lifesytle which, unfortunately, is being actively encouraged in some places at the moment.

5. We do not want drug addiction to be encouraged by the Government with the supply of needles because with the nature of the drug

culture needles are bound to be shared, or sold to raise cash to buy further drugs.

6. A massive research programme funded substantially by Government working in collaboration with the private sector, should be initiated to try to discover a cure for AIDS and a vaccine to stop it spreading.

7. Contraceptives should be made available for married couples only. NHS subsidy for the contraceptive pill should be stopped. The whole thrust of DHSS and NHS policy must be to encourage chastity before marriage, and fidelity and faithfulness within marriage.

8. The advice given by the DES to the governing bodies of schools who, under the 1986 Education Act will be responsible for determining sex education curriculum in state schools, should uphold the law, namely, "the value of family life". This means that teaching must reiterate that for public health reasons, if for none other, there is chastity before marriage and fidelity and faithfulness within marriage. It follows from our earlier recommendation regarding the recriminalisation of homosexuality that this would obviously be taught as illegal, undesirable and a public health risk.

9. Government support and, in particular, funds should be withdrawn from organisations which have adopted a clearly promiscuous propagandist position on sexual activities. We think in particular here, for example, of the Terrence Higgins Trust which is an organisation designed to present homosexuality as respectable, and the Family Planning Association who for a number of years have put forward ideas incompatible with morality and conducive to promiscuity. Conversely, we believe that Government support should be given to bodies promoting family values and to those offering Christian counselling services to help homosexuals refrain from their practices. An example of the former organisations should be the MEdical Education Trust and the National Campaign for the Family, whilst examples of the second organisations are Turning Point, Pilot, True Freedom Trust and Courage.

10. The Tax and Social Security System needs to be radically overhauled to promote and reward marriage.

We believe that the package needs to be viewed as a whole and to take individual elements only would not be effective or desirable. We also believe that it must be understood that it is in part the permissive society itself which has allowed the creation of a disease as horrible as AIDS. We strongly recommend members of the Select Committee to read the article in *The Times* of Thursday, 20 November by Ronald Butt — "Making Capital out of AIDS."

Sadly we believe that the Government's advisers on this issue are those very same people who have been responsible for spreading the permissive society message through the DHSS, NHS, DES and various other bodies including the Health Education Council, Family PLanning Association, etc. A clean sweep of these sort of people is going to be required and their replacement by those who uphold moral standards, preferably Christian moral standards, is going to be required before politicians are going to receive the correct advice on how AIDS can be handled as a public health risk, which is what at its simplest it is.

We suggest to the Committee that you have to recognise that a medical profession which can allow the slaughter of two and a half million children through the 1967 Abortion Act, and which is prepared to supply contraceptives to enable girls under the age of 16 to engage in promiscuous sexual activity which is bound to affect their health let alone their mental state, and which appears to condone homosexual practices and other abnormalities, eg the BMA in one of its recent books puts forward the proposition to teenager that they could experiment with bondage; then those in the medical profession who claim to speak on their behalf are no longer upholding high professional ethical standards which we came to expect from them. Fortunately there are still doctors in all areas of the profession who do understand the difference between right and wrong, good and bad, and moral and immoral. Increasing numbers of these doctors have been joining with us and other organisations because not only do they know that the action currently being advocated to deal with AIDS will be ineffective and is wrong, but also because they know that the advice being given to the public is incomplete. Not all the facts are being given, and that is one of the most disturbing features of the AIDS issue at present. Much is unproven and unknown. With something which is incurable and where there are many unknown elements, surely the action which should be taken needs to be particularly drastic until we can be more sure of the fullest extent of the danger to the whole population. Some examples of what we mean are that generally spokesmen on behalf of the Government or the medical profession say that they now believe that the 30 percent of AIDS carriers will become victims and will, therefore, die. This is an increase on the 10 percent figure which was being used only 12 months ago. In fact the most recent research based upon a full European study undertaken by Frankfurt University has shown that 75 percent of AIDS carriers will become victims and will also die within seven years. Another example of incomplete information being given concerns the possibility of the disease being spread through saliva. We now know that the virus can remain active for one week in water. This has led certain doctors to put forward the theory that it could be spread through kissing. There is also a view held by certain scientists that it may be spread through skin contact, and there are reports coming in from different parts of the world that it may even be transmittable via bare feet, for example.

Conservative Family Campaign are not claiming that these are facts. We are merely reporting what learned scientists or doctors consider are possible theories. They are saying that they are unproven. Our belief is that there we are faced with a public health danger for which there is no cure, then it is irresponsible on the part of Government to pretend that these possibilities do not exist and to try to rely on less radical measures than they would adopt if these possibilities turned out to be true.

We have not shirked in the past when dealing with problems such as scarlet fever, tuberculosis or other deadly diseases to restrict people's liberties and to impose what might be termed wartime conditions upon the population to help stop the spread or even eradicate a particularly virulent disease. AIDS is more virulent and more deadly than any of the other illnesses we have had to treat including smallpox, for example. It is absolutely incumbent upon the Government to act with vigour and determination.

Other countries are beginning to show a realisation of the application of normal public health measures. Switzerland has decided to make AIDS a notifiable disease. Certain countries such as the United Arab Emirates have decided to impose tests on foreigners entering their country, and certain countries have decided to turn away people they suspect of carrying the AIDS virus. These are only sensible precautions which the United Kingdom should adopt. Interestingly certain authorities within the UK do not appear to be taking such an unrealistic view of the possibility of AIDS being spread through means other than sexual activity. The Thames Valley Police Authority have already decided that their policemen should not use the normal mouth to mouth techniques when they undertake resuscitation. Certain advice issued by DHSS to nurses and doctors in hospitals also indicates that they are aware of the possibility that it might be spread in this way. If the advice is there for hospitals and the police, why one wonders do we not let the general public in on this information and concern?

The key area revolves around whether the Government is prepared
to make a moral stand on what is essentially a disease spread by
immoral behaviour. If the Government would unequivocally state
that monogamy is the cure and the means of prevention of the spread
of AIDS, then this would see a dramatic impact and lead to a significant improvement in other aspects of our life. Medically there is no
question that if one is chaste before marriage and faithful within
marriage and never indulges in any form of abnormal sex, then AIDS
will not be caught nor spread and will wither away. All medical
authorities agree on that.

We strongly believe, therefore, that the Government should adopt
a position of advocating chastity before marriage, and faithfulness
within marriage with all the means at its disposal. We are not sanguine
in b believing that this would automatically change everybody but we
think that cumulatively over the years it would have a favourable
effect. It has already been announced by the Secretary of State for
Social Services that the Government sees the AIDS issue as one requiring many years of work. The work must start now but on the right
basis.

We would comment that the advertising currently being used is
not on the right basis. It does not make an unequivocal statement
about monogamy. Instead it talks about the concept of "safe sex".
There is no such thing. It advocates that condoms be used and yet we
know that condoms used for anal intercourse which presently exist
may not be strong enough. We also know that even in normal vaginal
heterosexual intercourse a condom is only 96 percent efficient.

Conservative Family Campaign, therefore, believe that the current
advertising campaign is not only ineffective in curbing the spread of
AIDS and could be offensive and distasteful to some of the population
but could, in fact, be counter productive. By suggesting that there is
such a thing as "safe sex" impressionable young people might be
encouraged to engage in sexual activity before they would have done
otherwise. In a way it could be promoting the very permissiveness
which is one of the problems which lies behind the spread of AIDS.

VII. The Agony of Africa

The Editors

It is not difficult to see that most of the scientific and epidemiological studies presented so far in this book are directed toward (if not pointing at) the continent of Africa as the origin of the infectious agent which causes AIDS. We do not believe this is a conspiracy to apportion blame nor a politically motivated vendetta towards any special group or area of the world. Africa was not simply "chosen" as a scapegoat and it does not appear to be a whitewash of modern science. The data are carefully and rationally presented — and in the end it could be concluded that all roads lead to somewhere in central Africa but as yet for reasons unknown. However, we must stress, as we did in the very beginning, that the origin of the disease is not as important as how to control it and stop its spread.

One thing is certain from the scientific articles and letters — it cannot be stopped by denying that it exists. Important breakthroughs were achieved only when people suffering from AIDS came forward and volunteered for treatment, study and experimentation. Some African countries are now coming forward and saying quite openly that they do indeed admit that there is a problem within their borders and that they would like to invite assistance from whomever is willing to help. That is a beginning. In many cases that beginning is two to five years too late, but at least steps have been taken toward stopping the spread of AIDS in Africa.

Since this book is intended to be a documentary history of the early phases of the epidemic, we feel that it is only proper that we present some of the arguments of African writers in expressing their views on the work which was being done in the laboratories of the First World.

The year 1985 was probably the most crucial and vocal in the history of AIDS in Africa. The first article by Dr. Quinn and colleagues presented data from the late 70s and early 80s which pointed out that there was indeed a case for considering central Africa as a place (if not an origin) where AIDS had already progressed to large proportions. This paper, and hundreds of others in the scientific press, was important in the change of attitudes toward the disease in many African nations. However, at the same time we show how African researchers, governments and others were boycotting conferences and writing diatribes against what they felt was a new form of imperialism.

We hope that the final article "Imperial Bedroom" leaves you with the same sense of anger which it brought to us — and with it a resolve to do everything possible to help stop the spread of this killer disease.

AIDS in Africa: An Epidemiologic Paradigm

by Thomas C.
Quinn, Jonathan M. Mann,
James W. Curran and Peter Piot

Reprinted with permission from *Science, Vol. 234; 955-63.*
November 21, 1986

The acquired immune deficiency syndrome (AIDS) has become recognized as a global health problem. Cases have now been reported in 74 countries with more than 25,000 cases in the United States, nearly 3,000 cases in other countries of the Americas, more than 3,000 cases in Europe, and several thousand cases suspected and many more unrecognized in Africa. It is estimated that at least several million people worldwide have been infected with the causative agent, referred to as human T-lymphotropic virus type III/lymphadenopathy virus, or more recently as human immunodeficiency virus (HIV). As many as 10 to 30 percent of these HIV-infected individuals may develop AIDS within the next 5 to 10 years. With the present lack of a curative therapy or vaccine, this disease now ranks as the most serious epidemic of the past 50 years.

Although the immunopathogenesis of HIV infection is similar in most AIDS patients, the epidemiology and clinical features of the infection in different countries may vary, depending on cultural differences, endemic diseases, and other unidentified risk factors. In Africa, the different clinical features of AIDS and the difficulty in identifying the risk factors frequently associated with AIDS in the United States, such as homosexuality and intravenous drug use, have raised questions regarding the nature of the disease and the factors responsible for HIV dissemination in that continent. Here we review the epidemiologic and clinical features of AIDS in Africa and discuss the potential problems faced by public health officials in developing prevention and control strategies. Shortly after the recognition of AIDS in the United States, cases of the disease were identified among Africans residing in Europe. Immunologically, these cases were identical to AIDS cases in the United States, with marked depression of CD4 + lymphocytes and cell-mediated immunosuppression. Clinically, the African cases resembled Haitian AIDS cases with prominent gastrointestinal symptoms and opportunistic infections, such as oroesophageal candidiasis, cryptococcosis, toxoplasmosis, and mycobacterial infections. As of 31 March 1986, 177 cases of AIDS were reported among Africans residing in ten European countries. These cases originated from 24 African countries, mostly in Central Africa. In contrast to the European cases, African cases had a male to female ratio of 1.7:1, and 90 percent had no identifiable risk factors. Even among Europeans with AIDS and a recent history of travel to Africa, nearly 90 percent denied homosexuality or intravenous drug use.

These unusual epidemiologic features prompted a series of investigations in 1983 to determine the pattern of AIDS in Central Africa. During a 4-week period, 38 patients with AIDS and 20 patients with AIDS-related diseases were identified in a large general hospital in Kinshasa, Zaire. Cases were equally distributed among men and women; females with the disease were younger and more often unmarried than male AIDS patients; and clusters of AIDS cases among men and women were linked by heterosexual contact. In a simultaneous investigation of 26 cases in Kigali, Rwanda, 43 percent of the female patients were identified as prostitutes. The fact that there was no evidence of homosexual transmission or intravenous drug use indicated that the pattern of AIDS transmission was different, and that heterosexual contact might be an important factor in transmission.

Although the recognition of AIDS in Africa is consistent with the temporal occurrence of the disease in the United States, and Haiti, several case reports and retrospective serologic surveys of banked sera have suggested that HIV infection may have occurred earlier in Africa. The earliest serologic response to HIV was found in serum collected from Kinshasa, Zaire, in 1959. Sera from West and East Africa in the 1960's and early 1970's have also shown high prevalence of weakly positive specimens (for example, seropositivity in 1.4 percent of 144 children from Burkina Faso in 1963, and in 50 of 75 Ugandan children in 1972-73). However, serologic studies of HIV in Africa have been inconsistent because of problems in interpretation of the results from ELISA's and Western blot tests of banked specimens particularly from malaria endemic areas, and the validity of these data has been questioned.

While it is difficult to determine precisely when and where the first cases of AIDS or HIV infection occurred in Africa, retrospective studies on the frequency of certain clinical diseases as sentinel markers of AIDS indicate that there was a marked increase in cases in Africa during the late 1970's and early 1980's. Epidemic increases in chronic, life-threatening enteropathic illnesses were noted in the late 1970's in Kinshasa and in the early 1980's in Uganda and Tanzania, where this was referred to as "slim disease". In Rwanda, a marked increase in esophageal candidiasis was first noted in 1983 in a hospital where approximately 300 esophagoscopies had been performed annually since 1979. In Kinshasa, the annual number of cases of Kaposi's sarcoma diagnosed in a large public hospital tripled from 1970 to 1984, and the number of aggressive Kaposi's sarcoma cases increased eight times in 1981. Investigators in Zambia and Uganda also reported a marked increase in disseminated Kaposi's sarcoma starting in 1982 and 1983. Finally, careful surveillance of cryptococcal meningitis in Kinshasa showed a sevenfold increase in 1978-84 compared with the period in 1953-77. These studies suggested that while isolated cases of AIDS may have occurred in Africa earlier, it was probably rare until the late 1970's and early 1980's, a pattern similar to that in the United States and Haiti.

The geographic scope and intensity of AIDS and HIV infection in Africa is difficult to assess precisely. First, infectious disease surveillance capability is often limited because of weaknesses in the health infrastructure and inadequate resources. Second, the widely used CDC/WHO definition of AIDS requires sophisticated laboratory support for diagnosis of opportunistic infections and malignancies and exclusion of other known causes of immunodeficiency, and is not applicable to developing countries. Third, diagnostic services for opportunistic infections and for serodiagnosis of HIV infection are not yet generally available. Furthermore, serodiagnosis is complicated by the need for confirmatory testing because of the presence of possible cross-reacting antibodies. However, African countries in collaboration with international investigators are now attempting to address these issues so that a clear picture of the descriptive epidemiology of AIDS in Africa is gradually emerging.

On the basis of available information, it appears that Central Africa and, to a lesser degree, adjacent countries in East and Southern Africa, are most severely affected by HIV infection. HIV is being increasingly detected in areas of Africa previously thought to be free of infection, although, with few exceptions, the data are inadequate to distinguish between recent introduction of the virus and recent recognition or awareness of the problem. Investigators extrapolating from 1983 studies in Kigali, Rwanda and Kinshasa, Zaire, estimated the annual AIDS incidence in 1983 to be 800 per million and 170 per million population, respectively. AIDS surveillance has continued in Kinshasa were 332 cases were identified between July 1984 and February 1985, for an adjusted annual incidence of approximately 176 per million population. Since nearly all reported cases occurred among persons 20 years of age or older, the incidence for adult Kinshasa residents would be approximately 380 cases per million. Peak age-specific incidence of 786 per million and 601 per million were present among 30 — 39 year old men and women, respectively. While these surveillance data provided a preliminary estimate of the actual disease incidence in Kinshasa, a more reasonable estimate of the annual incidence based on the first 6 months of 1985 would be between 550 to 1,000 cases per million adults. However, these are probably minimal estimates since the data reflect only recognized and reported cases of AIDS in several hospitals within Kinshasa.

Surveillance data reflect some of the basic epidemiologic trends of AIDS in Africa. The sex ration of AIDS cases in Zaire was approximately 1:1.2. As in developed countries, AIDS in Africa primarily affects young and middle-aged persons. The mean age of AIDS patients in Kinshasa was 33.6 years, and men were significantly older than women. The sex and age distributions of 500 AIDS cases reflect patterns seen with other sexually transmitted diseases both in developed and developing countries in which incidence and morbidity rates are higher among younger women. Women with AIDS were more likely than men to be unmarried (61 vs 36 percent), and nearly one-third of the married AIDS patients had at least one previous marriage or "union libre". One-third of AIDS patients reported having at least one sexually transmitted disease during the 3 years preceding their illness. Twenty-nine percent of patients utilized traditional medical practitioner, and 80 percent reported receiving medical injections. Nine percent of patients received a blood transfusion during the 3-year period before onset of illness. These data do not allow for direct assessment of the risks associated with these activities, however, since no information was provided from a control population without HIV infection.

Prevalence of HIV antibody positive individuals in Africa: Though surveillance studies have been limited in Africa, serologic studies better indicate the extent of HIV infection throughout Africa. Thus far, serologic studies have indicated the presence of HIV antibody in persons in Burundi, Botswana, Central African Republic, Congo, Gambia, Gabon, Kenya, Malawi, Rwanda, Senegal, South Africa, Tanzania, Transkei, Uganda, Zambia, Zaire, and Zimbabwe. Seroprevalence rates among healthy populations in these areas range from 0.7 percent for blood donors in the Congo to as high as 18 percent for blood donors in Kigali, Rwanda. Seroprevalence rates among high-risk groups, such as female prostitutes, have been reported to range from 27 to 88 percent, depending on selection, socioeconomic status, and geographic location.

Longitudinal data on HIV seroprevalence in different populations are available from Kenya and Zaire. The increase in HIV seroprevalence among prostitutes in Nairobi from 4 to 59 percent between 1980 and 1986 demonstrates the rapid dissemination of HIV infection in a high-risk group in Africa, similar to that observed among homosexual men in San Francisco. The relatively low but steady increase in seroprevalence among pregnant women in Nairobi from 0 to 2 percent in 5 years and in Kinshasa from 0.25 to 8 percent within 16 years indicates the potential spread of HIV infection to the general population in these areas. Consistent with this apparent rate of increase in the general population, Mann et al., found in a follow-up study of 579 seronegative men and women working at a general hospital in Kinshasa from 1984 to 1985 that the annual incidence of HIV antibodies was approximately 0.75 percent.

Data on HIV seroprevalence from 5,099 healthy people (2,982 men and 2,117 women) in Kinshasa show a bimodal curve, with a peak prevalence under 1 year of age and among young adults aged 16 to 29 years old. While other factors may be influencing this distribution of HIV infection rates, this pattern is suggestive of a sexually transmitted disease with higher prevalence among younger sexually active women. A combination of passive antibody transfer and transmission of virus from mother to infant is probably responsible for the high seroprevalence in younger children under age 2. In a preliminary evaluation of the natural history of HIV infection in Africa, 67 seropositive individuals with no signs or symptoms of disease were enrolled in a study in Kinshasa in October 1984. Sixteen months later, one individual had developed AIDS and eight had developed generalized lymphadenopathy, giving annual progression rates of 1.3 per 100 person-years and 10.4 per 100 person years respectively. These data are remarkably similar to a San Francisco cohort of seropositive homosexual men in which approximately 1.3 percent progressed to

AIDS and 5.12 percent developed AIDS-related conditions each year. Thus even if further HIV infections were prevented, substantial numbers of AIDS cases can be anticipated in Africa during the next decade emerging from the pool of already infected persons.

In North America and Europe, transmission of HIV infection has been documented to occur through one or more of four modes: sexual contact, exposure to blood-contaminated needles, administration of infected blood or blood products, and passage of the virus from infected mothers to their newborns. In contrast to North American and European AIDS patients, African AIDS patients rarely report a history of homosexual activity or intravenous drug abuse. While it may be difficult to ascertain homosexual and drug history because of cultural differences, it is evident from the multiple studies performed in Africa by both national and international experts in sexually transmitted diseases that these two risk factors do not play a major role in HIV transmission in Africa. Available data suggest that heterosexual activity, blood transfusions, vertical transmission from mother to infant, and probably frequent exposure to unsterilized needles account for the spread of HIV infection and AIDS in Africa.

Heterosexual transmission: Several lines of evidence support the concept that HIV infection is transmitted heterosexually in Africa. In addition to the 1:1 male to female ratio among cases and the younger age and single marital status for female cases, case-control studies have also shown that AIDS patients have a significantly higher number of heterosexual partners than controls (mean of 32 vs 3), that male patients have had sex significantly more often with female prostitutes 81 vs. 34 percent), and that the risk of seropositivity increases significantly with the number of different sexual partners per year and with a history of other sexually transmitted diseases. In Africa, prostitutes show the highest infection rate (27 to 88 percent) and may have played an important role in the dissemination of HIV infection in Nairobi, since HIV antibody prevalence was initially higher in prostitutes in that city than in men with sexually transmitted diseases who frequented prostitutes.

Whereas male-to-female transmission of HIV has been increasingly documented in the United States and Europe, evidence of female-to-male transmission has been limited in the United States because of the relatively low number of infected women. In Africa, however, there is sufficient evidence to support bidirectional transmission of HIV. First, it may be possible for HIV to be transmitted bidirectionally among heterosexual contacts, since the virus can be isolated from semen as well as from cervical-vaginal secretions. Second, African male AIDS patients, as well as expatriate males with AIDS who previously lived in Africa, frequently report a history of sex with prostitutes, and the prevalence of HIV in male heterosexuals attending clinics for sexually transmitted disease is increasing, suggesting female-to-male transmission. Further evidence for such transmission comes from a household study of AIDS patients in Zaire in which HIV antibody was significantly higher among spouses and infants of infected mothers than in other household members or controls. In this study, 11 (3 men, 8 women) (61 percent) of 18 spouses of 3 female and 15 male AIDS cases were HIV antibody-positive compared to only 1 (3.7 percent) of 27 spouses of seronegative control patients, a statistically significant difference. Finally, several clusters of African AIDS cases have been identified in whom the chronology of events suggested both female-to-male and male-to-female transmission of HIV.

Risk factors associated with HIV infection in heterosexuals include number of sexual partners, sex with prostitutes, being a prostitute, and being a sexual partner of an infected person. Specific sexual activities, including anal intercourse reported by only 4 to 8 percent of female AIDS patients, were not associated with HIV infection in surveys in Kenya, Zaire, and Rwanda. In studies among Nairobi prostitutes, HIV seropositivity was significantly associated with current sexually transmitted diseases such as gonorrhea, genital ulcers, and syphilis. In another study in Zambia, seropositivity in men was also correlated with the presence of genital ulcers. These observations suggest that disruption of genital epithelial integrity caused by sexually transmitted diseases that are common in Africa may facilitate transmission of HIV during vaginal intercourse. Alternatively, the presence of these sexually transmitted diseases may be indicative of high-risk activities for HIV infection or of exposure to unsterilized needles for treatment of sexually transmitted diseases, and may not be directly related to transmissibility. However, in two studies of female prostitutes in Nairobi and Kinshasa, HIV seropositivity was directly associated with number of sexual exposures, independent of the frequency of needle exposures which was not associated with HIV seropositivity. The potential for HIV transmission by unsterilized needles, however, should not be underestimated, and further studies should be undertaken to assess risk associated with these factors and to develop effective means of prevention.

Perinatal transmission: As a result of heterosexual transmission, African women of child-bearing age are exposed to HIV. In 1985, the proportion of seropositive pregnant women was 2 percent in one maternity hospital in Nairobi and 8 percent in Kinshasa. As in U.S.

studies, maternal HIV infection appears to be strongly associated with seropositivity among infants in Africa. In an ongoing study of 44 seropositive children between the ages of 1 and 24 months in Kinshasa, 27 (61 percent) had seropositive mothers. Until prospective studies are performed, it will be unclear what percentage of these children acquired maternal HIV antibody passively as opposed to acquiring the virus perinatally. Nevertheless, it is clear from the high seropositivity among pregnant women that a substantial number of newborn children are being infected with HIV. The impact that this high seropositivity rate will have on the general health of these children and on the safety and efficacy of childhood vaccinations is unknown.

Injections: The use of unsterilized needles or other skin-piercing instruments for medical or ritual purposes (for example, scarification, tattooing, ear piercing, male or female circumcision, blood-brotherhood ceremonies) has potential for HIV transmission. In a seroprevalence study of 2,384 hospital workers in Kinshasa, significantly more HIV seropositive than seronegative workers reported receiving medical injections during the previous 3 years; among those reporting injections, seroprevalence was nearly twice as high for those with five or more injections compared with those receiving fewer than five injections. In a study of hospitalized seropositive children aged 1 to 24 months in Kinshasa who had similar medical problems, 16 born to seronegative mothers received significantly more injections compared with 222 seronegative children born to seronegative mothers. In addition, among adult patients with tuberculosis, HIV seropositives reported significantly more injections than seronegatives during the 5-year period prior to hospitalization. Similarly, a history of scarification in the previous year was significantly more common among 40 seropositive hospitalized children of 2 to 14 years old (25 percent) compared with 92 seronegative children of the same age and sex (25 vs 6.6 percent).

These data suggest that injections and scarifications are associated with HIV infection, but it is difficult to distinguish whether the association is truly causal, that is, provides a means of exposure to HIV, or secondary due to treatment for early symptoms of HIV infection or other illnesses, such as sexually transmitted diseases. The potential importance of HIV transmission by needles reflects several cultural factors in Africa that merit emphasis. Patients often express strong preference for parenteral rather than oral therapy. For example, in survey of 50 mothers in Kinshasa, 84 percent expressed the belief that parenteral medication is more effective than oral medication. Injections as well as scarifications may be administered in clinics or nonmedical sites by personnel inadequately trained in aseptic techniques. Financial and other practical constraints also lead to reuse of disposable equipment and to insufficient sterilization or use of contaminated needles and instruments. In contrast, the lack of association between HIV seropositivity and childhood vaccinations probably reflects the wider use of properly sterilized injection equipment in immunization programs, relatively small numbers of vaccinations received per child and the general absence of traditional healers in vaccination programs.

Transfusions: As with injections, patient expectations and medical overuse of blood transfusions may contribute to the potential spread of HIV through transfusions. In a recent review of transfusion practices in a large public hospital in Central Africa, over 90 percent of transfusions to adult patients involved only a single unit of blood. However, in a more careful analysis of indications for blood transfusions in children, over 70 percent to transfusions in one large hospital were for severe anemia associated with acute malaria. This may be a particularly difficult problem in some areas of Africa where malaria is highly endemic and frequently causes severe aneamia in children. Studies are needed to assess the present indications for blood transfusion in Africa and the risks of HIV transmission via transfusions.

Other modes of transmission?

There is no direct evidence yet for arthropod transmission of HIV in Africa, nor in the United States where HIV infection occurs in some areas of substantial arthropod densities. Recently, it was shown that HIV could be cultured from bedbugs 60 minutes after they had engorged on blood containing tissue culture supernatants from HIV-infected cells. Becker et al. using HIV molecular probes, also demonstrated genomic material of HIV within several insects from HIV-endemic areas of Africa. However, HIV could not be isolated from these insects, and, as with hepatitis B virus, it appears that prolonged survival and transmission of HIV by insects is unlikely. Because of the low titer of HIV in the blood of infected persons and the small amount of blood ingested by an insect, mechanical transmission of HIV by insect vectors seems unlikely, particularly in view of the fact that hepatitis B virus, which is more readily parenterally transmitted, has not been found to be transmitted by arthropods.

With estimates of several million HIV-infected people in Africa, it is evident that the virus has created a major health problem in that continent. Nearly 25 percent of adult and 10 percent of pediatric inpatients in several hospitals in Central Africa are HIV-seropositive, and the high prevalence rates of other infectious diseases endemic in Africa may result in further exacerbation of HIV disease. In addition, the morbidity and mortality caused by other infectious diseases may increase as a result of the underlying immunosuppression induced by HIV infection.

The recent rapid increase in urbanization in many parts of Africa has resulted in economic and sociological changes that have influenced behavior and severely affected the health infrastructure. Consequently, one cannot expect public health officials to upgrade blood transfusion services to prevent HIV infection when the proposed intervention is likely to cost, per person, approximately 30 times the annual per capita public health budget. In the United States, approximately $60 million was spend on blood-bank screening for HIV infection in 1985, a budget many times greater than the entire health budgets of many African countries. Similarly, one cannot hope to prevent reuse of disposable injection equipment when many hospital budgets are insufficient for the purchase of antibiotics. The costs of caring for ten AIDS patients in the United States (approximately $450,000) is greater than the entire budget of a large hospital in Zaire, where up to 25 percent of the pediatric and adult hospital admissions have HIV infection.

Nevertheless, in response to recent data on the AIDS epidemic, representatives from 45 African countries have developed, under the auspices of the African Regional Office of the World Health Organization, a plan of action for the prevention and control of AIDS. In November 1986, these representatives will reconvene in Brazzaville to discuss the following strategies. Each country will (1) establish a national AIDS committee that includes representatives from the health and social services and from communications, education, and other relevant governmental and nongovernmental sectors; (2) conduct an epidemiologic assessment of the burden of HIV infection and associated risk factors; and (3) institute a surveillance system for AIDS and HIV infection that includes serological surveys of selected populations, such as prostitutes and blood donors. Concomitantly, appropriate level of laboratory capability for the serological diagnosis of HIV infection will be established either in each country or through collaborative regional agreements. In addition, increased numbers of health care personnel will be educated in the recognition and management of HIV associated disease in hospitals and communities, with consideration being given to patient confidentiality, counseling, and ethical issues.

These strategies are expected to lead rapidly to the development of programs to halt the spread of the AIDS virus. For example, creative educational approaches are needed to prevent virus transmission through reductions in the number of sexual partners or through use of condoms. Changes in medical practices, including traditional practices are required to reduce transmission rates associated with injections, scarification, and blood transfusions. The screening of women of child-bearing age and counseling regarding contraception for HIV-seropositive women are necessary in order to interrupt perinatal HIV transmission.

To be successful, these programs will have to be integrated into existing health and educational programs and will require full support by the appropriate governmental agencies. However, many countries may lack the financial and other resources that will be required to build and sustain these activities on a long-term basis. Controlling the spread of the AIDS virus will thus require a major international commitment, not only in terms of providing financial help but also in providing scientific, educational, and technical assistance. With 74 countries of the world affected by the disease and several million people carrying the virus, worldwide cooperation is now a necessity.

Politics and Science Clash on African AIDS

by Colin Norman

Reprinted with permission from *Science, Vol. 230; 1140-42.*
December 6, 1985

Brussels: Not a single case of acquired immune deficiency syndrome has officially been reported from central Africa. Yet, according to a mass of evidence presented at a 2-day meeting (International Symposium on African AIDS, Brussels, Nov. 22, 1985) here, the incidence of the disease is rising sharply in some countries and the retrovirus that is widely believed to be the prime cause of AIDS has spread to an alarming extent in some regions.

The discrepancy between the official picture of the disease and the portrait emerging from clinical and epidemiological studies reflects deep political sensitivity, at times resulting in censorship. Some African governments apparently fear that adverse publicity about AIDS could discourage tourism and seriously disrupt their economies.

Such sentiments left an unfortunate mark on the meeting. At the last moment, several African researchers and some of their European coworkers cancelled their presentations. Some 50 Africans who did attend issued a statement that the papers presented "did not show any conclusive evidence that AIDS originated in Africa." And at an extraordinary press conference at the conclusion of the meeting, David Serwadda, a Ugandan researcher, berated the Western media for "conveying out of all proportion what is happening in Africa."

This political sensitivity is clearly hampering efforts to make sense of the complex puzzle of how, and to what extent, the disease and the AIDS virus are spreading in Africa. However, some elements are clear. In contrast to the United States, where AIDS has so far been confined largely to homosexuals and intravenous drug users, the disease appears to be spreading in Africa largely through heterosexual contact. It afflicts men and women in roughly equal numbers and, because the virus can be passed on to children before birth, more children in Africa are coming down with the disease.

Because the disease pattern appears to be so different, understanding African AIDS could be extremely important not only for Africa itself but also for the rest of the world. "If we are concerned about the public health of the peoples in Africa and all over the world, we cannot pretend that AIDS is not there," said Robin Weiss of the Institute of Cancer Research in London, at the opening of the meeting.

In spite of the lack of official reporting of AIDS in central Africa, it is clear that the disease is appearing in many countries. One early indication was the diagnosis of AIDS among Africans who had moved to Europe or were referred to European hospitals for treatment. According to Nathan Clumeck of St. Pierre University Hospital in Brussels, some 12 percent of European AIDS cases are in fact African patients from 21 different countries. In addition, new cases of AIDS or diseases that appear to be related to AIDS are showing up at an increasing rate in hospitals in parts of Africa. For example, Daniel Zagury of the University Pierre et Marie Curie in Paris, reported that antibodies to the AIDS virus were detected in 60 of 117 patients hospitalized at the university clinic in Kinshasa, Zaire, early this year. Some of the patients met all the currently accepted criteria for AIDS itself, while others were suffering from conditions such as intestinal disorders, pneumonia, dermatitis, and a variety of cancers.

Another paper, scheduled for presentation by a group from the same clinic in Kinshasa but which was withdrawn, reported that 93 patients with AIDS were seen there between October 1983 and December 1984.

Similarly, in a paper that was delivered, Anne Bayley of the University of Zambia School of Medicine in Lusaka reported finding a new form of Kaposi's sarcoma among some patients in 1983. It tends to afflict younger people than the classic form of the disease does, and it is far more aggressive and generally fatal. She saw 13 patients with atypical Kaposi's sarcoma in 1983, 22 in 1984 and 19 in the first 4 months of 1985 alone. Antibodies to the AIDS virus were detected in 91 percent of the patients with this aggressive form of the disease but in only 24 percent of those with the endemic form.

Many cases of what is known locally as "slim disease" have been reported recently from Uganda. Characterized by severe weight loss, it is generally indistinguishable from AIDS. A paper recently published in *The Lancet* by Serwadda and collaborators from Zambia and Britain reported that AIDS virus antibodies were detected in 63 of 71 slim disease patients in Uganda and noted that "an epidemic of [AIDS] is spreading in neighboring Rwanda and Zaire."

Since no central African countries are keeping their own records of AIDS cases — let alone reporting them to the World Health Organization — it is impossible to know what the incidence is. Moreover, it is clear that many cases of AIDS are likely to be diagnosed as other diseases because the spectrum of opportunistic infections is different in Africa from that in the United States and Europe.

For example, *Pneumosystis carinii* pneumonia, a tell-tale marker of AIDS in western countries, seems to occur much less frequently in African AIDS patients, while skin diseases, cryptococcal meningitis, and a variety of intestinal complications appear more frequently. For this reason, there was general agreement at the meeting — supported by the statement of the African representatives — that the definition of AIDS used in the West needs to be broadened for use in Africa.

The extent to which the virus itself is spreading in Africa is also a topic of intense debate — on both political and scientific grounds. What is becoming increasingly clear, however, is that it has reached alarming levels in some urban areas of central Africa but has not yet spread much in southern Africa.

— In a paper scheduled for presentation by Francoise Brun-Vezinet of the Hopital Claude Bernard in Paris, which was cancelled at the last moment, 7 percent of serum samples collected from prostitutes in Kenya in 1980 contained antibodies to the AIDS virus; by 1984,the proportion had risen to 51 percent. Their male customers also showed an increase in infection. Only 1 percent of a sample of men attending a clinic for sexually transmitted diseases had antibodies to the virus in 1980; by 1984, the proportion has risen to 13 percent.

— A study of prostitutes in Butare, Rwanda, indicated that 29 of 33 tested in 1984 had antibodies to the virus, and 27 were showing symptoms of generalized lymphadenopathy. Seven out of 25 men treated for sexually transmitted diseases who admitted contact with prostitutes also tested positive. In comparison, 12 percent of female controls and 17 percent of male controls showed signs of infection. According to Philippe Van de Perre, of the Hopital Saint Pierre, who presented that data, there was a high correlation between a history of infection by sexually transmitted agents and infection with the AIDS virus. Van de Perre and others found no correlation, however, with therapeutic injections, indicating that use of dirty needles may not currently be playing a major role in transmission of the disease. (A possible exception may be injections at clinics for sexually transmitted diseases.

— A second study in Rwanda indicated that 10.5 percent of a sample of 258 blood donations contained antibodies to the AIDS virus. The rate of infection appears to be higher in urban than in rural areas; 17.5 percent of a sample of young adults living in Kigali tested positive, compared with 3 percent of young adults from a rural area.

— Chris Williams of the University of Ibadan, Nigeria, reported that 7 percent of Nigerian blood donations tested positive for AIDS virus antibodies, although he claimed that there is no evidence for the disease itself is present in Nigeria.

Although there was little disagreement about the trends conveyed by these serological studies, there was considerable debate about how much weight should be put on the absolute numbers. One problem is that a relatively high rate of false positives occurs when African sera are tested by some of the commercially available kits. However, some researchers also reported high rates of false negatives. For example, Zagury said he isolated virus from 12 patients from Zaire who were producing no detectable antibodies, out of 84 tested.

Although the epidemiological picture is somewhat hazy, spread of the virus and the disease through heterosexual contact is clearly indicated. Even the statement by the African representatives acknowledged that "heterosexual promiscuity with multiple sexual partners is one of the high risk factors for AIDS and therefore the public should be informed." Many researchers believe the same message should be conveyed in the West.

* * * * * * * * * * * *

On January 4, 1988, The Centers for Disease Control reported 50,265 AIDS cases in the United States.

The Politics of AIDS in Kenya

by Alfred J. Fortin

Reprinted with permission from *The Third World Quarterly*
July, 1987

Let us at once state the necessary and the dramatic. There may at present be 10 million people in the world who have been infected by the AIDS virus. By 1990, according to the World Health Organization, there may be as many as 100 million. Over 100 countries have reported AIDS victims, including thirty African nations. But half of those estimated to be infected world-wide live in the eleven countries that comprise Central Africa, and it is there that 50,000 to several hundred thousand lives may already have been lost.

The African AIDS connection was first recognized in 1983 by physicians in Europe who reported AIDS-like illnesses among their African patients. These incidences prompted clinical studies by Western researchers in Rwanda and Zaire where people with similar illnesses and immunological problems were found. With the subsequent isolation of the human T-lymphotropic virus type III, now referred to as the human immunodeficiency virus (HIV), and the development of screening procedures to detect antibodies against HIV (the ELISA and Western blot techniques), further studies confirmed that African patients were suffering from the ill-effects caused by the same virus.

Estimates of the extent of those infected abound in the scientific and popular press even if they are at times difficult to prove with certainty. Yet despite the latitude that we may give to a sensationalist press and its exaggerations, the message is appallingly clear: if what is predicted does happen, then countries in the hardest-hit region, those touching the Great Rift Valley — Zambia, Uganda, Rwanda, Zaire, Burundi, Tanzania — face a serious challenge that may, in some cases, threaten their already fragile political and economic stability. In Lusaka, for example, 15 percent of the adult population, and 30 percent of all its men may be infected. Serological testing of healthy adults in Kigali, Rwanda has shown 18 percent are positive to HIV. In Bujumbura, the capital of Burundi, it is estimated that one out of every ten adults carries the AIDS virus; and in the Rakai area of southwest Uganda, one of the most heavily AIDS-stricken areas in the world, an incredible 30 percent of the population are estimated to be infected. For Central and East Africa, deadly AIDS statistics seem all too easily available and they seem to be getting worse all the time.

Kenya, while not untouched by the virus, has, according to most accounts, been relatively spared. Although high rates of infection among prostitutes have been reported, the overall prevalence of the disease in Kenya has been considerably lower than in neighbouring countries. But AIDS is in Kenya! And although Kenya is the country in the region best equipped to mount an effective prevention programme, it has failed in many respects to do so. Despite its comparatively well-developed medical infrastructure and working coterie of Western scientists, its efforts have fallen short of even the minimum requirements suggested by its statistics.

In January, 1985, under the headlines "Killer disease in Kenya" and "Horror sex disease in Kakamenga", the Kenyan press made public its first serious interest in the AIDS problem. In these stories, the press reported that in the Kakamenga District of Kenya four cases of AIDS had been diagnosed and that the patients had subsequently died. Later accounts contradicted the story, quoting a hostile district medical officer who claimed that the deaths were not due to AIDS but were simply extreme cases of skin cancer. Despite the confusion and the obvious need for clarification, relative silence followed until the Autumn of 1985 when Western press accounts began to focus sharply on the somewhat frightening implications of AIDS research in Central Africa. Realising the importance of these studies, the respected Kenyan magazine, The Weekly Review, took up the cause of informing the public. It issued a carefully worded summary of some of the material printed in the West, citing the numbers of AIDS victims reported in Zaire, Rwanda, Uganda and Kenya. In September 1985, under the growing public pressure caused by these reports, the Kenyan Ministry of Health unofficially let it be known that only 20 victims with AIDS had actually been diagnosed in Kenya since May 1985. Officially, however, the government continued to deny to foreign reports the presence of AIDS within its borders, until the now famous study of Kenyan prostitutes broke in the international press. In this study of 90 prostitutes in Nairobi, over half were reportedly infected with the

HIV virus and three-quarters of these women showed signs of significant illness. Kenyan leaders who had up to this point steadfastly avoided the health care implications of AIDS in the country, now became incensed by these disclosures and by others, which they conceived to be part of a Western racist campaign to exaggerate the prevalence of AIDS in Africa. Yet the immediate effect of this unwanted publicity was to wake up a somewhat lethargic Kenyan health officialdom, which until then (and still now) has tended to play down the AIDS threat.

In October 1985, Kenyan government leaders, concerned about jeopardising the local tourist industry (which generated 600,000 visitors in 1986) protested through the national press that the reports about AIDS in Kenya were alarmist and untrue. Americans and others in the West were being given the impression that AIDS was sweeping across Africa even though the virus had been documented in only "a handful of countries: Zaire, Rwanda, Burundi, and Uganda". Even the President of Kenya, Daniel arap Moi, was prompted to remark that the foreign press was conducting a "hate campaign" and urged wananchi (Kenyan citizens) to "turn a deaf ear to our enemies". This kind of reaction gained support in Kenya as Central Africa came increasingly under the scrutiny of the inquisitive Western scientific community, eager to answer critical epidemiological and clinical questions about the HIV virus. The international media, heady with the potential importance of the AIDS story, also began invading Central Africa in search of answers to questions of its own, questions that would invariably embarrass and call to account African health officials.

In November 1985, the New York Times quoted leading American scientists, Robert Gallo of the National Cancer Institute and William Haseltine of Harvard University, as arguing strongly, on the basis of early epidemiological studies, that the AIDS epidemic probably began in Africa. Kenyan officials were outraged and reacted swiftly to minimise the impact of these reports by confiscating the entire shipment of the 9 November 1985 issue of the International Herald Tribune in which reports began of Lawrence Altman's New York Times series on African AIDS research and its implications. The African offensive in Kenya to combat the Western "African origin" theory of AIDS then began in earnest. An editorial in Medicus, the official publication of the Kenya Medical Association, suggested the possibility that tourists from around the world had introduced AIDS into Africa, and complained of the West's apparent need for an African connection for every disease. One columnist of a major Kenyan daily went so far as to claim that infected foreigners were deliberately being sent to Africa as part of a global conspiracy of multinational drug companies to produce African "guinea pigs" for Western AIDS research.

The hostility of African governments including that of Kenya was also witnessed in the low attendance of African scientists and physicians at a major European conference, ostensibly about AIDS in Africa, which was held at about the same time. At this conference where 700 AIDS experts gathered from around the world to discuss the issues involved, only fifty delegates from African countries were present. These delegates, however, made the African position very clear in a joint statement challenging the contention that AIDS originated in Africa. They feared that "a blanket identification of Africans with AIDS could lead to large-scale discrimination against nationals of the continent elsewhere in the world". Indeed, later press accounts cited the case of two Zairian brothers who were expelled from a school in Brussels when it was reported to the authorities by their family doctor that they were carrying the AIDS virus. The tests were subsequently found to be incorrect. More recent reports of discussions over possible restrictions on world travel for citizens of infected ares have given a prophetic ring to these original fears. Yet, in addition to these legitimate concerns, it later became obvious that African governments were exerting significant pressure on both African and Western scholars and researchers not to participate in the sharing of AIDS information on Africa. These pressures included a number of increasingly restrictive government conditions concerning the conduct and publication of research on AIDS in African countries.

The image of AIDS held by the West was not easily digestible by Africans. Yet, the African defence against the "African origin" theory, and the consequent hostility to the West, went deeper than the fear of being stigmatised. It questioned the scientific and methodological grounds of the studies being undertaken, as well as the projections of AIDS casualties highlighted by the media. Gheorghiu Grigorieff argued against the theory in his book, *No to AIDS*, saying in part that non-African researchers did not take into consideration physiological differences between black Africans and their non-African counterparts, and that carrying the AIDS virus may possibly be part of Africans' normal haematological make-up. Furthermore, later scientific reviews of the early AIDS epidemiological surveys also confirmed African suspicions that the extent of seropositivity among the population may have been greatly overestimated.

More importantly however, the African response was in defence of an Africa that, as the local press was wont to say, was an easy target to shoot at. Countries such as Kenya which have little money to conduct their own studies, are consequently dependent on the West for information and research. Health budgets are stretched to their limits in fighting malaria, diarrhoea, cholera, malnutrition and other maladies more frequent in Africa. African politicians are also shrewd enough to know that Western science itself often comes to Africa with dirty hands. According to one Kenyan journalist; "The competition between research institutions for a share of research financing may also lead unscrupulous scientists to put forward half-baked theories in hopes of attracting funds. Quacks can easily thrive in Africa where they are far from more respectable researchers likely to cross-check their findings and methodology."

Yet, in spite of these initial denials, Kenya started to "open up" officially. In November 1985, in response to a question from a member of the Kenyan Parliament, the Minister of Health, Peter Nyakiano revealed that there had been 8 persons conclusively diagnosed as suffering from AIDS in Kenya and 14 others suspected as having the disease. Of the 22 patients only 10 were Kenyan. Seven of the 8 diagnosed patients had already died. The local press hailed this frankness as a welcome sign that the government had finally admitted that AIDS existed in Kenya and was possibly preparing to doing something about it. But the admission also drew some criticism. While Western newspaper articles may have been exaggerated or even racist in their implications, one Kenyan journalist complained that "African governments are to blame for creating an information vacuum by placing a lid on the AIDS problem."

Since the public explosion in the Autumn of 1985, the government has pursued a deliberate, although not necessarily vigorous, AIDS reporting and prevention policy. It agreed in late 1985 to report the incidences of AIDS to the World Health Organisation and has since held regular press conferences to up-date the information being given to the Kenyan public. An authoritative statement given when I was in Kenya came from the Director of Medical Services, Dr. Karuga Koinange, on 12 August, 1986. He reported that a total of 109 persons with AIDS had so far been diagnosed in Kenya. He explained that Kenya was diagnosing about 4 AIDS victims each month. Of the victims, 65 percent were in the western part of Kenya (Nyanza and western provinces), 30 percent were in central Kenya, and 5 percent were spread among the Rift Valley, and eastern and coastal provinces. Victims were equally distributed according to sex, about 30 percent were non-Kenyans, and only two were homosexuals.

But these numbers, it must be remembered, must be approached in the full knowledge of our ignorance of the hidden battles that have taken place, the silences imposed, and the sectional interest reflected in their construction and eventual public consumption. The problem with numbers is not just a technical one, exacerbated by the conditions of the African context. Numbers also reflect ideological, and political problems as well. In Africa, the numbers that constitute an important part of the "language of AIDS" are severely compromised by massive problems of appropriate diagnosis and diagnostic protocol, of basic and accurate record-keeping, of local cultural and political sensitivities, of the manipulations that are part of Western "grantsmanship", and, finally, of irresponsible and deliberate manipulation by official powerbrokers.

Certainly the government in Kenya can be criticised for being slow to take the AIDS epidemic seriously enough. The Ministry of Health still does not see AIDS prevention efforts as a national priority, although it claims to be monitoring the situation closely. But an important question remains in this AIDS numbers game beyond the problems inherent in diagnosis, record-keeping, and interpretation: Is the government, even given these limitations, reporting the incidence of AIDS and other relevant information honestly and thoroughly? Or to put it another way: Is the Kenyan Ministry of Health deliberately under-reporting the incidence of AIDS in Kenya?

There is some cause to suspect that this may be the case. In the announcement of August 1986 by the Ministry of Health referred to above, Dr. Koinange reported that there had been a total of 109 diagnosed persons with AIDS since 1985 averaging about 4 cases per month for the last twelve months. The reporting in all three national newspapers, The Nation, The Standard, and the Kenya Times was essentially the same, all carrying the statement without seriously questioning how those figures were formulated. No attempt was made to estimate the numbers of people who may be infected with the virus, although a central province dermatologist, Dr. Irungu Mwangi, announced that there were "300 confirmed carriers" of AIDS in Kenya. In my own direct conversations with researchers of the Kenya Medical Research Institute in Nairobi over 340 patients with clinical symptoms common to AIDS had tested as positive for AIDS antibodies in the first six months of 1986 alone. Add to this fact, probable government tampering with AIDS statistics and major gaps in the AIDS reporting system itself, and any numbers officially deriving from Kenya become highly suspect. In fairness to Kenyan officials, they are not alone in their hesitation to report on the incidence of AIDS. Jonathan Mann, head of the WHO's AIDS prevention efforts, suspects a "huge" under-reporting of AIDS by countries in general.

The lack of local press interest in problems of AIDS detection and prevention is remarkable, given the fairly open access of reporters to the Kenya Medical Research Institute. When it comes to AIDS, however, the truth seems to be that the Kenyan press has all but abdicated its role as public watchdog, and is under the control of government censors. There is no critical press in Kenya and any serious political opposition is clandestine or a mere product of the extensive rumour mill that forms part of any expression of discontent with the government. The press simply records and reports official statements. Typically, it does not analyse or evaluate the government's performance. This is not the case with the foreign press, however, who continue to keep the AIDS issue alive much to the consternation of public officials. Following President Moi's uncomfortable trip to the USA last March where he was haunted by press questions on human rights abuses in his suppression of the Mwakenya movement as well as on AIDS in Kenya, KANU National Secretary, Laban Kitele, threatened to censor all Nairobi-based foreign correspondents. He criticised all of these reports as an "orchestrated move by certain foreign powers and self-exiled Kenyan dissidents".

Some of the problems in press and government reporting are related to the absence of what may be called a politically active AIDS constituency. Unlike the USA with its highly organised, efficient and widespread "Gay Movement", there is no comparable group with the potential to galvanise, articulate and document AIDS activities in Kenya and other African states. These countries, to their detriment, have no similar catalyst to stimulate and keep objective their AIDS efforts. This gap is partly due to the contrasting constellation of AIDS victims in Africa as compared with the West. AIDS in the West primarily affects the homosexual population (70 percent of victims) unlike Africa, where the virus takes an equal toll of men and women. These factors to some extent explain the acceptance of the rather impoverished official response and corresponding lack of commitment in the face of this serious medical problem. This criticism does not necessarily entail a lack of sympathy for the massive problems that these agencies already face. The health issues they are confronting are enormous; cholera, malaria, accidents, poor medical care and facilities, and chronic shortages of essential supplies are all too frequent and demanding. Certainly, in the face of these problems, the difficulties in the way of obtaining the resources needed for an adequate AIDS campaign must seem overwhelming.

The Autumn of 1985 also witnessed the formation of the Kenya National AIDS Committee to assist the Ministry of Health in its prevention campaign. This committee which only meets every two months is made up of physicians and researchers. They began working in January 1986 on AIDS guidelines for heath care professionals and the public. The announcement of the formation of this committee came in the wake of a report that medical staff in a leading private hospital in Nairobi had refused to handle a diagnosed AIDS patient. Doctors from KMRI were called in to take the patient to Kenyatta National Hospital where most AIDS patients receive treatment. These guidelines were issued at the end of January 1986 to senior doctors in Nairobi and to those in provincial hospitals. A series of workshops for those physicians was also conducted by KMRI staff on the management of AIDS patients. A central unit for blood testing and patient profile make-up was established, and a cost analysis of screening the nation's blood supply was begun. In these guidelines confidentiality was stressed. However, keeping information confidential is jeopardised by an over-elaborate and loose system of reporting. Information on a confirmed AIDS diagnosis goes first to the director of the hospital involved, then the doctor, then presumably the patient. The guidelines also called for hospitals to set up AIDS registers as well as to establish hospital committees to oversee discharges of AIDS patients.

The government's public education campaign consists of periodic statements placed in the national media (both in Swahili and English) offering information about the conditions of transmission, and prevention measures. The Ministry has also distributed pamphlets and posters. They are not, however, easily accessible or available, and their distribution is often more discussed than seen. Posters have been reported to have been widely distributed in those areas reporting the highest incidence of AIDS victims, although I did not see any in Nairobi or Mombasa. The nature of the information has ranged between the over-technical and clinical to the vague and misleading, such as those by the Director of Medical Services, to refrain from "grazing in other pastures". The material bounces between confusing explanations of medical terminology to blatantly sexist references as to the unfortunate implications of AIDS for many sexual practices. Yet, there is important information being distributed also. However, it was only in August 1986 that any serious attempt was made to mention condoms in the prevention literature. That delay is somewhat understandable given their high cost and low availability, and the problem of their acceptance by men. These are major problems that still receive little attention in Kenya.

It is clear that there is much public concern about AIDS in Kenya. Letters to daily newspapers frequently request educational materials on AIDS. A public lecture on sexually transmitted diseases, held at Kerugoya Catholic Church in the central province attracted thousands of eager listeners. And the readiness of the press to report any "approved" detail of the epidemic reflects the commodity value of AIDS talk. But expressions of public sentiment in interviews and public comments have also included the negative, such as calls for the government to screen all foreigners for AIDS or to round up AIDS victims and put them in a "secret place". Then there is also the charge by Kenya's rising right-wing evangelicals that AIDS is "a clear sign of divine judgement in connection with homosexuality and drug abuse". The fact that these divine assessments fail to fit the reality of the African AIDS predicament appears to be of little consequence.

One troubling silence in the public discourse on AIDS in Kenya involves the pressing problem of blood supply for transfusion. Not surprisingly, the blood supply in Kenya is not adequately protected. Infections through contaminated blood may account for as many as 10 percent of all AIDS victims in Africa. It has been reported that screening the blood supply for AIDS patients is occurring in Nairobi and Mombasa, and that by March 1987, Kenya will, according to Dr. Koinange, become the first African nation to screen all blood for the AIDS virus. There are, however, many good reasons to be skeptical of this proclamation. There is, for example, a widespread lack of testing kits, complicated by a fast-moving blood supply, chronic blood shortages, and the absence of adequate blood reserves and storage facilities. These problems also prevent the storage of blood by those who themselves need to use it for forthcoming elective surgery. In addition, the tendency in African medical practice to transfuse blood more frequently, raises even higher the risk of the spread of infection. All of these problems plus the cost of such active screening are certainly demoralising, and have contributed to a feeble government response to the aspect of the AIDS crisis.

An additional problem is the transmission of the virus by the use of contaminated needles. Studies have already linked seropositivity with the number of injections received by patients. Infection via this route is a major problem both in legitimate medical facilities in Kenya and on the street. Sterilisation or re-usable (and even what are meant to be disposable) needles and syringes is poor, owing to shortages of supplies and equipment, inadequate staff education, non-existent monitoring procedures, and the high number of patients. Even more troublesome is the danger of infection due to injections given by a wide variety of local healers (and charlatans) living in the shanties and in the bush. The cultural preference given to the injection as a mode of treatment has spawned a host of profiteers at the grass-roots level. If one considers that an estimated 75 percent of the population use folk-healers as the first line of health defence, the possible magnitude of the problem becomes apparent.

But while the problems of AIDS prevention may receive little attention in the press, those of regulation are reported in great detail. It is now common knowledge that Kenyans who fail to report to the authorities that they may have AIDS are liable for arrest. Recently a man at the provincial hospital in Nyeri who was suspected of having AIDS, and transferred to Kenyatta National Hospital in Nairobi, left the hospital on his own before his diagnosis was completed. The police and medial officers arrested the man in his home and took him back to the hospital where he was eventually given a "conditional discharge". Another man in Nairobi was suspected of having AIDS and admitted to Kenyatta National Hospital. His relatives were not allowed to enter his room and after his subsequent death, his coffin was sealed and police and medical officers prohibited the public viewing of his body. In a similar incident, public health officials in Mombasa refused permission to transport the body of a man who had died and was suspected of having AIDS. The man had to be buried in Mombasa and not his home town. His family was instructed to have no more than eight people at his funeral.

In a more recent display of medical policing, 275 women were picked up by the police in two separate sweeps in Eldama and in Kisumu, Kenya. They were all tested for sexually-transmitted diseases including AIDS. These women faced criminal charges if they were tested positive on any STD. One should note that no similar sweeps were done on the men that frequented the bars where these women were picked up. The authorities claim the right to authorise these police hunts under the Kenyan Public Health Act, Section 17.

Recent press accounts have noted an increasing openness by African officials in discussions of the AIDS epidemic in their countries, and the WHO has become more aggressive in its efforts to engage African governments in AIDS reporting and prevention efforts. But Kenya's political leaders have continued to react fiercely to any direct or implied criticism of their dealing with AIDS. When it was reported in London press that Prince Charles would be carrying his own blood supply during his visits to Kenya, Malawi, and Swaziland, the President and several of his ministers condemned the "Malicious propaganda emanating from outside the country". This defensiveness has practical consequences for AIDS efforts in Kenya. The language governing this AIDS efforts is characterised by a number of major absences and silences. These gaps in the AIDS discourse in Kenya are conditioned by the environment of struggle found throughout Africa, which exerts a strong negative impact on attempts to combat AIDS on the continent. Contagion and prevention are cultural, social and political phenomena. Since AIDS preventive efforts fall mostly within the area of behavioural education, these gaps are all the more important since they blind us to a more thorough understanding of the social meaning of AIDS in Africa and the complex set of human processes which contribute to its spread.

I think it is safe to say that the language of AIDS in Kenya and in many other parts of Africa suffers from a lack of critical reflection and dialogue. At the local level, as I have indicated, frank, open, and honest discussion is smothered by the absence of a free press, the economic pressures exerted by tourism, and the politics of the Western scientific invasion of the area. These forces also operate at the regional and international levels but are further complicated by the politics of neocolonialism and the struggles of the Third World against the cultural and political penetration of the West. AIDS talk in this atmosphere becomes very complicated indeed, and is infused with political agendas which have little to do with the immediate goals of AIDS prevention.

But there are other silences that must be addressed, in the voices that make up the AIDS language itself. Sacrificed in the African discourse on AIDS, for example, is the voice of the victim. There is no literature, no popular media, no major group articulating this voice. There is, in other words, no visible response from those who suffer from this malady, no dialogue with those who can most directly communicate the meaning of this pain. What is the social and cultural experience of the illness for Africans? How can preventive measures reflect and adapt to his experience? Where is the communication and learning between the fields of medicine, culture and AIDS? How will compassion and understanding be created in the absence of this voice? There are indications that most Africans know very little about AIDS and its prevention. This is not just the result of the lack of AIDS brochures. It is the product of the historical, cultural and political gap between the First and Third Worlds. One can gain a small measure of appreciation of the issues here by considering the difficulties experienced even by AIDS activists in the USA in finding an effective bridge between the language of AIDS prevention and that of homosexuality and intimacy. With the silence is lost the potentially positive efforts that comes when AIDS victims speak out.

There are, in addition, other victims silenced or ignored in the AIDS language of Kenya. Current AIDS talk reinforces heavy discrimination against women in Kenya and in other African countries. Given the male-oriented bias of the medical community, as well as the lack of an active AIDS constituency, AIDS talk becomes part of an arsenal of reasons to harass, abuse, and exploit the victims of the booming sex trade, namely, poor and disadvantaged women. The medical policing of these women proceeds with almost total disregard for due legal process and basic civil liberties. The weight of science and medicine now contributes to an already poor human rights record for women, and the AIDS language does nothing to reflect the suffering of these victims.

Finally, the African AIDS situation is further complicated not only by the political struggles but by the cultural ones as well. The language of AIDS in Africa is one derived from the West. It is a transplanted language that is dependent on the West for its meaning and continued development. It speaks in Western symbol and with a voice that was born from that cultural cosmology. It is not indigenous to Africa and thus is blind to the African world of meaning. For example, there are cultural practices, traditional rituals including a host of communal eating and drinking practices, that seem to be coming under what may be called the negative influence of AIDS preventive efforts. These practices are coming increasingly under review by anthropologists and social scientists who are moved by their concern over the potential for transmission of HIV. Where these practices are intact, they are fundamental to community bonding and the meaning of social life. Yet, they are all falling victim, justifiably or not, to both the negative impact of Western inspection, and the public's fear of contracting the AIDS virus. This fear is in part generated by the media, and other sources of information which rely on Western reports. A prevention language insensitive to this potential runs the real risk of contributing significantly to the deterioration of the everyday symbols of communality specific to those areas of Africa involved.

Given the richness of the cultural diversity of the African continent, the language of AIDS should be a polyphony of voices aware of the many dimensions and problems that this epidemic presents. Yet, at root, the basic preventive strategy should be one that addresses the voices from below, that is, from those who suffer. This singularly important hermeneutic point cannot be neglected. It alone poses the critical question, namely, what would an AIDS prevention pro-gramme look like from the social, political and cultural word-view of those most directly affected? This kind of strategy cannot be ade-quately represented in the current monopoly of AIDS research by Western medicine. While certainly indispensable for efforts to stop the spread of AIDS, this monopoly precludes an analysis sympathetic to different cultural symbols of meaning, and often fails to recognise its own conventional origins and limited perspectives. It is difficult to avoid the conclusion that the silence of voices from below, for whatever reasons, presents a major obstacle to the effectiveness of AIDS prevention efforts in Africa.

Sense and Nonsense on AIDS

Editorial in *West Africa*
February 9, 1987

AIDS — the almost always fatal stage of infection of the deadly HIV virus —has been described, with justification, as the great scourge of the 20th century. In the short period since it was first diagnosed, the numbers of its victims have risen alarmingly, as has, the number of countries where it can be found. While, despite intense research, very little is yet known about its origins, and there is still no cure, it is now known that it can very easily be spread through established social practices, which perhaps accounts for the panic that reigns wherever it is mentioned. In several countries however, especially the developed ones, unreasoning panic is gradually giving way to more organised responses; special facilities are being provided to take care of victims, and public information campaigns aimed at prevention have been started.

Along with these worthwhile campaigns there is another campaign, of a more despicable nature, whose sole aim seems to be to trace the origin of AIDS to Africa. Although it is known that the disease first manifested itself among the homosexual community of the United States, all kinds of "experts" are proposing an African origin, without saying what possible links there could be between American homosexuals and Africa. This propaganda campaign which uses the suspect opinions of so-called experts, who if they were so expert should have been more cautious in reaching conclusions about a subject which they, as well as other people, apparently know so little about, has assumed increasingly racist tones. Thus the British government announces an intention to test visitors arriving from Africa for AIDS (and not those from America), the British Medical Association warns, and then recants on the high risk of blood donated by anyone who may have had a sexual relationship with a black Africa, and countless articles and television programmes are being run which use what amounts to abuse of statistics to insinuate that there is a higher prevalence of AIDS in certain parts of Africa than anywhere else.

It is all nonsense of course, even if the West, with its overwhelming domination of information media succeeds in making this blatant misinformation fashionable. One fact which the campaign cannot get over is that the disease first appeared in America. Those who argue a prior existence in Africa, where they claim it was previously wrongly diagnosed, are still to offer any explanation of the link with America, and not Europe which has had and continues to have a longer and more extensive contact with Africa. They have an even harder task explaining why a disease of such virulence as AIDS is now known to be, had not long ago wiped out the populations of the accused countries, where without exception medical facilities and services are poor. They also have to explain why they have become so alarmingly susceptible since the American manifestation.

And one cannot easily discount the suggestion that AIDS is the product of germ-warfare research gone dangerously wrong. The Western media dismiss the suggestion as Soviet propaganda, and yet all the evidence points to a new disease. Even the campaign to blame it on Africa cannot date its emergence before the 1970's; and some in Africa are beginning to wonder whether the ongoing campaign is not an attempt to divert enquiry from the possibility that some previously unknown germs may have been tested on Africans.

The most unfortunate effect of the current campaign has been to put Africans on the defensive about AIDS. Whereas African governments, in line with the efforts being made elsewhere, ought to be engaged in campaigns to educate their citizens about the dangers and ways to avoid infection, they are now more occupied fending off the calumny. For them it seems more important to prove that there is no AIDS in their countries. The reason is obvious, AIDS still inspires so much panic that it frightens off visitors.

In the meantime, the urgent public education campaigns have been deferred. Given the acute poverty of the continent only a few of the countries can afford the cost of importing equipment for diagnosing and treating AIDS. In such circumstances prevention would be of critical importance, but even here, very little, it seems, is being done. Blood transfusions, one of the known ways of transmitting the infection, are still being given without screening; people of easy virtue, whose association with tourists may have been the route by which the disease reached Africa, still do not apparently believe that there is a grave danger, and their ignorance is matched almost everywhere by that of their compatriots. While people elsewhere are taking action to control the spread of the deadly disease, Africans are still not being given sufficient warning of a risk which could become even more disastrous than anything the continent's detractors had imagined. Some may wish to derive some comfort from the declaration: "There is no AIDS here". The truth of course is that it will get there, if it hasn't already. And the sooner governments begin to take that reality more seriously, the better for their threatened citizens.

The Spread of Racism

by Richard Chirimuuta,
Rosalind Harrison
and Davis Gazi
Reprinted with permission from *West Africa*
February 9, 1987

The widely held belief that the AIDS virus originated in Africa has had disturbing consequences for black people in Africa and abroad. The proposal from the British Foreign Office that people from certain African countries wishing to enter the United Kingdom should be screened for AIDS; the description of black people as AIDS carriers in National Front propaganda in the normal course of racist abuse, and the damaging effect of loss of revenue from tourism in countries where tourism is a major industry are all consequences of a hypothesis that has been proposed and accepted by medical scientists. The uncontrolled sexuality of black people is a continuing theme of racist mythology used, for example, to justify the lynching of thousands of innocent black people in the southern United States, and when AIDS first appeared in black people, it changed overnight from a "gay plague" to an imported Haitian and then an African disease. Many black people view the Haitian and African connections with a profound skepticism that is now finding increasing scientific support.

The British Medical Journal recently published (27 Sept, 1986) the most important challenge to date to the hypothesis that the virus responsible for AIDS originated in Africa. A group of West German researchers tested serum samples from 6,015 people in nine African countries including Kenya, Uganda and Zaire where AIDS is not a serious problem. The samples were collected between 1976 and 1984, and the authors concluded that "these data show that fewer than one in 1,000 subjects were seropositive for AIDS at the time of sampling before 1985 and do not support the hypothesis of the disease originating in Africa." Ironically researchers from another country famous for its espousal of racial superiority, South Africa, produced similar results, whilst American, British, French and Belgian scientists have published a plethora of articles proposing and supporting an African origin to AIDS.

It is most unfortunate, particularly for the Africans who are now regarded as the AIDS scourge of the world, that a hypothesis that has not withstood the normal process of scientific challenge and investigation is now so widely accepted as established scientific fact. It is inevitable that the mass media on an issue of such great public concern will at times misrepresent and distort the facts. In this instance, though, the medical scientists themselves must bear the greatest responsibility for propagating the "AIDS from Africa" story.

During the short history of AIDS there has been not one, but two attempts to attribute the source of the disease to black people. When the Centers for Disease Control in Atlanta reported in 1982 that approximately five percent of AIDS cases in the United States were Haitian immigrants, Haitians were soon considered the source of the American epidemic. There was no scientific evidence for a Haitian origin when it was proposed, nor could any be found on subsequent investigation. As Port au Prince, the capital of Haiti, was a popular resort for American homosexuals in the late 1970's it is probable that AIDS was an imported and not an exported disease. In spite of the lack of scientific evidence, anti-Haitian hysteria was whipped up by the popular press. Healthy Haitians throughout the United States were sacked from their jobs and evicted from their homes, and Haitian criminals were even put in separate prisons.

Although the Haitian hypothesis collapsed, the idea of black people as the source of AIDS was too attractive to abandon. It was now argued (British Medical Journal, August 1984) that the AIDS virus originated in central Africa, and had been present there for many years — an "old disease of Africa". No scientific evidence was available to support this hypothesis, which contained some striking inconsistencies. Increased cultural contacts between Americans and Africans was offered as the reason for the initial appearance of the disease in the United States, but there was no attempt to explain how European slave traders and colonists of previous centuries avoided their just desserts and escaped infection. To explain how AIDS had previously escaped medical attention, an analogy was made with Lassa fever, an acute febrile illness of short duration first described in a missionary nurse in north-eastern Nigeria. Despite initial alarm surrounding this disease, it soon became apparent that subclinical infection was common. AIDS is a progressive, wasting disease that often kills the patient slowly, and doctors practicing in tropical Africa during the 1960's and 1970's do not accept that cases even in distant rural areas could have escaped their attention.

Undaunted and armed with this new hypothesis, there followed another "scramble for Africa" by European and American doctors looking for the source of AIDS. Arriving in Africa after the American and European epidemics were well under way, they gathered startling evidence. Flying teams of French and Belgian doctors in a few weeks found numbers of patients with symptoms and signs of AIDS. Blood tests revealed that up to 50 percent of the population of some areas had been infected with the AIDS virus, although few if any of these people showed any clinical evidence of the disease. The medical world was largely convinced that the African origin of AIDS became a fact. But how well does the evidence stand up to critical assessment?

First, some of the evidence has been anectotal and circumstantial. Cases of AIDS in patients originating from central Africa were confirmed in the early 1980's soon after the syndrome was recognised in America and Europe. Although many of these patients had been resident in Europe for years, the possibility that they may have contracted the disease in Europe was not considered. A few cases of patients from, or working in central Africa who died of mysterious, AIDS-like illnesses in the 1970's were presented retrospectively as evidence that AIDS was present in Africa before the American and European epidemics. Such clinical evidence without laboratory confirmation is of dubious quality, as AIDS-like cases before the late 1970's were also reported in Western countries, and insect-transmitted tropical diseases such as visceral leishmaniasis can be difficult to distinguish from AIDS.

Secondly, a type of tumour called Kaposi's sarcoma (KS), which occurs in one-third of patients with AIDS, was previously rare in Europe but common in some parts of tropical Africa. Although proponents of the African hypothesis argued this could be evidence for the longstanding presence of the HTLV-III virus in Africa, no association between endemic African Kaposi's sarcoma and AIDS has been found. Researchers in Zambia, in a report in the Lancet (Feb. 1985) concluded: "Although the endemic form of KS has long been known in Zambia, the typical aggressive form first appeared in 1983. . . . These results are further evidence of the emergence of a clinically typical form of KS in Africans which resembles that seen in American patients with AIDS and which is associated with HTLV-III infection ... suggesting that this virus is new to Zambia...."

Thirdly, there is the serological evidence, the blood tests for AIDS antibodies that the German research now challenges. The most commonly used test for AIDS, the rapid and economical enzyme-linked immunosorbent assay (ELISA), is known to produce false positives, that is, cases of patients giving a positive result without having the disease. In Europe and America this false positive rate is low and the test is useful for screening blood and organ donors. The German researchers found that approximately 10 percent of blood samples collected between 1976 and 1984 were positive with the ELISA test, but only 0.07 percent were actually found to have AIDS antibodies when more specific tests were made. The most probable explanation for the high false positive rate is cross-reaction of the ELISA reagent with antibodies to malarial parasites. Positive ELISA tests in blood collected in Africa prior to the American epidemic and no longer be considered as evidence for the African hypothesis. Similarly the high rate of ELISA positive in some parts of Africa provides thoroughly misleading information about the current rate of HTLV-III infection. The German researchers conclude that the African AIDS epidemic started at the same time as, or even later than, the epidemics in American and Europe.

Although the high rate of false positives has confused the picture, it is now becoming clear that th risk groups for AIDS in central and eastern Africa are the female prostitutes and relatively wealthy promiscuous men who travel widely, the very people most likely to acquire a disease introduced to, rather than originating from the continent. This is contrary to the expectations of the AIDS researchers and conflicts with the hypothesis of an old African disease. Rather than confront the lack of evidence for any African origin, proponents of the African connection have quietly shifted their ground. AIDS, it is claimed, is no longer an old African disease but a new disease that originated in Africa about 10 years ago.

It is little wonder that black people view much AIDS "research" (for want of a better word) with resentment and increasing anger. Recognition of an equal sex incidence of AIDS in Africa was accompanied by entirely unsubstantiated assertions that Africans indulged in frequent anal intercourse, or that "primitive African tribes" had intercourse during menstruation. A recent study of applicants for military service in the United States found a ratio of affected men to women of 2.5 to 1 nationwide, whilst in New York metropolitan area the ratio was nearly equal. They concluded that the AIDS virus is transmitted very efficiently through normal heterosexual contact. The widespread use of condoms by prostitutes in the West but not in Africa is one more reasonable explanation for the slower spread of the AIDS virus to heterosexuals in Western countries than bizarre speculations about the sexual activities of Africans.

We would like to believe that the uncritical acceptance of the African connection was a simple error of judgement but it seems far more likely that the AIDS researchers, the medical experts, the media and the public at large are affected by the insidious and frequently unrecognised disease of racism. How else can we explain the rubbish that was published by respected scientific journals such as The Lancet, in the following example arguing that the African swine fever virus was responsible for AIDS: "Perhaps an infected pig was killed and eaten either as uncooked or undercooked meat. One of the people eating the meat who was both immunocompromised and homosexual would be a pivotal point, allowing for the disease to spread to the vacationing "gay" tourists in Haiti". (Note that Haitians are homosexual but the Americans are gay.) How else can the abandonment of scientific methods and the persistence in the attempts to attribute the source of AIDS to black people be explained?

After all that has been written about AIDS in Africa we should remind ourselves that over 90 percent of cases of AIDS in the world are in the United States and Western Europe (WHO Chronicle 1985). The notion that AIDS is an African disease is entrenched in the minds of doctors and public alike, but scientists are only now urging caution. Dr. J.J. Jefferies, a leading British virologist, criticised a teaching video produced by the Leichestershire Health Authority in the following way: "Many people are curious as to the origin of the virus, but without further evidence it seems unfair to perpetuate the suggestion that the virus was taken by Haitian migrants from Zaire to Haiti." We have seen a greater willingness to believe a hypothesis inspired by racism than a search for scientific truth. Let us hope that the truth now prevails.

Breadwinners and the Poor are Most Vulnerable

Jon Tinker
Reprinted with permission from *People*
October 1987

There are growing signs that AIDS is hitting preferentially at the poor: at both the impoverished ethnic minorities within the rich, white societies, and at the poor nations of Asia, Latin America, the Caribbean — and most of all in Africa.

In March this year, the Panos Institute convened a consultation at Talloires in the French Alps of all the main bilateral, multilateral and voluntary development agencies, to discuss the development implications of AIDS. Participants included the heads of WHO and of UNICEF, of the Canadian and Swiss aid agencies, and of the Red Cross League, and senior officials from a score more agencies. Our unanimous conclusion was that the development impacts of AIDS were still largely unforeseen, but likely to be immense.

Most of the leading official and voluntary development agencies have since started to address AIDS as a development issue. Panos is playing its part, in a continuing collaboration with the Norwegian Red Cross. One of our major projects, in association with Imperial College, London, is research into the probable epidemiological, demographic and economic effects of AIDS epidemics. Of about 52,000 cases of AIDS officially reported to WHO, 36,000 are in the United States. This sounds as if the US has the biggest AIDS problem by far. Not so. Based on figures officially reported to WHO by governments, the United States has 15 cases of AIDS per 100,000 population. But the Bahamas has recorded 37 cases per 100,000 population, French Guyana 71 cases, and Bermuda 98 cases. In Europe, Switzerland has reported the most cases: 3.6 per 100,000. France comes next with

3.0, then Denmark with 2.9. Compare that with the Congo's 14 AIDS cases per 100,000, Rwanda with 12, Uganda with 7, Tanzania with 5.

All these Third World figures are substantially higher than those for the US and Europe. All the African figures are certainly under-reported. All of them are from countries where even in the cities not everyone has access to a doctor. All of them are countries with health services which are grossly underfunded, rudimentary by our rich-nation standards. Infection with the AIDS virus in some central African countries, among urban people in the sexually-active age groups, already ranges from 5 to 20 percent equally among men and women. In a number of east and central African cities, from 5 to 25 percent of women attending urban prenatal clinics are now carriers of the virus. These women have at least a 50/50 chance of passing the virus to their babies; half of these infected infants will die before their first birthdays, and the rest within a year or two. The development implications are profound. Consider first the obvious, direct economic costs of health care: a single bloodtest in the Third World retails for about $4, one machine for testing blood samples costs up to $15,000, a hundred condoms, a year's supply for one person, costs $5 wholesale, and a great deal more over the counter of a shop.

Compare those figures with the annual health budget of many African countries: well under $5 per capita. By 1991, now only four years away, the US Surgeon General estimates that the annual health costs of treating AIDS patients will have reached at least $8 billion; a figure of Pentagon-like dimensions, which will strain even America's vast resources and humanity. The far less well-equipped health services of Burundi and Zaire, of Brazil and Haiti, are facing an AIDS epidemic that is, or will soon be, as bad if not worse. Deaths from AIDS in developing countries will mainly be in the breadwinning age-groups: 20-40 years old. This is in marked contrast to most other diseases and illnesses, which largely kill the very young and the old. In the Third World, the people stricken by AIDS are those who support the young and the old, the disabled and the sick. Deaths in this breadwinning age group will change the dependency ratio — the number of dependents which each surviving worker must support.

The deaths from AIDS will (apart from infants) be overwhelmingly among the active labour force, the women and men who hoe the fields and weed the crops. Each surviving farmer will have more dependents to support. Her poverty will become greater, not less. She will be forced into more, not less environmental damage. Much African subsistence agriculture is labour-limited, especially during planting and seeding after the rains. AIDS epidemics, causing many deaths among active rural women and men, may significantly reduce output. Since at the same time the dependency ratio will be increasing, food shortages may well result.

A number of the developing countries already affected by AIDS rely heavily on tourism for foreign exchange. Last year, Gambia's tourist bookings were badly affected when a British newspaper incorrectly reported that a second AIDS virus, not detectable by tests then available, was widespread in that country. The 1987 edition of Fodor's guide to Kenya, as part of a generally accurate and helpful section on AIDS, contains the sentence: "Doctors speculate that in some African countries the infection rate may be 30 percent of the *total* population." Now this is complete nonsense. In *no* African country are the figures even half that, and in Kenya they are almost certainly well under one-tenth the figure quoted by Fodor. The publication of such an exaggeration in a widely-read and respected tourist guide is bound to be harmful to Kenya's tourist industry — its biggest single dollar-earner.

Tourists are *not* at risk from AIDS, in Kenya or anywhere else, unless they engage in unsafe sex (which is after all a strictly voluntary activity), or unless they receive medical treatment involving unscreened blood or unsterilized needles. Tourism is a highly competitive business, where customers switch easily from one destination to another. It is understandable why some Third World countries which rely heavily on tourism have so far been cautious about publicizing their AIDS epidemics. But tourists' fears of AIDS are real, and these countries may need to mount factual information campaigns to reassure them by publicizing when hospitals in resorts do start to screen blood, for example.

In countries where trained manpower is in short supply, as is especially the case in Africa, some companies and industries may face massive losses of key personnel. In one central African mining town, 68 percent of a small sample of skilled male mineworkers were carrying the virus last year. Contract workers in mining or cash-crop agriculture may also be vulnerable. Many work far away from their families, for months at a time, and many among them use prostitutes or casual sex. AIDS epidemics in these industries could affect mining production, earnings of foreign exchange, and ultimately international commodity prices. In many developing countries, employers traditionally help with medical charges, hospital care, and sick pay. One mining corporation in central Africa has concluded from the present levels of the virus among its workforce that its sick pay policy could bankrupt it within a few years.

AIDS epidemics may also have significant effects on foreign investment in the Third World. Transnationals, and other investors with the
possibility of switching investment away from a country with a major
AIDS epidemic, are likely to be affected by considerations such as
reduced local markets, the cost of sick pay for employees affected by
AIDS, higher premiums for health and life insurance, and an unwilling-
ness of expatriates or their families to be transferred there.

Secondary and higher education in Third World countries with
major AIDS epidemics may also be affected. In Lusaka, for example, a
small number of blood samples last year suggested that 6 percent of
high school students, and 10 percent of university students, were
infected. These people are Zambia's future doctors, teachers, engi-
neers and administrators. Losing them will limit the nation's development for a generation.

Regular and irregular armed forces have historically had high levels
of sexually transmitted disease. The same is true of AIDS. The military
authorities of the US, UK, Belgium, France, USSR and Cuba are already
seriously concerned about the risks of AIDS infection among their
troops. Guerilla wars probably involve especially high sexual contact
rates. There are indications that guerilla action in Ethiopia,
Mozambique, Angola, Nicaragua and elsewhere is linked with growing AIDS epidemics.

In too many Third World countries, the army is the ultimate source
of political power. The impact of AIDS is going to be felt far beyond
the health sector in the Third World. It is going to threaten every
aspect of development: tourism, industry, agriculture, balance of pay-
ments, the supply of trained doctors and administrators, even political
stability.

How is the international community reacting to this crisis? The
development of education programmes, both in developed and developing countries, has been remarkable and encouraging in recent
months. Rwanda and Brazil already have government run education
campaigns, for example, and the leaflets produced by the Kenyan Red
Cross are some of the best in the world.

Uganda's campaign centres round the slogan "Love Carefully": so
much more socially responsible than the narrowly self-protective US
and European concept of "safe sex".

The national and international leadership on AIDS education given
by President Museveni of Uganda, and more recently by President
Kaunda of Zambia, has been extremely important. So far, the reaction
of donor countries to WHO's appeals for funds to tackle AIDS has

been excellent. But this money appears largely to have been subtracted from other accounts in existing development assistance budgets. And it is a drop in the ocean compared with what will be needed in two, five, ten years' time.

In the United States, AIDS was at first an illness of relatively affluent and educated gay men. Now, it is more and more becoming a problem for the Black and Hispanic minorities. Of all the US AIDS cases reported by September 1986, 25 percent were among Blacks, who make up only 12 percent of the US population, and 14 percent were among Hispanics, who make up 6 percent of the population. Today, Black and Hispanic Americans appear several times more likely to pick up the AIDS virus than whites. These ethnic minorities are likely to be poorer than the white majority; they are more likely to be involved in high-risk activities such as prostitution or intravenous drug abuse; and they are far less likely than whites to be reached by current education campaigns.

And just as the poorest in our rich societies are likely to suffer disproportionately from AIDS, especially as epidemics spread into the heterosexual community, so are the poorest likely to be disproportionately vulnerable in developing countries. The global underclass, those who live in rural and urban shantytowns and squatter settlements, whose families are split apart by poverty, who cannot afford condoms and are not reached by family planning advice, who often cannot read, who have little or no access to health clinics, whose medical needs have to be satisfied by street-corner injections, who may have to sell their very blood to buy food, whose daughters and sons are more likely to be driven into prostitution, who are least likely to be reached by education campaigns — this global underclass will be disproportionately affected by AIDS, just as Blacks and Hispanics already are in New York and Miami. AIDS is not a series of disconnected national epidemics, but a worldwide pandemic. Our international response to it has so far focussed mainly on the rich and the white.

Imperial Bedroom

Julie Burchill

Reprinted with permission from *New Society*

February 20, 1987

**The white man has been copulating with the natives
of faraway places as long as he has been killing them.
Now *they* can do both to *him* at once.**

Although written 20 years before, it was very fitting that Joe
Orton's diaries were published last year; Year One AA. (Before
Christ, Anno Domini, After AIDS.) The most regular feature of
this journal is the incredible ease and speed with which Mr. Orton
buggers the boy children of Morocco — for a small fee. A *very* small
fee. But then, they were Third World babies.

AIDS has proved a catalyst that shows up a lot of sloppy thinking;
about the minority always being right-on, about sexism, racism and
that most icky of isms, tourism. Of course there is no reasonable way
one can continue to refer to AIDS as a "gay plague" (but that being so,
homosexuals *must* stop screaming "persecution!" every time anyone
says something judgmental about AIDS; they must learn to let go of
their latest chip). But the fact does remain that homosexuals were the
people who brought AIDS into this country.

AIDS was brought here by homosexuals, British and American, who
had had their beady eyes caught by advertisements in the gay press
which told them in so many words how cheap and easy it was to have
a holiday in the sun of Haiti or Morocco — and have a native thrown
in for the price of a pina collada. That this is so should be a matter of
great shame and regret to our homosexual community. (Sue me).

Since the early seventies, several dubious homosexual ideas have
been indulged by liberals who would have blanched and ordered 20

Hail Fidels to heterosexual practitioners. They were indulged because they were a persecuted minority and thus always right. In the
same way white liberals don't dare question scummy behaviour towards women from the Rastafarian and Asian immigrants for fear of
being called racist. (The volubility with which our Rastafarian and
Asian communities have begun to speak out against homosexuals in
the eighties will prove a big stumbling ground to white liberals as they
decide *which* minority to back.)

Enlightened people have long dismissed heterosexual dances as
"meat racks." Yet few things other than Smithfield are more Meat
Marketing Boardish than a gay disco. Appreciation of youth and beauty in a woman by a man has long brought catcalls of "sexist" — yet
youth and beauty score higher in Heaven than anywhere on earth.
Liberals despise the macho, heterosexual heroes like Rambo and
Cobra; but the homosexual worship of the strongman, from Genet
and his adored nazis onward, is never questioned. Incredibly, some
advertisements for gay discotheques stipulate "No swastikas"; very
admirable, I'm sure, but that this needs to be stipulated in the first
place is amazing.

Only the political lesbians, not burdened by heterosexist guilt, have
tackled this dubious ideological itch, and are now more alienated
from their male counterparts than at any time — homosexual men
have much more in common with heterosexual men that with your
average monogamous, politically pure lesbian. A year or so ago, the
Camden GLC girls and the homosexuals were at each others' throats
when a community centre which the feminists had just persuaded
local Asian women to frequent was the venue of a Gay Skinhead disco.
The Asian women, terrified by the boots and insignia that in real life
threaten them so monstrously, took flight and were never seen again.
Despite the Gay Skinheads screams about "rights," that other minorities might have rights not to feel threatened by white men seemed to
have escaped them yet again.

But the most criminally and now fatally neglected grey area has
been that of sexual tourism — or sexual imperialism, to use a word
enlightened people are fond of applying to others. Many a manly
velour chest has been beaten about the vile practice of sex tourism to
Indo-China — Anthony Mighella even wrote a play about it. But one
expects that from the Japanese and German businessmen who do it.

What I find less understandable is how the homosexual community
has justified to itself the homosexual package tours advertised in such
anti-racists, anti-imperialist publications as *Gay News* (of course one
doesn't expect political analysis from *Throb* or *Zipper*, but *Gay*

News?) to such countries as Morocco and Haiti — countries where poverty, torture and repression of the people easily matches that of South Africa. After a recent AIDS benefit at Heaven, groups of gay men joined the candlelight vigil outside South Africa House; yet if South Africa were a little more to the north of the continent, and if it had going black before AIDS hit, the same homosexuals who protest against the exploitation of blacks by white men might easily have gone there on holiday, making whores out of the same people whose liberation they call for.

A standing cock has no conscience, said some old literary lecher; this maxim has never found a sadder demonstration than with those homosexuals who at home are supporters of the oppressed and abroad the buyers of boys who sell themselves only to alleviate the wretchedness of their families. (If they were naturally so inclined, they wouldn't need paying — ask any callgirl.) People who fiercely defend the right of immigrants in Britain to preserve their culture and traditions completely ignore the fact that there is absolutely no way a Moroccan Muslim or Haitian Catholic boy's upbringing says that homosexuality and promiscuity and the fatal mating of the two in the life of the rented boy is anything but a shameful perversion of all culture and tradition. Homosexuals can give any wicked hiss-boo hetero a run for his American Express card when it comes to racism, imperialism and sexism — they're just racist, imperialist and sexist to their own sex.

The whole issue of tourism is a sticky one, and one that westerners seem singularly inept at looking at clearly — eyes bedazzled by that midday sun that makes such mad dogs out of Englishmen. Footloose liberals who shake their heads at the breaking up of communities by heartless architects in Britain continue to frequent foreign hotels whose creation scattered the indigenous people irretrievably.

Yet *no* people are born to serve, despite what greedy third world dictatorships advertise in the international glossies; and *no one* likes a tourist. In London we come right out and snigger at the lumpy euros and Yanks who clog up our beloved West Wonderland; in Paris they come *right* out and refuse to let any but a small minority of tables in good restaurants to tourists at peak season. In other countries they are more polite, which is probably why the tourist is still touchingly sure that the natives are friendly. Whites assume ethnics are friendly in the same ignorant way they assume they're sexually uninhibited, whereas in fact the whole of the non-white world is bound tight in taboos and tribal superstition. We misread their good manners in the same way.

Countries become tourist servicers like people become prostitutes — because they have no other choice. Britain is trying to do it right now, and having a most traumatic time too; it's no job for a man. Nothing emasculates a country like tourism — it took tourism to turn the Spanish, once the proudest, most politically advanced peasants in Europe, into a nation of dumb waiters. And it took a Franco to take them there — repressive countries always make the best tourist traps, because the people are so used to kow-towing. It is no accident that those third world cities that now specialise in tourism were originally westernised by the American troops whose "rest and recreation" bases they became. The white man has been going to faraway places with strange-sounding names and copulating with their bemused inhabitants as long as he has been going there and killing them. At last, in one, they have found a way of doing both to the white man at once.

The Anglo-Asian politicos have a great saying when faced with English complaints about their presence: We're here because you were there." AIDS is here because white men were there, screwing those wretched people royally, in both senses of the word. Now they've got *their* fist up *our* fundament. And it's going to hurt like hell. It's going to hurt like Haiti.

* * * * * * * * * * * *

By 1992, some epidemiologists estimate that there could be from 30,000,000 to 90,000,000 cases of AIDS worldwide!

VIII. Afterword

The Editors

AIDS seems to have been almost designed to confuse policymakers. It challenges the two 20th century taboos of sex and death. By definition, it is going to begin in those groups which are most sexually active, which includes gay men and prostitutes who are for many members of society, unpopular or despised. The virus breaks down the barriers with which the immune system normally prevents infection; the disease raises the walls which separate minorities from the rest of society. To compound our problems, the incubation period of the infection is uniquely long and, for example, the time between infection and the first symptoms of AIDS is often longer than the terms of most elected representatives in a democracy.

Medical science has done a great deal to unravel the natural history of AIDS, but the answers which scientists give to questions are often expressed as probabilities; health workers have become infected with AIDS but it is so rare as it need not be a substantial worry if routine preventive measures are taken. Unfortunately, the itch for incontravertible and un-nuanced truth by the public has become a rash, especially in America, and freak cases of HIV transmission, although there are indeed unusual methods of transmission, are likely to continue to hit the headlines.

The worldwide pandemic of AIDS will be contained if society can accommodate to those groups whose high risk behavior makes them the first victims of the disease. On the other hand, if gay men, IV drug abusers and prostitutes, many of which groups also belong to racial minorities in the US, are pushed out of society, then there will be no chance of halting the spread of the disease.

AIDS has opened a window on the sexual behavior of the gay community for the rest of society; gay men do have many more partners than heterosexual men and some groups have developed surprising erotic practices. IV drug users are fed by criminal pushers, they inhabit the most dangerous and unpleasant areas of inner cities, but are they criminals or have they chosen the wrong remedy to cure the afflictions of a brutal life? Prostitutes are ruthlessly exploited by their pimps and sometimes needlessly harrassed by authorities.

The problem is that AIDS is incurable and is spread by a private action. The only weapons available are education to change peoples' behavior and the use of condoms and spermicides whenever an individual believes that he or she may be exposed to the risk of HIV infection. However, these strategies can only work if they are promoted in a style that is acceptable to the group and with the sincerity and respect which is basic to the transmission of any piece of life and death information.

In 1905, the cause of syphilis was discovered, and one year later the Bossaman test was devized. As with AIDS, as with syphilis, the understanding of the disease was turned against those that suffered from it, It was more than just a suggestion that all cases of sexual transmission were a self-inflicted illness. With the double standard which is so often applied to sexual behavior, a category of patients was "invented" who were the "innocent victims" of the disease. A whole fantasy pathology of "casual transmission" was devized, and hysterical physicians suggested that everything from pens to toilet seats could spread the disease. In 1918, the US Navy solemnly removed the knobs off the doors of warships because handling the door furnitue was one imagined way the disease could be spread among the innocent.

Compulsory screening for syphilis was introduced in 1915 in some states because policymakers and politicians wanted to "know" who was the innocent bystander and who the culpable victim.

In Biblical times and throughout the Middle Ages disease was universally interpreted as a punishment for some sin in the patient or their ancestors. When the Conquistadores took smallpox to the New World the holocaust of death among the Indians was merely seen as proof that they belonged to an inferior race.

The 20th Century is coming dangerously close to linking illness with inferiority and when modern medicine removes the sick from the family and places themn in a high-technology hospital in a way they help sustain this belief.

AIDS has made the challenge of treating those with the disease with respect and love doubly difficult because it is, and must, change the rules of sexual behavior. The slogan of the swinging 60s, that any sex activities between consenting adults is acceptable has been overturned. A miserable fragment of RNA is challenging the remarkable and complex set of behaviors built into the one meter of DNA found in each human cell which determines our anatomy and our behavior and makes us what we are. In a way, AIDS is a paradigm of many of the other great problems that face us in the 20th century — can we bring our behavior, whether it is our innate aggression or our exploding populations, under control so that we meet the needs of the modern world and not of our hunter/gatherer superstitous-ridden ancestors.

Suggested Further Reading

Books

AIDS and the Third World, Panos Dossier 1, Panos Institute, London, 1987

Fettner, A. and Check, W. *The Truth About AIDS,* Henry Holt, N.Y., 1985

Langone, J. *AIDS: The Facts,* Little, Brown, N.Y., 1988

Baker, J. *Everything You Must Know About the Killer Epidemic of the '80's,* R & E Publishers, N.Y., 1986

Cahill, K. *AIDS: The Epidemic,* St. Martin's Press, N.Y., 1983

Slaff, J. and Brubaker, J. *The AIDS Epidemic,* Warner Books, N.Y., 1985

Jennings, C. *Understanding and Preventing AIDS,* Health Alert Press, Cambridge, MA, 1986

Douglas, P. and Pinsky, L. *The Essential AIDS Fact Book: What You Need to Know to Protect Yourself, Your Family, All Your Loved Ones,* Pocket Books, N.Y., 1987

Ulene, A. *Safe Sex in a Dangerous World,* Random House, N.Y., 1987

Peabody, B. *The Screaming Room: A Mother's Journal of Son's Struggle with AIDS,* Avon, N.Y., 1987

Kubler-Ross, E. *AIDS: The Ultimate Challenge,* Macmillan, N.Y., 1987

Pearson, C. *Goodbye, I Love You: The True Story of a Wife, Her Homosexual Husband and a Love Honored for Time and All Eternity,* Random House, N.Y., 1986

Sourkes, B. *The Deepening Shade: Psychological Aspects of Life-threatening Illness,* Univ. of Pittsburgh Press, Pittsburgh, 1982

Siegal, F. and Siegal, M. *AIDS: The Medical Mystery,* Grove Press, N.Y., 1983

Brandt, A. *No Magic Bullet: A Social History of Venereal Disease in the United States Since 1880,* Oxford Univ. Press, Oxford, 1987

Fortunato, J. *AIDS: The Spiritual Dilemma,* Harper & Row, N.Y., 1987

Pearsall, P. *Superimmunity,* McGraw-Hill, N.Y., 1987

Weiner, M. *Maximum Immunity,* Pocket Books, N.Y., 1986

Altman, D. *AIDS in the Mind of America,* Doubleday, N.Y., 1986

Sontag, S. *Illness as Metaphor,* Farrar, Straus & Giroux, N.Y., 1986

Corless, I., *AIDS: Principles, Practices, and Politics,* Hemisphere, N.Y., 1987

Institute of Medicine, National Academy of Sciences: *Confronting AIDS: Direction for Public Health Care and Research, National Academy Press, Washington, D.C., 1986*

Witt, M.D. (ed), *AIDS and Patient Management: Legal, Ethical, and Social Issues,* National Health Publ., Owings Mills, Md., 1986

Articles

Acquired Immunodeficiency Syndrome, Plan of action for control in the African Region, *WHO Weekly Epidemiological Record,* 1986; 61

Agbabiaka, T., The AIDS pestilence and Africa. *African Concord,* Jan. 15, 1986; 123

AIDS, Deadly but hard to catch, *Consumer Reports,* Nov., 1986

Arno, P.W., The Nonprofit Sector's response to the AIDS epidemic: Community-based services in San Francisco, *American Journal of Public Health,* 1986; 76

Bach, M.C., Possible drug interaction during therapy with Azidothymidine and Acyclovir for AIDS, *New England Journal of Medicine,* 1987; 316

Baker, J.L., Kelen, G.D., Sivertson, K.T., Quinn, T.C., Unsuspected human immunodeficiency virus in critically ill emergency patients, *Journal of the American Medical Association,* 1987:257

Barbour, S.D., Acquired immunodeficiency syndrome of childhood, *Pediatric Clinics of North America,* 1987; 34

Barre-Sinoussi, F., and Chermann, J.C., The etiiologic agent of AIDS, *Mount Sinai Journal of Medicine,* 1986; 53

Bernstein, L.J., and Rubenstein, A. Acquired immunodeficiency syndrome in infants and children, *Progress in Allergy,* 1986; 37

Bigger, R.J., The AIDS Problem in Africa, *The Lancet,* 1986; 79-83

Booth, W. AIDS and insects, *Science,* 1987; 237

Bove, J.R., Transfusion-associated hepatitis and AIDS, *New England Journal of Medicine,* 1987; 317

Brahams, D., Human immunodeficiency virus and the law, *Lancet,* 1987; 2

Brookmeyer, R., and Gail, M.H., Minimum size of the acquired immunodeficiency syndrome epidemic in the United States, *Lancet,* 1986; 2

Burke, D.S., Brandt, B.L., Redfield, R.R., et al., Diagnosis of human immunodeficiency virus infection by immunoassay using a molecularly cloned and expressed virus envelope polypeptide. Comparison to Western blot on 2707 consecutive serum samples, *Annals of Internal Medicine,* 1987; 106

CDC, Antibody to human immunodeficiency virus in female prostitutes, *MMWR,* 1986; 35

CDC, Apparent transmission of HTLV-III from a child to mother providing health care, *MMWR,* 1986; 35

CDC, Human immunodeficiency virus infection in transfusion recipients and their family members, *MMWR,* 1987; 36

CDC, Recommendations for assisting in the prevention of perinatal transmission of human T-lymphadenfotropic virus type III/lymphadenopathy-associated virus and acquired immunodeficiency syndrome, *MMWR,* 1985; 34

CDC, Self-reported changes in sexual behaviors among homosexual and bisexual men from the San Francisco cohort, *MMWR,* 1987; 36

CDC, Tuberculosis and AIDS — Connecticut, *MMWR,* 1987; 36

CDC, Update: Public Health Service workshop in human T-lymphotropic virus type III antibody testing — United States, *MMWR;* 34

Chaisson, R.E., Moss, A.R., Onishi, R., Osmond, D. and Carlson, J.R., Human immunodeficiency virus infection in heterosexual intravenous drug users in San Francisco, *American Journal of Public Health,* 1987; 77

Cleary, P.D., Barry, M.J., Mayer, K.H., et al., Compulsory premarital screening for the human immunodeficiency virus: Technical and public health considerations, *Journal of the American Medical Association,* 1987; 258

Coolfront Report: A PHS plan for prevention and control of AIDS and the AIDS virus, *Public Health Reports,* 1986; 101

Curran, J.W., The epidemiology of prevention of the acquired immunodeficiency syndrome, Annals of Internal Medicine, 1985; 103

Dengler, R., Thomssen, H., Volkman, M., and Emmerich, B., Chronic Epstein-Barr virus infection and human immunodeficiency virus infection, *Annals of Internal Medicine,* 1987; 106

DeVita, V.T., Broder, S., Fauci, A.S., et al., Developmental therapeutics and the acquired immunodeficiency syndrome, *Annals of Internal Medicine,* 1987; 106

Drew, W.L., Is cytomegalovirus a co-factor in the pathogenesis of AIDS and Kaposi's sarcoma? *Mount Sinai Journal of Medicine,* 1986; 53

Fischinger, P.J., Gallo, R.C. and Bolognesi, D.P., Toward a vaccine against AIDS: rationale and current progress, *Mount Sinai Journal of Medicine,* 1986; 53

Fischl, M.A., Dickinson, G.M., Scott, G.B., et al. Evaluation of heterosexual partners, children and household contacts of adults with AIDS, *Journal of the American Medical Association,* 1987; 257

Fleming, D.W., Cochi, L.L., Steece, R.S., and Hull, H.F., Acquired immunodeficiency syndrome in low-incidence areas. How safe is unsafe sex? *New England Journal of Medicine,* 1987; 317

Francis, D.P. and Petricciani, J.C., The prospects for and pathways toward a vaccine for AIDS, *New England Journal of Medicine,* 1985; 313

Gillon, R., Testing for HIV without permission, *British Medical Journal,* 1987; 294

Goedert, J.J., What is safe sex? Suggested standards linked to testing for acquired immunodeficiency syndrome, *New England Journal of Medicine,* 1987; 316

Goodacre, T.E., Health professionals' attitudes toward AIDS and occupational risk, *Lancet,* 1987; 1

Gostin, L. and Ziegler, A., A review of AIDS-related legislative and regulatory policy in the United States, *Law, Medicine and Health Care,* 1987; 15

Hardy, A.M., Allen, J.R., Morgan, M. et al., The incidence rate of acquired immunodeficiency syndrome in selected populations, *Journal of the American Medical Association,* 1985; 253

Ho, K.H., Ochs, H.D., Dufford, M.T. and Wedgwood, R.J., Perinatal infection with human immunodeficiency virus, *New England Journal of Medicine,* 1987; 317

Kamani, N. and Krilov, L., AIDS in the spectrum of HIV infection in children, *Pediatric Review Communications,* 1987; 1

Martin, J.L., The impact of AIDS on gay male sexual behavior patterns in New York City, *American Journal of Public Health,* 1987; 77

Matthews, G.W., and Neslund, V.S., The initial impact of AIDS on public health law in the United States — 1986, *Journal of the American Medical Association,* 1987; 257

McCray, E., Occupational risk of the acquired immunodeficiency syndrome among health care workers, *New England Journal of Medicine,* 1986; 314

Medley, G.F., Anderson, R.M., Cox, D.R. and Billard, L., Incubation period of AIDS in patients infected via blood transfusion, *Nature,* 1986; 328

Meyer, K.B., and Pauker, S.G., Screening for HIV: Can we afford the false positive rate? *New England Journal of Medicine,* 1987; 317

Mitsuya, H. and Broder, S., Strategies for antiviral therapy in AIDS, *Nature,* 1987; 325

Morgen, K.B., Counseling and HIV: Test results and risk reduction, *Maryland Medical Journal,* 1987; 36

Navia, B.A. Jordan, B.D. and Price, R.W., The AIDS dementia complex: I. Clinical features, *Annals of Neurology,* 1986; 19

Ostrow, D.G., Psychiatric and neurologic aspects of AIDS, *International Review of Neuroscience,* 1986; 29

Padian, N., Marquis, L, Francis, D.P., et al. Male-to-female transmission of human immunodeficiency virus, *Journal of the American Medical Association,* 1987; 258

Peckham, C.S., Senturia, Y.D., and Ades, A.E., Obstetric and perinatal consequences of human immunodeficiency virus infection: A review, *British Journal of Obstetrics and Gynecology,* 1987; 94

Ranki, A., Krohn, M. and Allain, J.P., Long latency precedes overt seroconversion in sexually transmitted human immunodeficiency virus infection, *Lancet,* 1987; 2

Redfield, R.R., Wright, D.C., and Tramont, E.C., The Walter Reed staging classification for HTLV-III/LAV infection, *New England Journal of Medicine,* 1986; 314

Salk, J., Prospects for the control of AIDS by immunizing seropositive individuals, *Nature,* 1987; 327

Sandstrom, E., Antiviral drugs for AIDS. Current status and future prospects, *Drugs,* 1986; 31

Scott, G.B., Fischl, M.A., and Klimas, N., Mothers of infants with AIDS: Evidence for both symptomatic and asymptomatic carriers, *Journal of the American Medical Association,* 1985; 253

Shepard, F.A., Fanning, M.M., Duperval, R., et al., A guide to the investigation and treatment of patients with AIDS and AIDS-related disorders, *Canadian Medical Association Journal,* 1986; 134

Steinbrook, R., and Lo, R., Ethical dilemmas in caring for patients with acquired immunodeficiency syndrome, *Annals of Internal Medicine,* 1985; 103

Taylor, J.M., Schwartz, K. and Detels, R., The time from infection with human immunodeficiency virus to the onset of AIDS, *Journal of Infectious Diseases,* 1986; 154

Valenti, W.M., AIDS update: HTLV-III testing, immune globulins and employees with AIDS, *Infection Control,* 1986; 7

van der Graaf, M., and Diepersloot, R.J., Transmission of human immunodeficiency virus: A review, *Infection,* 1986; 14

Ward, J.W., Deppe, D.A., Samson, S., et al., Risk of human immunodeficiency virus infection from blood donors who later developed the acquired immunodeficiency syndrome, *Annals of Internal Medicine,* 1986; 256

Winkelstein, W., Samuel, M., Padian, N.S., et al., The San Francisco Men's Health Study: III. Reduction in human immunodeficiency virus transmission among homosexual-bisexual men, 1982-86, *American Journal of Public Health,* 1987; 77

Wofsy, C.B., Human immunodeficiency virus infection in women, *Journal of the American Medical Association,* 1987; 257

Yarchoan, R., and Broder, S., Development of antiretroviral therapy for the acquired immunodeficiency syndrome and related disorders, *New England Journal of Medicine,* 1987; 316